H.E. Takahashi (Ed.)

Spinal Disorders in Growth and Aging

With 206 Figures, Including 3 in Color

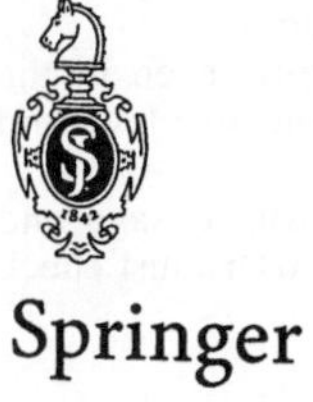

Springer

Hideaki E. Takahashi, m.d., ph.d.
Department of Orthopedic Surgery
Niigata University School of Medicine
Asahimachi-dori 1-757, Niigata, 951 Japan

ISBN 978-4-431-66941-8 ISBN 978-4-431-66939-5 (eBook)
DOI 10.1007/978-4-431-66939-5

Printed on acid-free paper

Originally published by Springer-Verlag Tokyo in 1995

Preface

This volume contains the papers presented at the International Symposium on Spine and Spinal Disorders in Growth and Aging held in Niigata on November 22–23, 1992. The symposium commemorates the 75th anniversary of the foundation of the Department of Orthopedic Surgery, Niigata University School of Medicine.

The purpose of the symposium was to investigate the field of spine and spinal disorders in growth and aging. Topics ranged from osteoporosis, other metabolic bone diseases, and deformity of the spinal column to degenerative spinal disorders and heterotopic ossification with resultant myelopathy. Spinal manifestations of systemic and local diseases were also included. Symptoms of spinal disorders in both the lower and upper extremity were presented and biomechanics and bone mineral measurement of the spine were also discussed.

The organizing committee would like to thank the following for their sponsorship and support of this international symposium: Japan Osteoporosis Foundation, Japan-North America Medical Exchange Foundation, Japan-Russia Medical Exchange Foundation, Niigata Prefectural Government, and Niigata City Government. We deeply appreciate their support and contributions to the success of the symposium.

The chairman of the organizing committee is most grateful for the contributions and support of the International Advisory Committee, Dr. B.D. Burr (USA), Dr. H.M. Frost (USA), and Dr. R.R. Recker (USA); the Local Advisory Committee, Dr. S. Kono (Prof. Emeritus of Niigata University) and Dr. T. Tajima (Prof. Emeritus of Niigata University); and the members of the organizing committee, Dr. Y. Watanabe (Yamagata University), Dr. K. Ibaraki (Ryukyu University), and Dr. H. Norimatsu (Kagawa Medical School).

The chairman would like to express gratitude to Dr. M. Sofue and Dr. Y. Dohmae and the current members and alumni of the Department of Orthopedic Surgery, Niigata University School of Medicine. The chairman owes a deep debt of gratitude to Miss Maria Homma, who provided excellent secretarial support. Finally, the chairman would like to thank the staff of

Springer-Verlag Tokyo for their patience and continuous efforts in compiling the manuscripts for the publication of the book.

HIDEAKI E. TAKAHASHI
Chairman
Organizing Committee

Contents

Part IV. Pathogenesis, Diagnosis and Treatment of Ossification and Degenerative Spine

Part V. Pathogenesis and Treatment of Osteoporosis and Rheumatoid Arthritis

Part I.

Spine and Spinal Deformity in Growth and Aging

The Optimization of Spinal Arthrodesis

MARC ASHER[1]

Key Words. Spinal arthrodesis, spinal deformity, scoliosis

Introduction

Spinal arthrodesis is currently the most widely used surgical means of stabilizing the deformed and mechanically insufficient spine. It may be accompanied by direct or indirect decompression and/or realignment by positioning, mechanical, or destabilization methods. Very often, arthrodesis is supplemented by internal fixation that may be utilized in the realignment as well as the immobilization of the spine.

For many years, we have conducted various studies, mostly clinical, aimed in some way at the common goal of optimizing spinal arthrodesis. These studies can be categorized into four general areas: (1) three-dimensional analysis of spinal deformity, (2) implant research and development, (3) advanced surgical technique development, and (4) improvement of bone healing.

A major stimulus to this line of study has been the continuing influence of Paul Randall Harrington (Kansas, AB '35, MD '38) through the establishment of the Mary Alice and Paul R. Harrington Distinguished Professorship of Orthopedic Research and the contribution of his papers to the Harrington Archives. Also important was the influence of our late colleague, Rae Rodney Jacobs (Wheaton, BA '58; Buffalo, MD '62) who labored diligently in the same area.

Many who have contributed to these studies are acknowledged in the references.

[1] University of Kansas Medical Center, Kansas City, KS 66160-7387, USA

Three-Dimensional Aspects of Spinal Deformity

In 1979, a diagnostic radiology group headed by Dr. Arthur DeSmet began developing a method for the three-dimensional analysis of spinal deformity. This was based on three standing radiographs: one posteroanterior and two obliques (45° right and left). The waists of T1 through L5 vertebrae were digitized on each of the three views, and their centers were determined. Thus, the spine could be displayed in the conventional coronal and sagittal plane and viewed in any intermediate plane between these two, as well as from the top. The in vivo spatial resolution was 1.0 mm (+0.3 mm). Because the transverse plane angular position of the vertebral body was less accurate, the measurement was not included in the final program. However, the transverse plane angular position was reflected in the vertebral segment position.

Two hundred and ten patients with adolescent idiopathic scoliosis were studied. This led to the publication and presentation of seven articles and book chapters [1–7] and six abstracts [8–13] between 1981 and 1992. Some of the observations were as follows. During the pilot development studies, it was determined that the conventional coronal plane Cobb measurement was essentially equivalent for posteroanterior and antero-posterior exposures [4]. Trunk thoracic kyphosis was not found to correlate with Cobb curvature severity [6]. The global top, cephalad-caudad, view suggested that in progressive scoliosis a posterior-to-anterior flattening of the spine occurred (Fig. 1) [5]. An

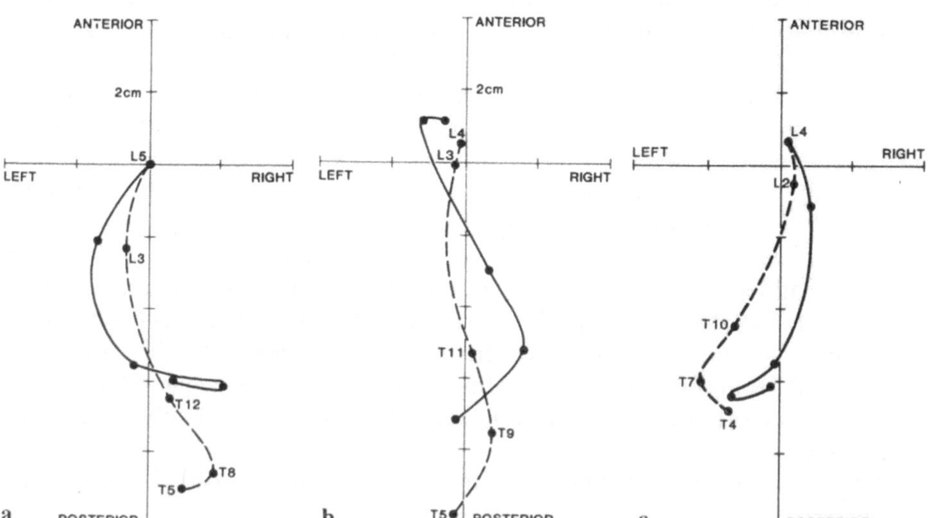

Fig. 1a–c. Line drawings showing apical and end vertebrae of the scolioses in patients VI(**a**), X(**b**), and XI(**c**). The initial (*dashed line*) and follow-up (*solid line*) curves are superimposed to clarify the patterns of progression. The *closed circles* on the solid-line curves correspond to the same vertebral levels indicated on the dashed-line curves. (Reprinted with permission from [5])

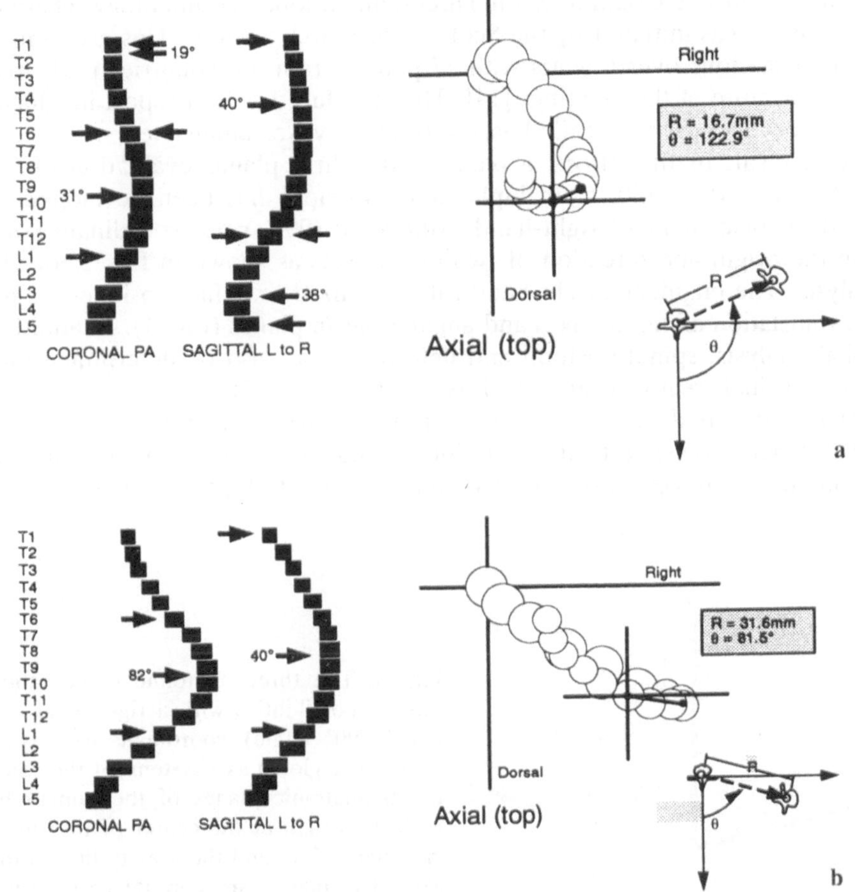

Fig. 2a,b. Coronal, sagittal, and axial plane views of the thoracolumbar spine illustrating the relationship of the apex vertebra to the upper end vertebra **a** in a 25-year-old female with a 31° King-Moe type IV curvature and **b** in a 14-year-old female with an 82° King-Moe type IV curvature. (Reprinted with permission from [7])

attempt to update scoliosis curve patterns on the basis of a 3-D classification suggested a much wider variety of curve patterns than had previously been suspected [13]. Finally, cross-sectional study of right thoracic scoliosis deformities was supportive of Perdriolle's suggestion that they evolved in the transverse plane as a clockwise torsion, with the apex vertebra moving in an anterior-to-posterior arc in relation to the upper end vertebra (Fig. 2) [7].

As a result of these three-dimensional studies, it was realized that we did not well enough understand the clinically relevant parameters most helpful in the diagnosis and management of adolescent idiopathic scoliosis. The need for a scientifically based terminology was recognized by many others as well. Thus, in 1989 an ad hoc Committee on Three-Dimensional Terminology, chaired by Ian Stokes, was initiated by the Scoliosis Research Society. This group met on eleven occasions over 6 years with 37 people from ten countries participating in one or more of the meetings [14]. They produced a draft report in which the framework for a scientifically based terminology was enunciated.

As a result of this effort, a plan for the three-planar evaluation of spinal position and deformity from biplanar radiographs has been developed. It is based on placement of right-hand orthogonal (90° angle) coordinate systems with the origin and direction of two of the axes as shown in Fig. 3 for global analysis. The engineer's right-hand rule is utilized to define positive and negative translation along the axes and angulations in planes (Fig. 4). In addition to global analysis, spinal position and deformity may also be determined on the basis of spinal, regional, and local axis systems (Fig. 5).

Five of the six degrees of freedom of motion may be measured directly from the biplanar X-rays: vertical translation, mediolateral translation, coronal plane angulation, anteroposterior translation, and sagittal plane angulation. The

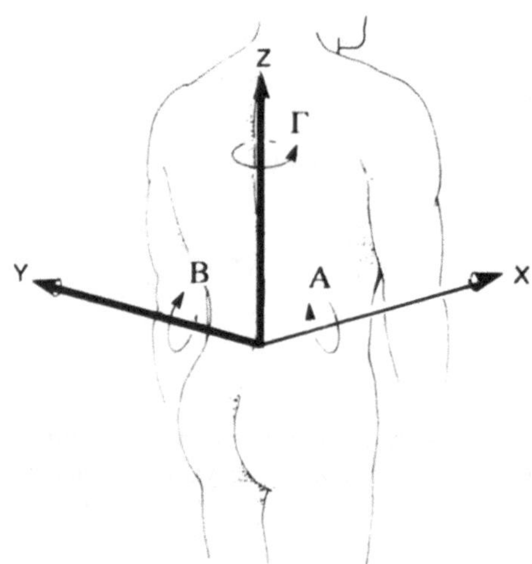

Fig. 3. The three anatomic planes and six motion possibilities with a right-hand orthogonal (90° angle) coordinate axis system. Shown is a global axis system for the conventional anatomic planes of the human body with the origin at the center of the superior end plate of S1 and the gravity line as the Z axis. The planes are coronal (YZ), sagittal (XZ), and transverse or axial (XY). Positive directions of translation and angulation are indicated by *arrows*. Translation and angulation may occur in each plane. (Partially redrawn from [39])

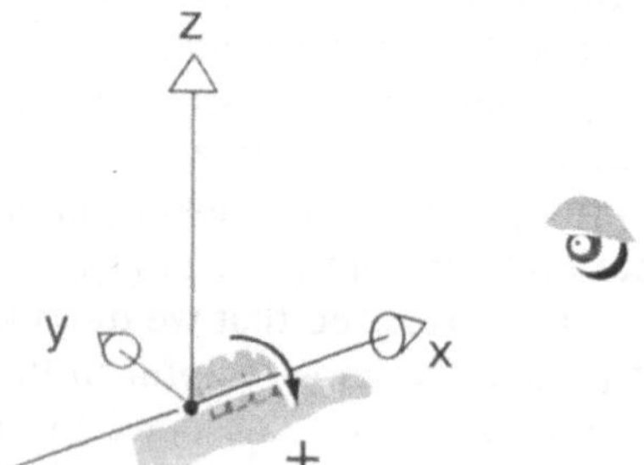

Fig. 4. Senses (positive and negative) of translation along axes and angulations around axes are defined by the engineer's right-hand rule in which the thumb points in the positive translational direction and the curled fingers define the sense of the angular position/motion (positive being counter-clockwise when viewed down the axis towards the origin)

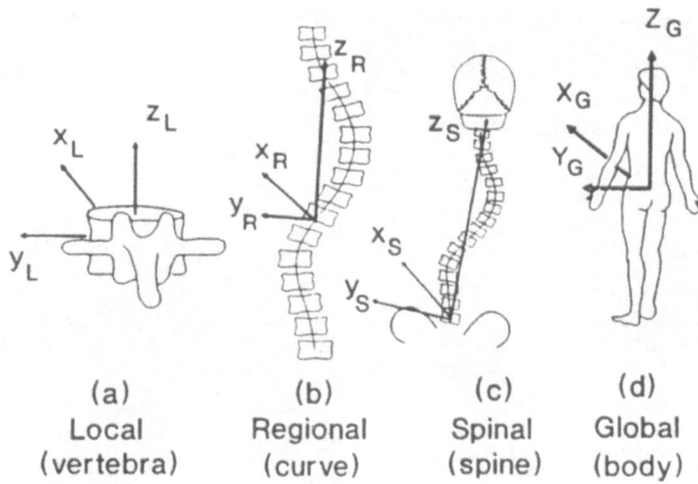

Fig. 5. Global, spinal, regional, and local application for measurement of spinal deformity (Reprinted with permission from [14])

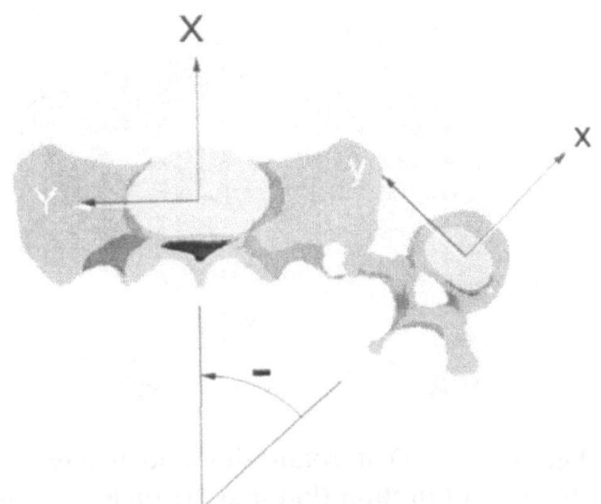

Fig. 6. Drawing of cephalad to caudad view of scoliosis apex vertebra, approximately T8, in relation to the sacrum illustrating the transverse plane angular position of T8 in relation to the sacrum

degree which cannot be measured directly from the biplanar radiographs, transverse plane angulation (Fig. 6), may be measured with some accuracy using the method of Perdriolle [15]. This makes it possible to measure all six degrees of freedom of motion from biplanar radiographs (Fig. 7a,b).

To control the volume of data being evaluated, it is essential to pick key landmarks for analysis. They seem to be the following vertebral bodies: T1, L1, S1, end/inflection vertebrae, apex vertebrae, neutral vertebrae (lowest caudal), and stable vertebrae. By connecting these points, spine lines can be developed and traced onto a coronal and sagittal plane gridwork sheet which has the normal spine alignment. This greatly simplifies the analysis procedure by eliminating the intervening vertebra since it is assumed that they can be anticipated to follow the spine line.

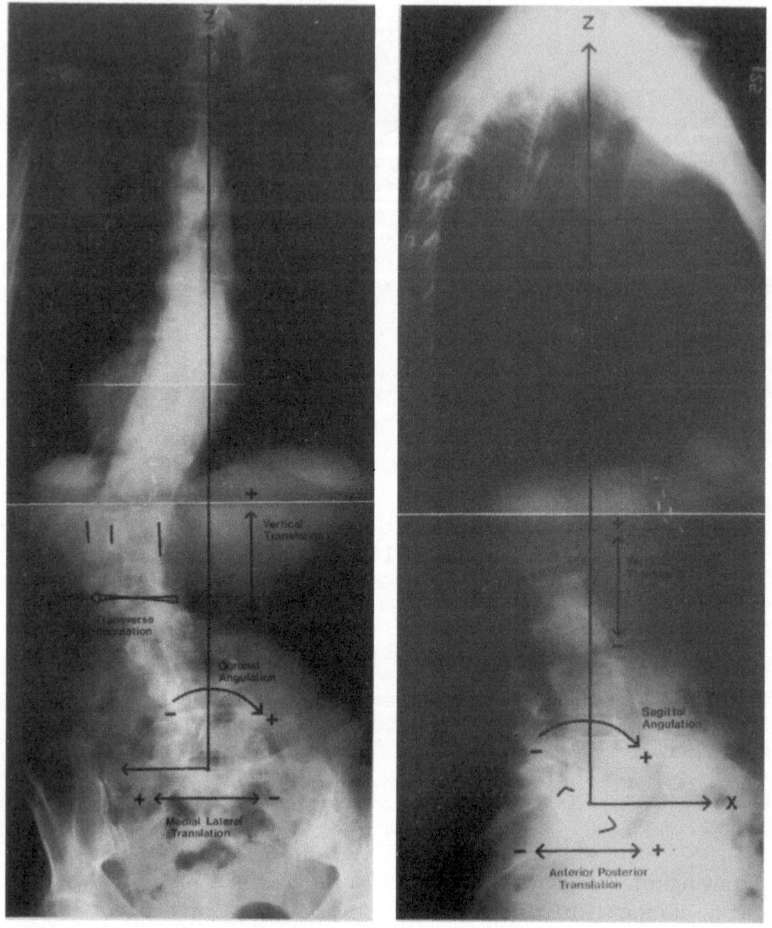

Fig. 7a,b. **a** Posteroanterior and **b** lateral radiographs illustrating the five degrees of freedom of motion that may be measured directly on biplanar radiographs and the sixth degree of freedom of motion, transverse plane angulation, that can be measured indirectly on the coronal plane view

A grid facilitating the three-planar analysis of biplanar radiographs has been created. It includes a preliminary selection of what seem to be the most valuable measurements (Fig. 8). It is stressed that this grid is preliminary and continuing refinement is anticipated.

Three Planar Analysis of Biplanar Radiographs: Grid Worksheet

	MEASUREMENT	Global	Spinal	Regional	Local
TRANSLATIONS	Vertical		T1 - S1	Intersegmental	Compression
	Mediolateral	T1 (C7) Apex Inflection (End)			
	Anteroposterior	T1 (C7) L1			
ANGULATIONS	Coronal	Pelvic obliquity T1 Lower end vertebrae	Pelvic obliquity	Cobb	Wedging Rib-vertebral angle
	Sagittal	Sacrum		Intersegmental "Cobb"	Wedging
	Transverse	Apex & end vertebrae			

05/21/93 MAA/jb

Fig. 8. Sample of important measurements utilized in the three-planar analysis of biplanar radiographs

Implant Research and Development

Because of long-standing frustration with the available spinal implants, a full-scale effort to develop a new option was begun in January 1985. Out of our work came the Isola Spine Implant System [16–21]. The design objectives were minimal internal and external profile, simplicity, versatility, VSP compatibility, dimension standardization, and user-friendly instrumentation. Isola is completely compatible with the Variable Screw Placement (VSP) System; together they form a comprehensive dorsal thoraco-lumbosacro-iliac implant system, applicable in the full range of ages, deformities, and mechanical insufficiencies.

The components of the Isola Spine Implant System are illustrated in Fig. 9. Those anchoring to bone include posts, screws, hooks, and wires. To accommodate the anatomical reality of variable lamina and transverse process thickness, there are a family of variable throat-height hooks. Since screws are the most stable of all implant anchors (that portion of the implant system which affixes to bone), considerable emphasis has been placed on screw fixation, particularly in the thoracolumbar, lumbar, sacral, and pelvic areas. The longitudinal members are 6.35-mm (1/4-inch) and 4.76-mm (3/16-inch) rods, as well as hybrid longitudinal members. Both closed and open connections are available. The closed connections utilized with hooks feature a drop entry design, facilitating placement on bone while located on the longitudinal members (rods). There are transverse, bypass, and tandem connectors and washers.

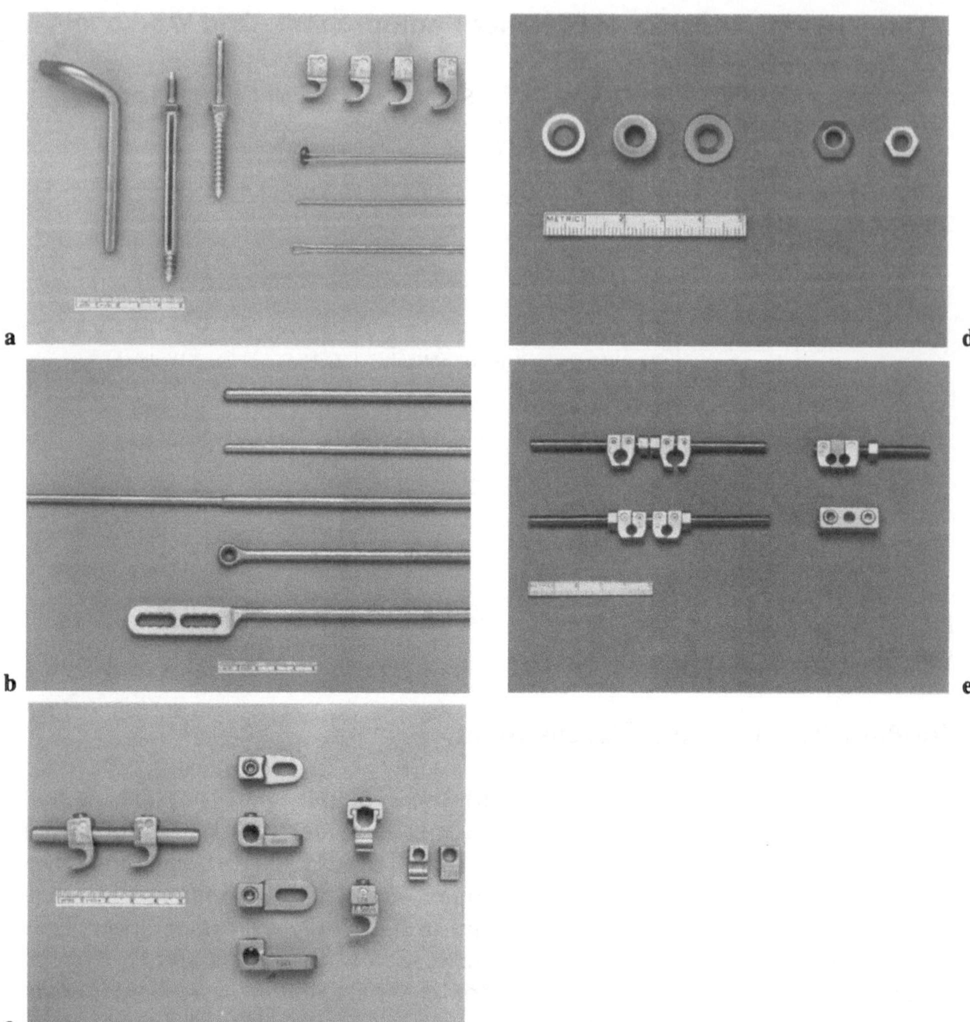

Fig. 9a–e. The implant component categories consist of anchors (attachments to bone), longitudinal members, longitudinal member to anchor connectors, longitudinal member to longitudinal member connectors, and accessories. The anchors **a** which are posts, screws, hooks, and wires, are shown *left* to *right* and *top* to *bottom*. The longitudinal members **b** are shown top to bottom and consist of 4.76-mm (3/16-inch) and 6.35-mm (1/4-inch) smooth rods, as well as hybrid, eye-rod, and plate-rod combinations. The longitudinal member to anchor clamp connectors may be closed or open **c**. Shown *left* to *right* are closed V-Groove Hollow-Ground (VHG) connections with the drop entry feature for placement while on a longitudinal member. Next are the slotted connector, the open connection, and split connection. The rod to rod connectors **d** include transverse connectors for connecting rods on opposite sides of the spine. These are shown on the *left* in the 6.35-mm version with the nuts medially placed (*above*) and in the 4.76-mm version with the nuts on the outside (*below*). On the right top is a 4.76-mm dual

Taken together the system provides for six degrees of freedom of motion connection of the anchors to the longitudinal members.

Smooth rods were chosen to improve fatigue life. Connection strength to the rods is enhanced by the VHG (V-Groove, Hollow-Ground) design that: produces wedge action gripping of the rod along with capture on four sides, accommodates sagittal plane rod contour, and produces superior flexion-extension bending strength by distribution of internal forces at opposite ends of the rod connection. The components, connections, and a number of resulting constructs have been subjected to substantial static strength, stiffness, and fatigue testing [18,21–25]. Proper rod contouring and alignment of connections, use of recommended set screw and nut tightening sequence and magnitude, and transverse connection [22] are very important to assure maximum construct stability and strength. Clinical needs result in implant constructs that are stiffer than the human spine [26] in some motions. The possible adverse effects of stiff implants on the bypassed bone have been studied in vivo [27,28]. Bone mineral loss of the bypassed bone in the range of 14%–20% does not increase after 3 months. One explanation for the lack of further bone loss may be that enough loosening at the bone-implant interface with time occurs to relieve some of the stress shielding effects of implants on the bypassed bone.

The application objectives are three-dimensional spinal alignment, six degrees of freedom of motion load application and resistance, sequential segmental application, maximum motion segment preservation, and liberal use of supplemental techniques to improve spinal realignment. These objectives are achieved utilizing five placement concepts: (1) the development of foundations, defined as two or more anchors through which corrective forces can be applied to the spine; (2) force couples in which forces applied in opposite directions provide a rotational moment; (3) anatomically contoured longitudinal members to assure proper realignment of the spine; (4) variable position connections which allow some initial and even residual spine longitudinal member mismatch to permit capture and manipulation to reduce the mismatch; and (5) stable, strong, and durable constructs that are stiff enough to secure the aligned position of the spine but not so rigid as to cause unwanted side effects, beyond those that may be encountered by fusion alone.

Clinical realization of these objectives and refinement of these concepts have occurred through the following: (1) small custom series in 1985–86 and 1988–89; (2) an investigational new device (IDE) study under the auspices of the United States Food and Drug Administration in which 383 patients aged 5–75 years with a variety of pathologies were enrolled by 11 centers and received Isola implants from 19 surgeons between April 1989 and September 1992; and (3)

◄

(bypass) connection for adjoining rods side to side and on the *bottom right* is a tandem connector for connecting rods end to end. From *left* to *right*, the accessories **e** consist of 3.0-mm and 5.0-mm thick washers, a 15° wedge washer, a 9.53-mm (3/8-inch) hex acorn nut, and a 7.94-mm (5/16-inch) hex nut. Some components are from the Variable Screw Placement System, and all are compatible with each other

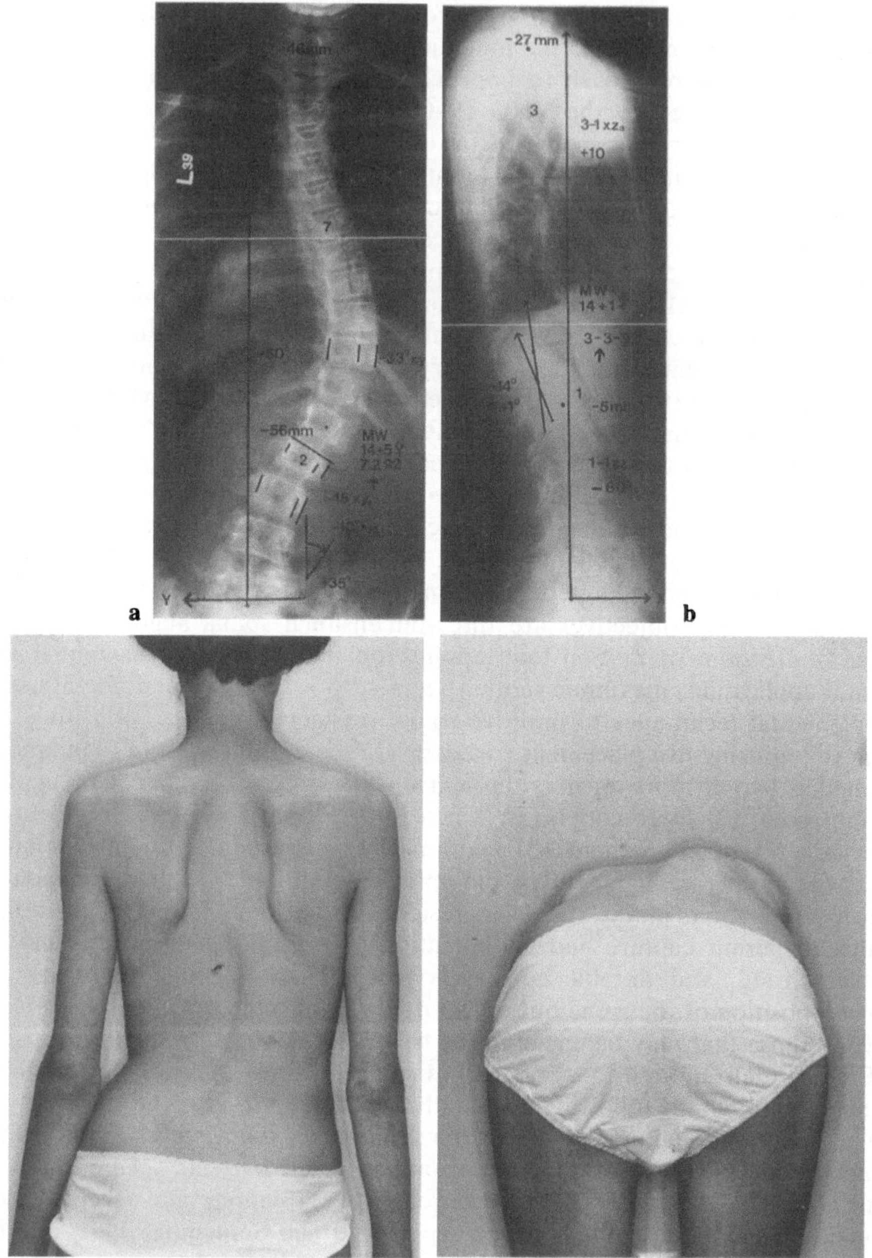

Fig. 10a–h. Preoperative standing posteroanterior **a** and lateral **b** radiographs and clinical photographs (**c** and **d**) of a 14-year, 5-month-old female with adolescent idiopathic scoliosis treated along the principles outlined. Postoperative posteroanterior **e** and lateral **f** radiographs and clinical photographs (**g** and **h**) are shown

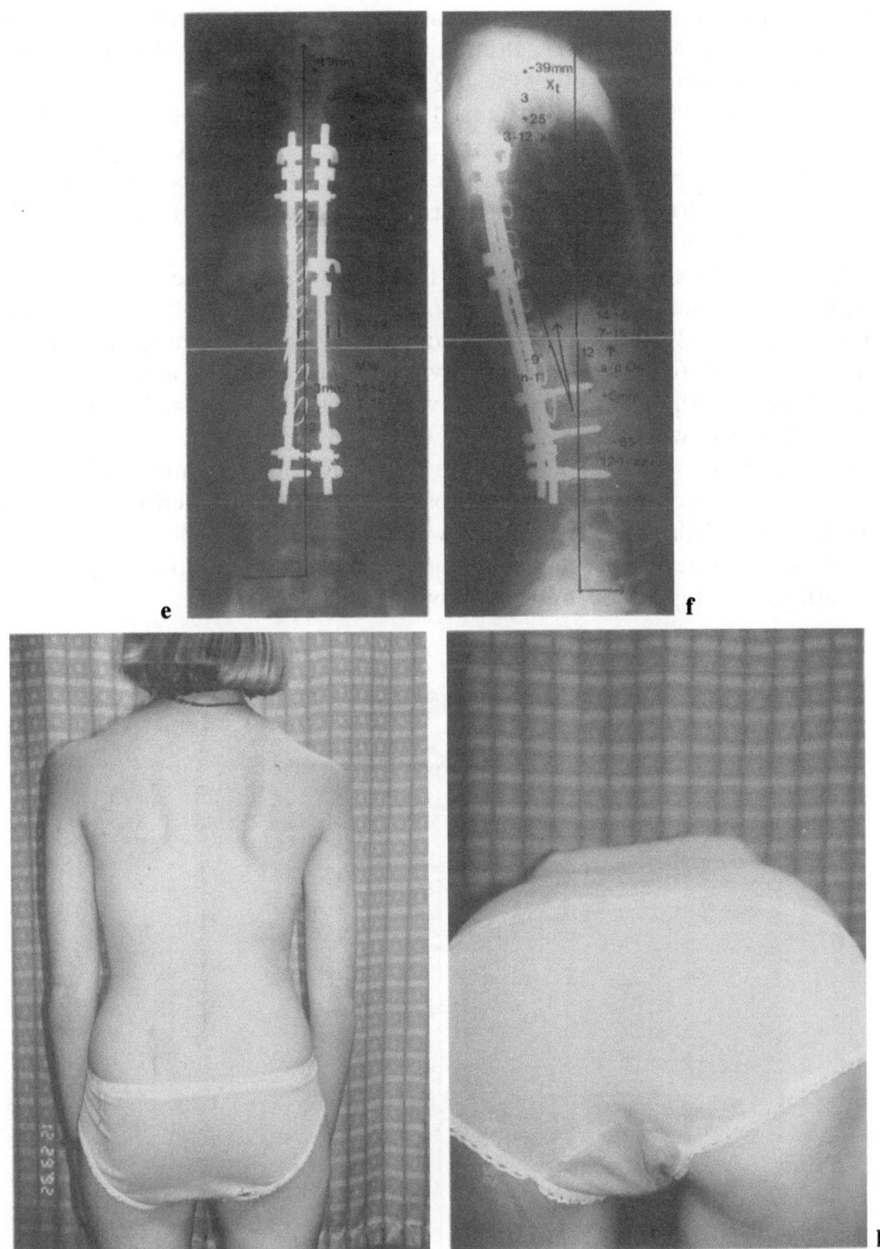

Fig. 10. *Continued*

broader utilization as components have been approved and made available, principally since March 1991. Preliminary results from the IDE study show a fusion rate of approximately 90% at 2 years' follow-up.

In a January 1991 through August 1992 series of consecutively instrumented idiopathic scoliosis patients, the average correction of the Cobb measurement was 70% in 25 patients with an average age of 14 years, 11 months. The preoperative instrumented curves averaged 57° (range 30–105°) [29]. A typical example is shown in Fig. 10.

These objectives and concepts of the Isola system have been particularly helpful in correcting severe pelvic obliquity in the cerebral palsy patient. Between May 1989 and July 1991, a consecutive series of ten sitting tetraplegia cerebral palsy patients with spinal pelvic obliquity of 20° or more was operated on posteriorly [30]. Their average age was 14 years, 9 months. The preoperative pelvic obliquity, which averaged 42°, was 6° postoperatively, thus achieving an 86% correction, which at an average follow-up of 17 months held steady at 82%. The average preoperative scoliosis of 78° was corrected to 30° postoperatively, for a 63% correction which was maintained at 67% at follow-up. No supplemental anterior surgery was done and no postoperative immobilization was utilized. A typical example is shown in Fig. 11.

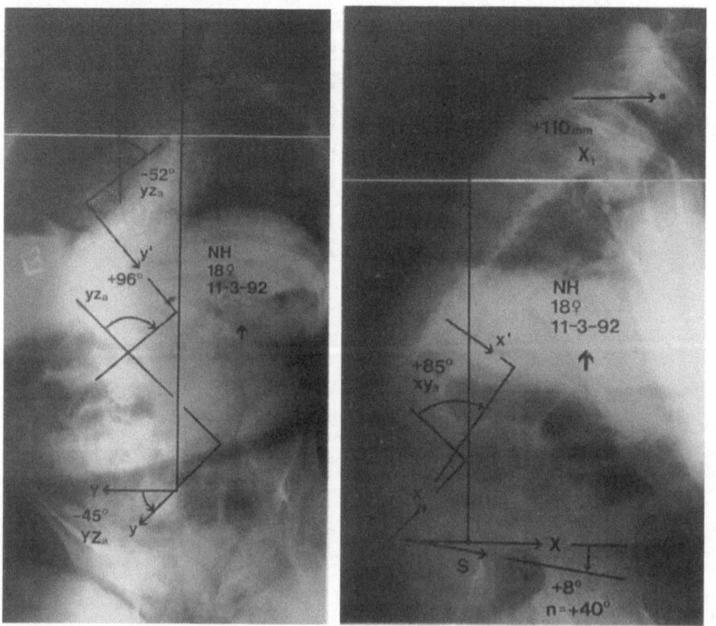

Fig. 11a–f. Preoperative sitting posteroanterior **a** and lateral **b** radiographs and clinical photograph **c** of an 18-year-old female with paralytic scoliosis treated along the principles outlined. Postoperative anteroposterior **d** and lateral **e** radiographs and clinical photograph **f** are shown

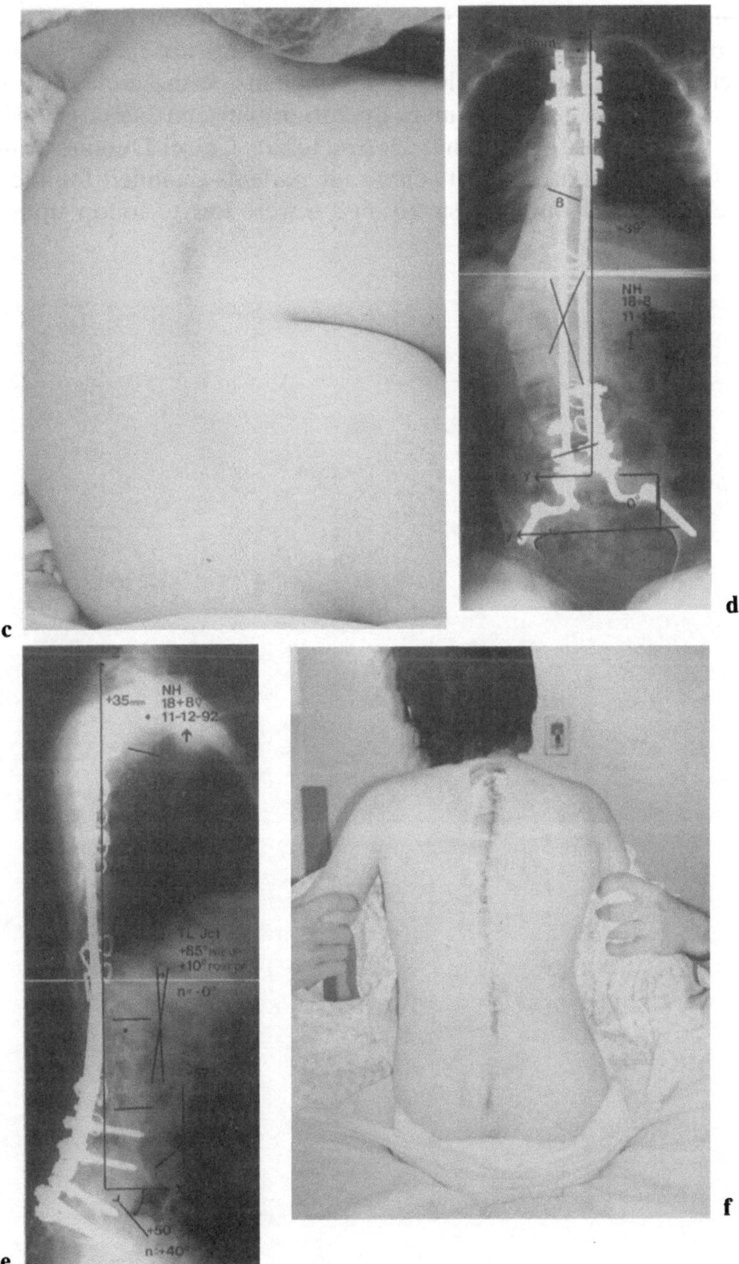

Fig. 11. *Continued*

To learn the incidence and outcome of dorsal spinal implant removal for pain in patients operated for idiopathic scoliosis, we recently conducted a retrospective study which included all patients with adolescent idiopathic scoliosis who received their primary operation between January 1981 and July 1989 and were treated with either Harrington or Cotrel-Dubousset instrumentation [31]. One hundred and twenty-four patients qualified for the study; 15 had to be removed from analysis because 6 were lost to follow-up at less than

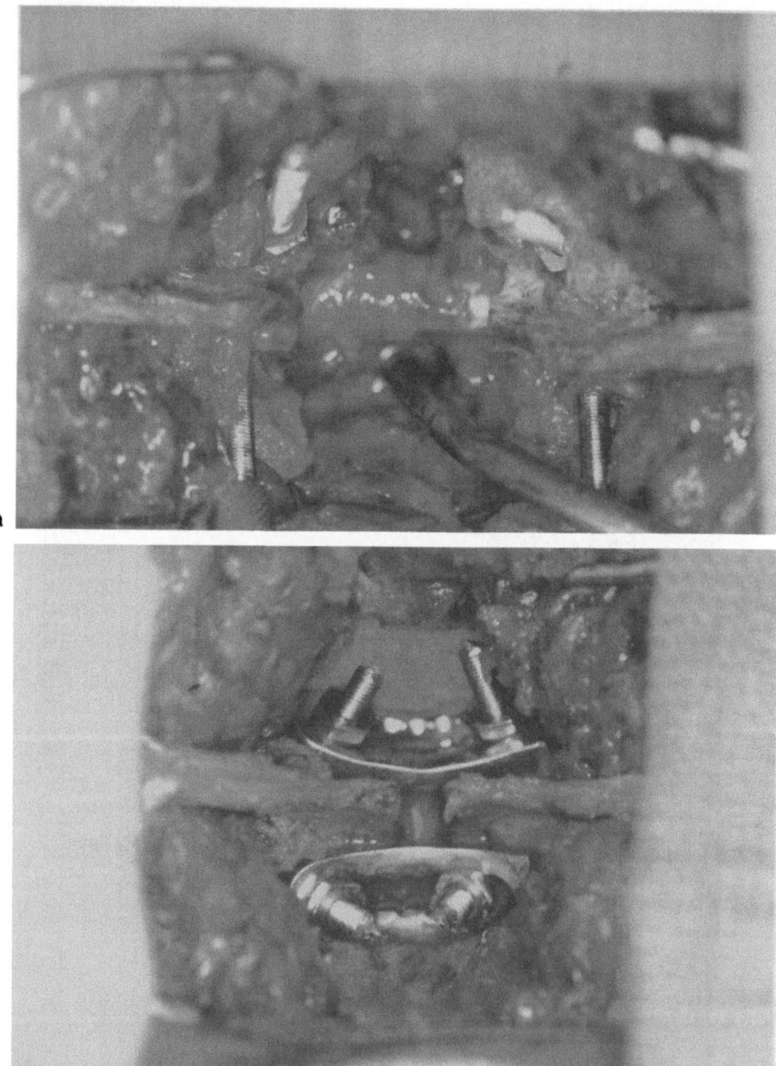

Fig. 12a,b. Dog eggshell extension osteotomy of the lumbar spine, with the head to the left. **a** After osteotomy and **b** after osteotomy closure

24 months, 7 had known pseudarthrosis, and 2 had been revised for other reasons. This left 109 patients with an average follow-up of 56 months (12–133 months) for study. Sixty-two had received Harrington instrumentation and 47 C-D instrumentation. Twelve patients underwent implant removal for the problem of late or persistent mid-line and/or parascapular pain. Eleven of the 12 experienced 75% or more relief of symptoms and would undergo the procedure again. The other patient had a fracture through the inflexion level fusion mass at 4 weeks postoperatively. Although apparently healed, outcome assessment for this patient remains uncertain. The removal incidence was slightly higher for C-D instrumentation (7 of 47) than for Harrington (5 of 62). The most frequent observation recorded at the time of removal was corrosion at component connection sites. Because of concern about this finding, alternative materials are being explored.

The increased complexity of the C-D instrumentation appeared to be well justified as there were no pseudarthroses in the 47 patients with that instrumentation compared to 7 patients of 62 receiving Harrington instrumentation (10%). Of course, the latter patients were done earlier in the series.

Advanced Surgical Technique Development

Spinal deformity is often too severe and too stiff to be managed by positioning or mechanical realignment techniques. Consequently, an effort has been made to safely apply destabilization methods to facilitate realignment.

A principal proponent of this approach has been Dr. Charles F. Heinig, who, in 1974, began to develop techniques of spinal destabilization specifically for short, sharp, stiff kyphotic deformities [32]. The procedure, now known as the eggshell procedure, results in a closing osteotomy of the spine, hinging on the anterior longitudinal ligament and anterior portion of the anterior column. All are performed posteriorly.

To analyze and understand Heinig's technique, we developed a canine model which has been very helpful in avoiding the pitfalls of the procedure [33] (Fig. 12). We have been able to utilize it clinically on several occasions, all with gratifying angular correction and none with serious complications. A typical application is shown in Fig. 13. A further application of this approach has been a posterolateral decompression of severe burst fractures. Dr. Heinig and Dr. Behrooz Akbarnia [34] have been strong advocates of this usage. Instruments have been developed to facilitate these procedures (Fig. 14).

Improvement of Bone Healing

There seems to be widespread consensus that autograft remains far superior to allograft. As a result, we use autograft whenever possible. Furthermore, we have observed that cortical cancellous autograft may be superior to cancellous

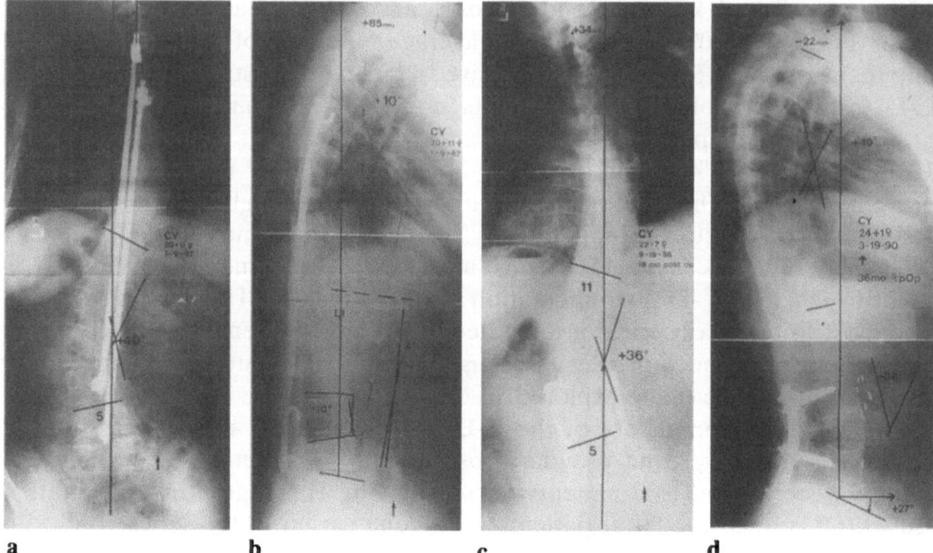

a b c d

Fig. 13a–d. Preoperative standing posterior **a** and lateral **b** radiographs of a 21-year-old female with flat back syndrome following prior instrumentation and fusion for idiopathic scoliosis. Posteroanterior **c** and lateral **d** radiographs following L4 eggshell osteotomy and second stage anterior interbody arthrodesis

autograft for anterior and middle column repair. However, it has been well recorded in the literature that autograft harvest is a source of considerable morbidity. To understand our patients' morbidity and identify areas that could be improved, we studied a consecutive series of 261 patients having iliac crest autograft harvests [35]. Although no serious perioperative complications were encountered, 10% of the 190 patients surveyed long-term had major complications of seromas, unslightly scars (one requiring revision), and chronic pain limiting activity (three patients), while an additional 39% indicated they either had some sensory dysesthesia or were unhappy with their scar. These findings were much higher than had been recorded at clinical follow-up. We believe they are minor problems, but also remain aggravations.

To refine autograft harvest technique, we have focused on improving exposure and closure. To limit sensory dysesthesia, we have attempted to place our graft incision precisely (Fig. 15a,b) and to spread the subcutaneous layer bluntly, allowing space for the sensory nerves to be retracted and, when obvious, identified and preserved. During closure, we have tried to relieve skin tension by providing a four-layer closure (Fig. 16), but a follow-up study will be necessary to determine the effectiveness of this approach. In the meantime, autograft remains our mainstay.

To move into the future and eliminate the need for autograft, Dr. H. Clarke Anderson, the Mary Alice and Paul R. Harrington Distinguished Professor of Orthopedic Research, and his team have been pursuing biological materials

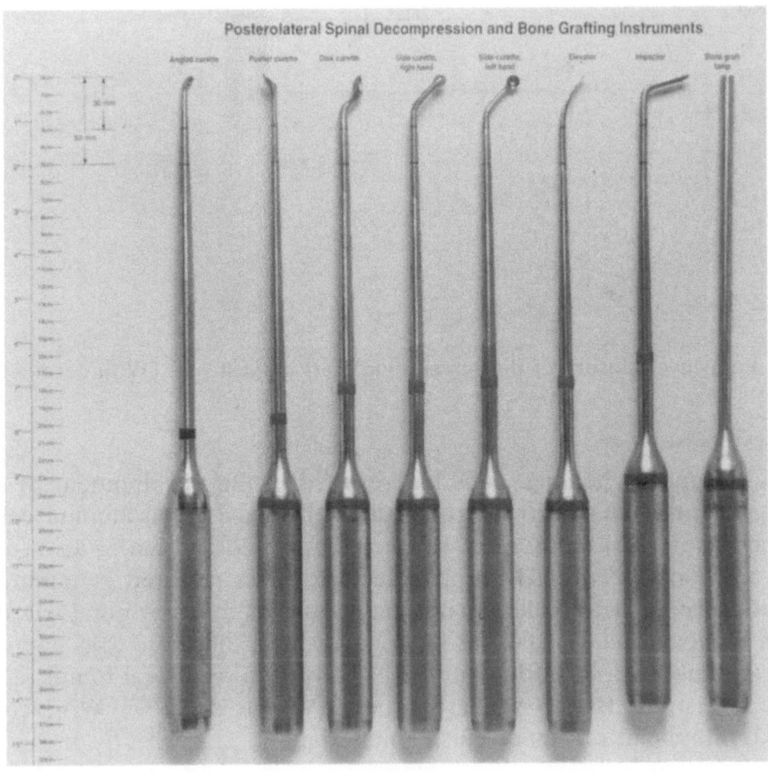

Fig. 14. Posterolateral dissection and decompression instrumentation set

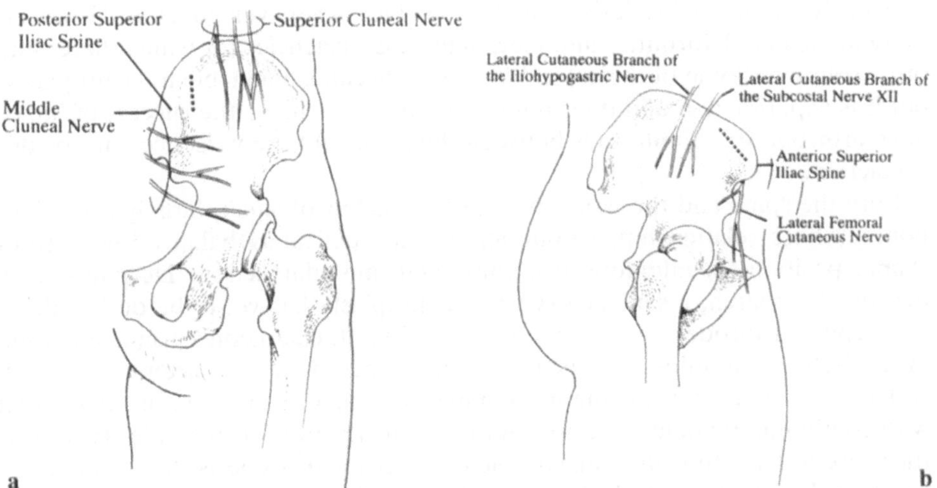

Fig. 15a,b. Incision location for posterior **a** and anterior **b** iliac crest bone graft removal. (With permission from [35a])

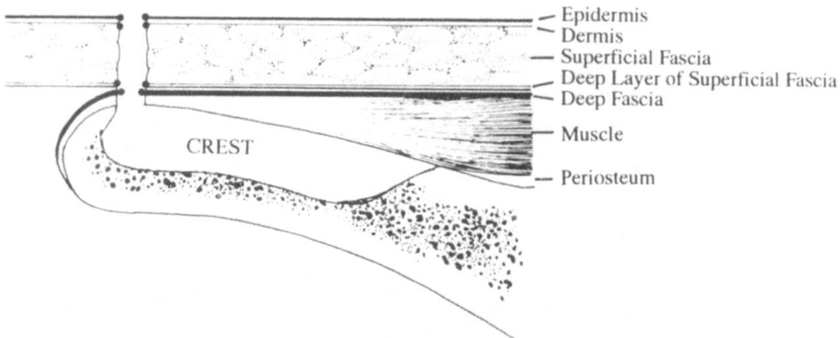

Fig. 16. Four-layer closure of iliac crest bone graft harvest site. (With permission from [35a])

that could improve healing. This has resulted in the development of a bone-inducing agent (BIA) derived from cultured Saos-2 osteosarcoma cells [36]. These cells were first cultured in 1975 from an osteosarcoma of an 11-year-old female and have been easily propagated and mass cultured at minimal cost. Implanted live or dead cells do not cause tumors and are not toxic to nude mice. A highly enriched BIA has been harvested from these cells and is active despite minimal matrix production by the cells. In a recent rat femur segmental defect repair study, BIA was clearly superior to autograft [37]. Work continues on the development of this promising material.

Discussion

Obviously, spinal arthrodesis should be avoided whenever possible. However, there are spinal deformities and mechanical insufficiencies for which there is no other solution. Some of these conditions may become amenable to arthroplasty, but it is experimental and does not seem likely to achieve the success of hip or knee arthroplasty. Similarities between the spine and the wrist account for this prediction.

Both the spine and the wrist consist of a number of small, largely cancellous bones, whose relationships to one another are delicately balanced because of shape, position, ligamentous restraints, and muscular action. Despite over a decade of research, a satisfactory wrist arthroplasty has yet to be designed.

As spinal arthrodesis seems likely to remain in the surgeon's armamentarium indefinitely, continuing efforts to optimize the procedure seem warranted. Reliable methods of achieving it are improving rapidly, and it seems likely that with continuing refinement, a fusion rate of nearly 100% is possible. However, there are at least four inherent problems in spinal arthrodesis that can only be minimized, not eliminated. Three of these problems deal with the junctional zone: motion and load concentration, malalignment, and stiffness mismatch.

The fourth relates to fusion stiffness and strength. All are associated with load concentration. Research continues on dealing with these problems [38].

Finally, no discussion of the optimization of spinal arthrodesis would be complete without acknowledging the critical importance of patient selection for arthrodesis. Research in this area is ongoing in a number of centers around the world. While most patients with spinal problems can be managed without surgery, when it is needed, optimization is essential. In conclusion, as a result of our studies and those of many other researchers, spinal arthrodesis continues to be improved as a therapeutic method.

Summary. For more than a decade, we have been conducting a series of studies focused on optimizing spinal arthrodesis. These studies can be categorized into four major areas: (1) three-dimensional analysis of spinal deformity, (2) implant research and development, (3) advanced surgical technique development, and (4) methods of promoting improved bone healing. The studies were briefly reviewed and an attempt made to place them into context. While spinal arthrodesis may eventually be partially replaced by arthroplasty, there are several reasons to believe that it will not be completely eliminated.

Acknowledgments. The author wishes to thank Jan Brunks and Barbara Funk for their assistance with this manuscript.

References

1. Jeffries BV, Tarlton MA, DeSmet AA, Dwyer SJ III, Brower AC (1980) Computerized measurement and analysis of scoliosis. Radiology 134:381–385
2. DeSmet AA, Tarlton MA, Cook LT, Fritz SL, Dwyer SJ III (1980) A radiographic method for three-dimensional analysis of spine configuration. Radiology 137:343–34
3. DeSmet AA, Cook LT, Tarlton MA, Asher MA (1981) Assessment of scoliosis using three-dimensional radiographic measurements. Automedia 4:25–348
4. DeSmet AA, Goin JE, Asher MA, Scheuech HG (1982) A clinical study of the differences between the scoliotic angles measured on PA and AP radiographs. J Bone Joint Surg 64A:489–493
5. DeSmet AA, Tarlton MA, Berridge AS, Asher MA (1983) The top view of analysis of scoliosis progression. Radiology 147:369–372
6. DeSmet AA, Asher MA, Cook LT, Goin JR, Scheuech HG, Orrick JM (1984) Three-dimensional analysis of right thoracic idiopathic scoliosis. Spine 9:377–381
7. Asher MA, Cook LT, DeSmet AA (1992) Axial (transverse) plane evolution of the right thoracic idiopathic scoliosis deformity. In: Dansereau J (ed) International symposium on 3-D scoliotic deformities. Gustav Fischer Verlag, Berlin Heidelberg New York, pp 198–205
8. DeSmet AA, Fritz SL, Asher MA (1981) A method for minimizing radiation exposure from scoliosis and radiographs. Orthop Trans 5:33
9. Asher MA, DeSmet AA, Tarlton MA, Cook LT, Scheuech HG, Orrick JM (1982)

Sagittal plane alignment of the spine in females with right thoracic idiopathic adolescent scoliosis. Orthop Trans 6:7–8
10. Asher M, DeSmet A, Goin J, Orrick J (1984) Single major thoracic and double major thoraco-lumbar idiopathic scoliosis curve separation: Lumbar curve analysis. Trans 30th Annual Meeting Orthop Res Soc 9:366
11. Asher M, DeSmet A, Orrick J (1986) Three-dimensional analysis of the effect of dorsal instrumentation on right thoracic idiopathic scoliosis. Orthop Trans 10:26
12. Asher M, DeSmet A, Whitney W, Orrick J, Cook L, Bramble J (1987) Changes in spinal alignment resulting from spinal deformity orthoses in patients with adolescent idiopathic scoliosis. Orthop Trans 11:105–106
13. Asher M, DeSmet A, Cook L, Orrick J (1988) Classification of adolescent idiopathic scoliosis curve patterns: A three-dimensional analysis. Orthop Trans 12:260
14. Stokes IAF (1994) Three-dimensional terminology of spinal deformity. Spine 19: 236–248
15. Perdriolle R (1979) La Scoliose, Maloine SA, editeur. Paris
16. Asher M, Strippgen W (1986) Anthropometric studies of the human sacrum relating to dorsal transsacral implant design and development. Clin Orthop 203:58–62
17. Asher M, Carson WL, Heinig C, Strippgen W, Arendt M, Lark R, Hartley M (1988) A modular spinal rod linkage system to provide rotational stability. Spine 3:272–277
18. Asher MA, Strippgen WE, Heinig CF, Carson WL (1990) Isola Spinal Implant System: Principles and Practice. AcroMed, Cleveland, Ohio
19. Asher MA, Strippgen WE, Heinig CF, Carson WL (1992) Isola spinal implant system: Principles, design, and applications In: An HS, Cotler JM (eds) Spinal instrumentation. Williams and Wilkins, Baltimore, pp 325–351
20. Asher MA, Strippgen WE, Heinig CF, Carson WL (1992) Isola spinal implant system. Semin Spine Surg 4:175–192
21. Asher MA, Strippgen WE, Heinig CF, Carson WL (1993) Spinal instrumentation: Emphasizing application during the first two decades of life. In: Weinstein S (ed) The Pediatric Spine. Raven, New York, pp 1619–1658
22. Carson WL, Duffield RC, Arendt M, Ridgely BJ, Gaines RW (1990) Internal forces and moments in transpedicular spine instrumentation–the effect of pedicle screw angle and transfixation—the 4R-4bar linkage concept. Spine 15:893–901
23. Carson WL, Redman RS, Richards K (1991) Bending stiffness and strength of VSP, Isola, CD, TSRH, and Luque longitudinal member to bone screw connection subconstructs. Trans Scoliosis Research Society Annual Meeting, Minneapolis, Minnesota, September 24–27
24. McCord DH, Cunningham BW, Shono YU, Myers JT, McAfee PC (1992) Biomechanical analysis of lumbosacral fixation. Spine 17:S235–S243
25. Cunningham BW, Sefter JG, Shono YU, McAfee PC (1993) Static and cyclical biomechanical analysis of pedicle screw constructs. Spine 18:1677–1688
26. Schultz AB, Ashton-Miller JA (1991) Biomechanics of the human spine. In: Mow VC, Hayes WC (eds) Basic orthopaedic biomechanics. Raven, New York, pp 337–374
27. Smith KR, Hunt TR, Asher MA, Anderson HC, Carson WL, Robinson RG (1992) The effect of a stiff spinal implant on the bone-mineral content of the lumbar spine in dogs. J Bone Joint Surg 73-A:115–123
28. Dalenberg D, Asher M, Jayaraman G, Robinson R (1993) The effect of a stiff spinal implant and its loosening on bone mineral content in canines. Spine 18:1862–1866

29. Asher MA (1992) Instrumentation constructs and application sequences for idiopathic scoliosis. Poster exhibit presented at the 27th Annual Meeting of the Scoliosis Research Society, Kansas City, Missouri, September 22–26
30. Asher M, Orrick J (1992) An improved technique for the correction of severe pelvic obliquity in the cerebral palsy patient. Poster exhibit and paper presented at the European Spinal Deformities Society Annual Meeting. Lyon, France, June 17–19
31. Shobe J, Asher M (1993) The incidence and outcome of dorsal spinal implant removal for pain in patients operated for adolescent idiopathic scoliosis. Presented at the Seventh Annual North American Spine Society Meeting, Boston, MA, July 8–11, 1992; GICD, Lyon, France, June 15–16, 1992; Annual Meeting of Pediatric Orthopaedic Society of North America, White Sulphur Springs, West Virginia, May 2–5
32. Heinig CF (1984) Eggshell procedure in segmental spinal instrumentation. In: Luque E (ed) Segmental spinal instrumentation. Slack, New Jersey, pp 221–234
33. Asher M, Lark D (1991) Eggshell procedure in the dog: A means of technique development. Orthop Trans 15:245
34. Akbarnia B (1991) Posterolateral decompression in the treatment of spine fractures. Video J Orthop 6:3
35. Banwart JC, Asher MA (1991) Is iliac crest donor site morbidity overstated? Presented at Sixth Annual North American Spine Society Meeting, Keystone, Colorado, July 31–August 3, paper #28, pp 288–289
35a. Banwart JC, Asher MA, Hassanein RS (1995) Iliac crest bone graft harvest donor site morbidity. Spine 20:1055–1060
36. Anderson HC, Sugamoto K, Morris DC, Hsu HHT, Hunt T (1992) Bone-inducing agent (BIA) from cultured human Saos-2 osteosarcoma cells. Bone and Miner 16:49–62
37. Hunt TR, Hsu HHT, Morris DC, Schwappach JR, Lark RG, Anderson HC (1993) Healing of a segmental defect in the rat femur using a bone-inducing agent (BIA) derived from a cultured human osteosarcoma cell line (Saos-2). Proceedings of the 39th Annual Meeting, Orthopedic Research Society, February 15–18, San Francisco, California, p. 489
38. Craven TG, Carson WL, Asher MA, Robinson RG (1994) The effects of implant stiffness on the bypassed bone mineral density and facet fusion stiffness of the canine spine. Spine 19:1664–1673
39. ISO 2631-1978 Guide to evaluation of human exposure to whole body vibration, 1978

Spinal Rotation in Congenital Scoliosis

SEIICHI ISHIKAWA and J. RICHARD BOWEN[1]

Key Words. Congenital scoliosis, spinal rotation, spinal deformity, posterior spinal fusion

Introduction

Congenital vertebral anomalies induce a variety of spinal deformities such as congenital scoliosis, congenital kyphosis or lordosis, spina bifida, spinal instability, diastematomyelia, spinal stenosis, and Klippel-Feil syndrome. The development of these congenital vertebral malformations and their natural history and outcome are still poorly understood.

Development and maturation of the spinal column occur throughout both the prenatal and postnatal periods. The prenatal period is divided into the embryogenic stage (the first eight weeks of gestation) and the fetal stage (from eight weeks gestation to birth). Many congenital defects of the spine result from abnormalities during the embryogenic period [1–3].

In the normal development of the spinal column, the notochord and somites are formed at 3 gestational weeks. The notochord induces the formation of the neural plate, the serial segmentation of the vertebral centrum, the prenatal morphologic development of the skeleton, and the neuromuscular elements [1]. The somites form paired mesodermal segments within the paraxial mesoderm and separate into dermatome, myotome, and sclerotome. The somites grow dorsolaterally around the notochord and form alternating dense and loose zones. The dense zones develop into the intervertebral disks, the ribs, and the bony neural arches [2]. The loose zones form the centrum of the vertebrae. As these mesenchymal vertebral columns develop, the notochord gradually

[1] Alfred I. duPont Institute, 1600 Rockland Rd., Wilmington, DE 19803, USA

regresses, and toward the end of the embryogenic period, primary centers of enchondral ossification develop within each vertebral segment [1,2].

Failure of the spine in the embryo or fetus to develop properly or to differentiate will lead to congenital vertebral anomalies. Based on roentgenographical morphology, Winter has proposed two basic concepts of pathogenesis in defining most of the anomalies: defects of segmentation and defects of formation [4]. These concepts are well accepted, even though the origin and the developmental sequence of spinal anomalies remained uncertain. Tsou and associates have proposed a classification of congenital vertebral anomalies that is based on specific defects, pathogenesis, and time of origin in embryonic or fetal development. In their theory, certain types of anomalies occur during the embryogenic period and the others occur during the fetal period [5]. Watterson et al. reported that notochord removal in developing chick embryos resulted in abnormal vertebral body development [6]. Shapiro and Eyre found abnormal spatial arrangement in congenital scoliotic spines in a histopathologic study [7], and supported the hypothesis of abnormal notochord induction. Other theories suggest that generalized disorders of the structural protein collagen or abnormal distribution of intersegmental arteries at the levels of anomalies may be responsible for the formation of congenital vertebral malformations, but the definite mechanism is still controversial [8–10].

In past decades, much attention has been given to understanding the development and natural history of congenital vertebral anomalies; however, many questions remain. This chapter will discuss the natural history and outcome of spinal rotation in congenital scoliosis.

	Type of Congenital Anomaly					
			Hemivertebra			
Site of Curvature	Block Vertebra	Wedged Vertebra	Single	Double	Unilateral Unsegmented Bar	Unilateral Unsegmented Bar and Contralateral Hemivertebrae
Upper thoracic	<1° – 1°	★ – 2°	1° – 2°	2° – 2.5°	2° – 4°	5° – 6°
Lower thoracic	<1° – 1°	2° – 2°	2° – 2.5°	2° – 3°	5° – 6.5°	6° – 7°
Thoraco lumbar	<1° – 1°	1.5° – 2°	2° – 3.5°	5° – ★	6° – 9°	> 10° – ★
Lumbar	<1° – ★	<1° – ★	<1° – 1°	★	> 5° – ★	★
Lumbo sacral	★	★	<1° – 1.5°	★	★	★

No treatment required   May require spinal fusion   Require spinal fusion

★ Too few or no curves

Fig. 1. Representation of the natural history of congenital scoliosis in 251 patients. (Reprinted with permission from [14])

Curve Progression and Spinal Rotation in Congenital Scoliosis

Many articles have described the natural history of the lateral curve in congenital scoliosis [11–24] and, to our knowledge, the report of McMaster and Ohtsuka is the most definitive [14]. They propose that the rate of deterioration and the ultimate severity of the curve depends on both the type of anomaly and the site in the spine at which it occurrs. In addition, they demonstrated the median yearly rate of deterioration without treatment for each type of congenital scoliosis in each region of the spine (Fig. 1) and that, furthermore, lateral curvature and rotation of the spine may develop in both areas of anomalous vertebrae (as congenital scoliosis) and areas of normal vertebrae (as noncongenital or compensatory scoliosis). They also reported that the noncongenital curvature may become more rigid, more severe, and more rotated than the congenital curve, and that it may contribute to the overall deformity [14].

In recent years, our concept of the three-dimensional aspects of scoliosis has been changing. In the past, the spinal deformity in congenital scoliosis was considered a two-dimensional deformity such as a lateral curvature, kyphosis, or lordosis. As progress has been made in our understanding of the natural history of congenital scoliosis, attention has been focused on the spatial alignment and rotation of the vertebral bodies (Fig. 2).

The fundamental treatment of a progressive lateral curvature in anomalous vertebrae (congenital scoliosis) is posterior spinal fusion, which halts the pro-

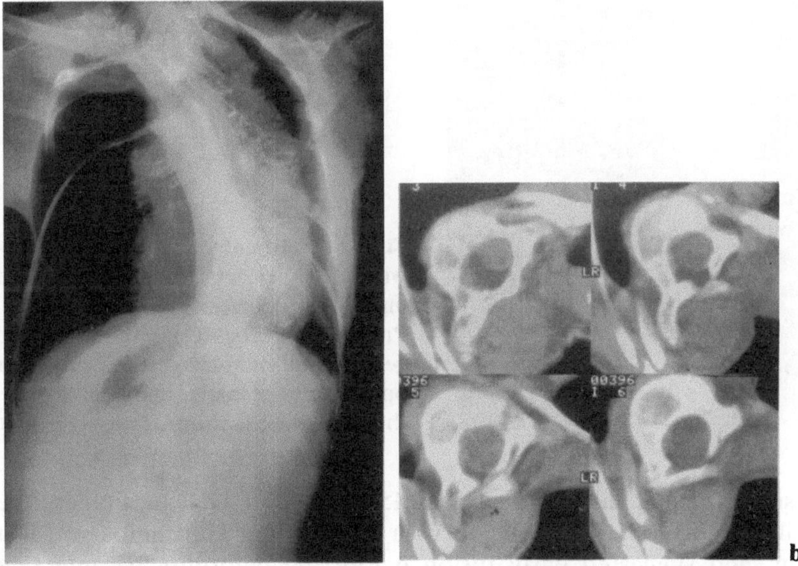

Fig. 2a,b. a Roentgenogram of a 14-year-old female showing a significant spinal rotation. **b** CT scan showing spinal rotation at the thoracolumbar region

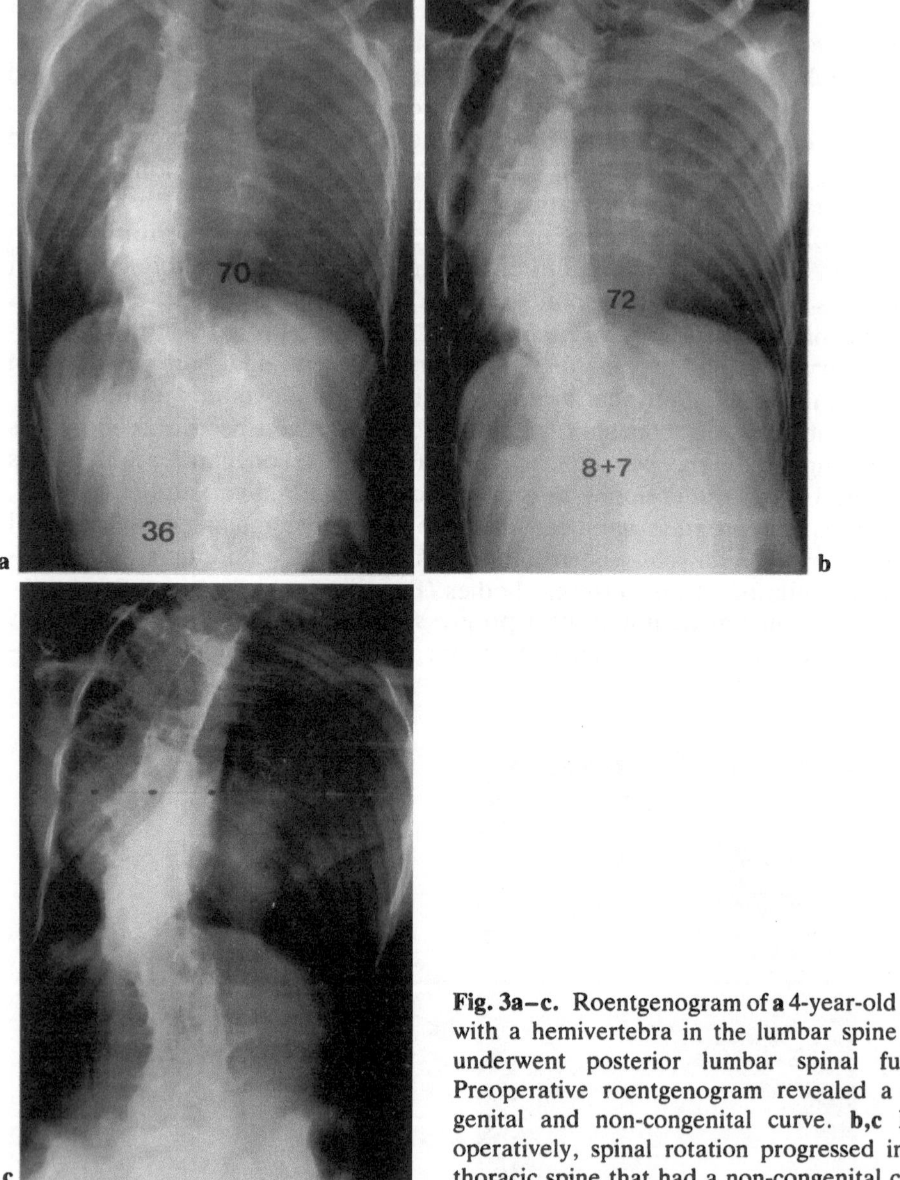

Fig. 3a–c. Roentgenogram of **a** 4-year-old male with a hemivertebra in the lumbar spine who underwent posterior lumbar spinal fusion. Preoperative roentgenogram revealed a congenital and non-congenital curve. **b,c** Postoperatively, spinal rotation progressed in the thoracic spine that had a non-congenital curve

gression of curve magnitude [12,13,15,16,18–27]. Hall et al. described good results of posterior spinal fusion with and without Harrington rod instrumentation, and suggested early fusion before the deformity became severe and required excessive correction [27]. Winter et al., in multiple studies, have written that posterior arthrodesis of the spine is satisfactory for most patients

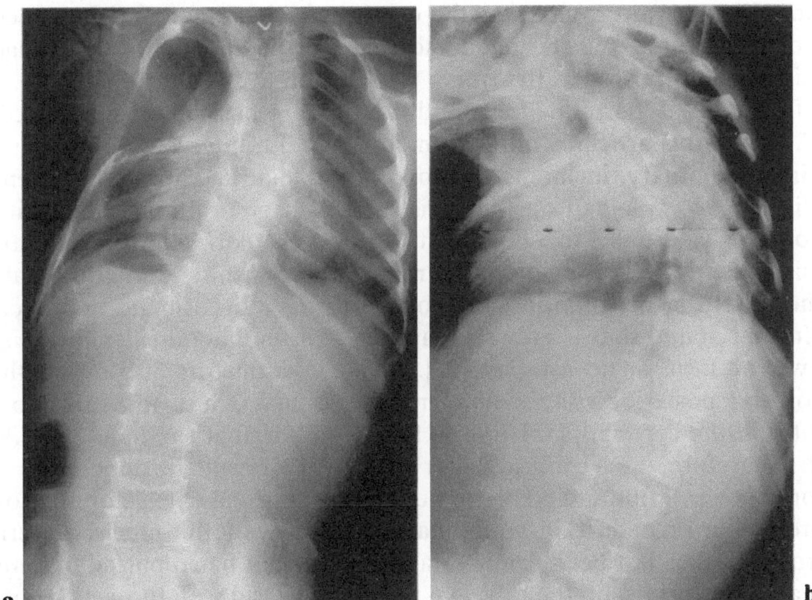

Fig. 4a,b. Roentgenogram of **a** patient who underwent posterior spinal fusion for a unilateral bar in the thoracic spine. **b** Twelve years after surgery, this patient had a bending of the fusion mass and spinal rotation

with congenital scoliosis; however, postoperative bending of the fusion mass in immature patients may occur [18–24]. They thought the reason for bending was a growth discrepancy between the convex and concave sides of the curve, but did not explain spinal rotation.

In recent years, the effects of arthrodesis on spinal growth has been a greatly debated topic [11,16,20,25,26,28–33]. Young patients with the most remaining growth at the time of arthrodesis should have the greatest potential for growth-related deformities [20,29,30,32]. Theoretically, the posterior fusion area does not grow longitudinally; however, vertebral body growth could result in curve progression, spinal rotation, or lordosis, which is not frequently seen [19,21,31]. Recently, postoperative progressive spinal rotation or bending of the fusion mass emerges as a major cosmetic problem (Figs. 3 and 4). Postoperative vertebral rotation with curve progression was described by Hefti and McMaster, who reported a series of 24 patients with a mean age of 10 years who underwent posterior spinal arthrodesis for infantile or juvenile idiopathic scoliosis [30]. Postoperatively, there was a mean 9-degree loss of correction, an increase in vertebral rotation, and a worsening rib hump deformity. Dubousset et al. reviewed 39 cases of posterior spinal fusion performed in children (Risser I) for idiopathic and paralytic scoliosis, and termed this combined effect of postoperative loss of correction and increase in vertebral rotation as the crankshaft phenomenon [29]. They pointed out that examples of bending in Winter's textbook demonstrate rotation as the crankshaft phenomenon. More recently, Terek et al. reported that this phenomenon occurred in patients with congenital scoliosis who had postoperative curve progression [32].

Roaf stated that lateral bending and rotation are basically linked in scoliosis [34]. Although his article is more than 30 years old, interesting statements are made in his summary, including the observation that the entire phenomenon of scoliosis can be explained on the basis of a primary rotational deformity and that rotation is usually the dominant factor, that correction and control of scoliosis depends on correction of the rotational deformity, and lastly that even a slight reduction in rotation can produce a marked cosmetic improvement. Roaf further stated that if growth is arrested on the lateral sides of the spine, there will be little or no rotation [35]. Other investigators also report that an anterior and posterior convex hemiarthrodesis may cause the spine to grow straighter in the coronal plane and to lessen the original rotation [22,25,28,33, 35,36]. Therefore, as a surgical intervention to prevent postoperative spinal rotation, both anterior and posterior hemiarthrodesis may be a more reasonable and preferable procedure in young patients; however, the precise criteria for this procedure has not been firmly established. Piggot has reported resection of the heads and necks of the ribs on the concave side of throacic idiopathic curves. He showed that if growth is arrested at the rib head on one side, some degree of asymmetry of vertebral growth will follow, as the vertebrae must grow into the position of rotatory deformity toward the side of growth arrest. Once rotation has appeared, the growth plates of the vertebral bodies are situated asymmetrically in such a way that they are subject to relative compression on the side from which they are rotated. Retardation of longitudinal growth will occur on this side, giving rise to lateral curve [36].

Alfred I. duPont Experience of Spinal Rotation in Congenital Scoliosis

Between 1946 and 1985, 242 patients with congenital scoliosis (who did not have myelomeningocele, spondylolisthesis with scoliosis, spondyloepiphyseal dysplasia, Scheuermann's kyphosis, or congenital kyphosis) were treated and the first 100 consecutive cases were evaluated [37]. There were 72 females and 28 males. Seventy-nine of the patients had been treated operatively, whereas 21 patients had been treated by nonoperative means. The mean age at diagnosis was 6 years (range, birth to 18 years), and the mean follow-up period was 10 years (range, 1–34 years) from the time of first visit. Seventy-eight patients had reached skeletal maturity by their final visit. The type of congenital scoliosis was cataloged according to the classification of MacEwen, Moe, and Winter [12,13,22,26,38]. Vertebral anomalies resulting from failure of segmentation included unilateral bar, unilateral bar with contralateral hemivertebrae at the same level, and bilateral failure of segmentation (block vertebrae). Failure

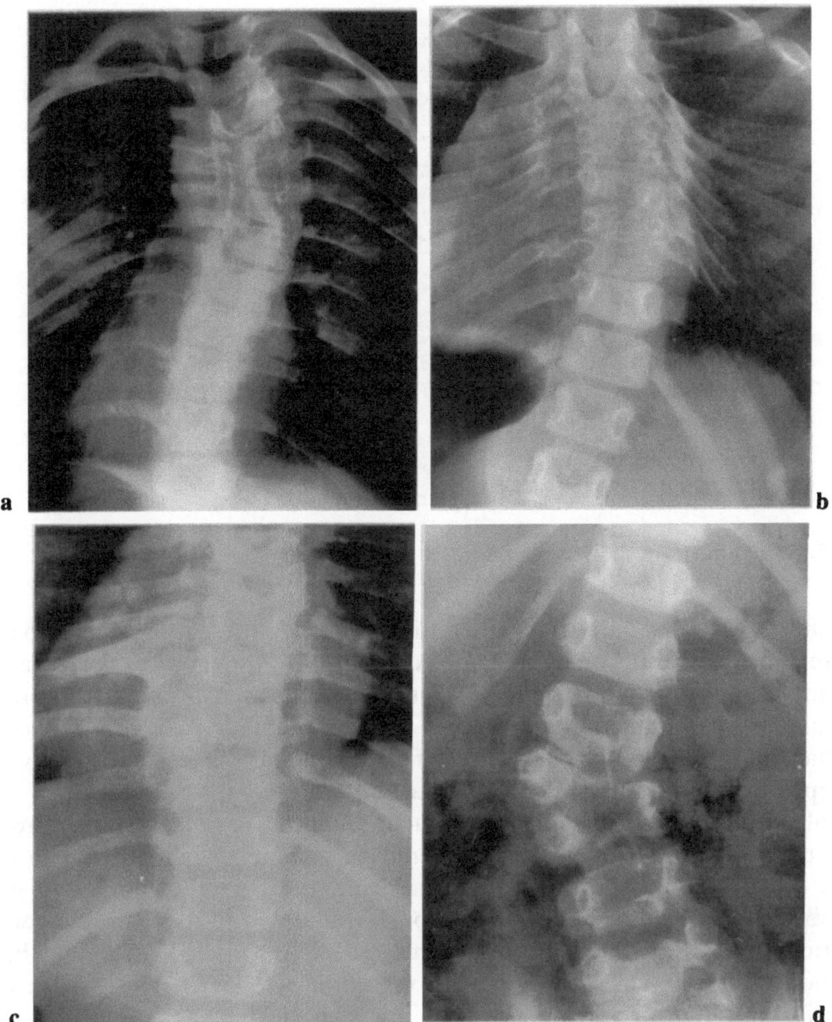

Fig. 5a–f. Roentgenogram of **a** unilateral bar, **b** nonsegmental vertebra (block vertebrae), **c** a hemivertebra nonsegmented on its superior surface, **d** a hemivertebra nonsegmented on both sides, **e** wedged vertebra, **f** unclassified vertebra

of formation of the vertebral body resulted in incarcerated hemivertebrae, nonincarcerated hemivertebrae, semisegmented hemivertebrae, nonsegmented hemivertebrae, or wedge vertebrae. Complex anomalies consisted of vertebral anomalies that were too diverse for classification (Fig. 5).

The area of congenital scoliosis was also catalogued according to the site of the apex of the curve, which frequently coincided with the site of the anomaly. A curve whose apex was inclusively between the second and sixth thoracic

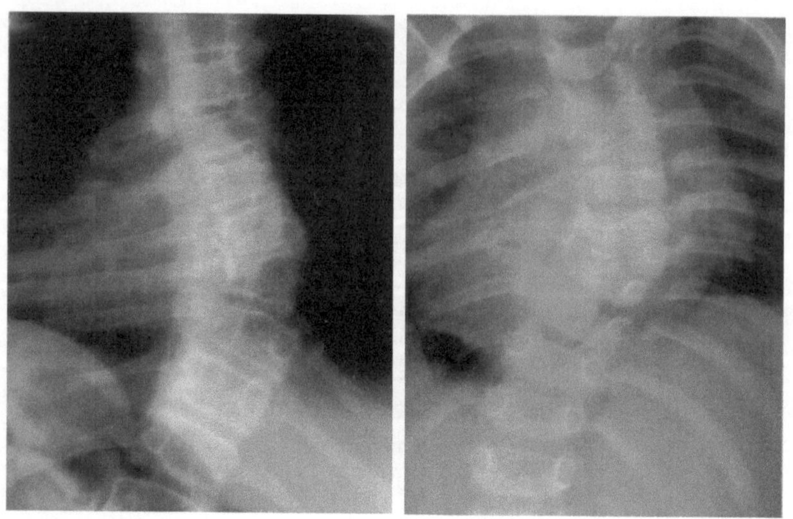

Fig. 5. *Continued*

vertebrae was considered an upper thoracic curve. A curve whose apex was located inclusively between the seventh and eleventh thoracic vertebrate was considered a lower thoracic curve. A curve with its apex at the 12th thoracic or 1st lumbar vertebrae was considered a thoracolumbar curve. The apex of a lumbar curve was between the 2nd and 4th lumbar vertebrae, inclusive, and the apex of a lumbosacral curves was at the 5th lumbar vertebrae.

Only curves with congenital vertebral anomalies were measured according to the guidelines set forth by Cobb for measuring the magnitude of the lateral curve [39] and by Perdriolle for measuring the vertebral rotation [40]. In several instances, information had to be extrapolated to measure the vertebral rotation because of the abnormal vertebrae. This entailed assuming that the location of the pedicles of the apical vertebrae was in line with those of the superior and inferior vertebrae.

Seventy-nine of the patients had been treated by nonoperative means. The indications for operation were the magnitude of the curve at the time of presentation and the increase in curve magnitude over time. Halofemoral traction was used for preoperative correction in 9 cases and Cotrel traction was used in 15 cases. The surgical technique was a bilateral Moe-type facet joint arthrodesis, bilateral decortication, and grafting with autogenous iliac bone graft [41]. Six patients underwent Harrington rod instrumentation in addition, which was their surgeon's choice. In all instances, the fusion levels included at least the vertebrae in the measured Cobb angle.

There was a total of 119 congenital curves. Thirty-nine cases showed failure of segmentation, 38 cases showed failure of formation, and 7 cases were complex (unclassifiable), for a total of 84 single curves. Thirteen cases had double curves and three cases had triple curves.

Unilateral Bar

There were 35 cases of unilateral bar. Average follow-up for all patients with a unilateral bar was 10 years, at which time, the average age of the patients was 19 years. Three patients were treated nonoperatively. For the three patients treated nonoperatively, the average initial curve magnitude was 27 degrees, and at follow-up it was 57 degrees. The average initial spinal rotation was 5 degrees, and at follow-up, two of the patients had 30 degrees of rotation; in one patient the rotation could not be measured. Thirty-two patients were treated by posterior spinal arthrodesis. The average age at the time of fusion was 10 years. Twenty-nine patients had posterior spinal fusion without instrumentation. The average initial curve magnitude was 51 degrees. The average preoperative curve magnitude was 60 degrees, and at follow-up it was 54 degrees. The average initial spinal rotation was 9 degrees, and preoperatively it was 14 degrees; at follow-up, it was 27 degrees.

One patient was treated with anterior and posterior arthrodesis; the initial curve magnitude was 35 degrees, preoperatively it was 32 degrees, and at follow-up it was 34 degrees. This patient's initial spinal rotation was 0 degrees, and at follow-up it was 15 degrees. Another patient was treated with resection of the contralateral hemivertebrae and posterior spinal arthrodesis. The initial curve magnitude was 63 degrees, and the preoperative curve magnitude was 65 degrees. This progressed to 87 degrees at the time of follow-up. The initial spinal rotation was 15 degrees, but 0 degrees at the time of operation. No follow-up measurement could be made because the apical vertebra had been resected. One patient had Harrington rod instrumentation in addition to the posterior spinal arthrodesis. The initial curve was 52 degrees, and 62 degrees at the time of operation; at last follow-up it was 36 degrees. No rotation was observed in this patient until at follow-up, at which time it measured 15 degrees.

Block Vertebrae

There were four cases of block vertebrae and the average follow-up was 16 years, at which time the average age was 24 years. Three patients were treated nonoperatively. The average initial curve magnitude was 4 degrees, and at follow-up it was 13 degrees. One case was treated by posterior spinal arthrodesis. This patient had an initial and preoperative curve magnitude of 30 degrees, which measured 34 degrees at follow-up. No rotation was observed at any time in any patient with block vertebrae regardless of the treatment given.

Hemivertebrae

There were 20 cases of segmented hemivertebrae. The average age at follow-up was 21 years. Four cases were incarcerated and treated nonoperatively. The average initial curve magnitude in these four cases was 19 degrees, and at the time of follow-up it was 27 degrees. No rotation was present at the initial visit; however, at the time of follow-up, the average rotation was 13 degrees. There were six cases of nonincarcerated segmented vertebrae. At follow-up, the average rotation was 23 degrees. Two cases were treated nonoperatively. In these two patients, the average initial curve magnitude was 22 degrees, and at the time of follow-up it was 36 degrees. Again, no rotation was measurable at the initial visit. Four cases were treated with posterior spinal arthrodesis. The average initial curve magnitude was 39 degrees, preoperatively it was 44 degrees, and at follow-up it was 38 degrees. The average initial rotation was 15 degrees, preoperatively it was 22 degrees, and at follow-up it was 26 degrees.

There were nine cases of nonincarcerated semisegmented hemivertebrae. The patients' average age at follow-up was 20 years (range, 17–24 years). One of these patients who had been treated non-operatively, had a curve of 47 degrees at the initial visit and 57 degrees at the last follow-up. There was no measurable rotation at either visit. Eight cases were treated with posterior spinal arthrodesis. The average initial curve magnitude was 38 degrees, preoperatively it was 41 degrees, and at last follow-up it was 32 degrees. The average initial rotation was 6 degrees, preoperatively it was 5 degrees, and at follow-up it was 11 degrees.

There was one case of a nonincarcerated nonsegmented hemivertebra, which was treated with posterior spinal arthrodesis. This patient was 17 years old at follow-up. The initial curve magnitude was 31 degrees, preoperatively it was 30 degrees, and at follow-up it was 30 degrees. There was no measurable rotation until follow-up, at which time it measured 15 degrees.

There were ten cases of multiple hemivertebrae, of which one case was treated nonoperatively. The initial curve magnitude was 40 degrees and 66 degrees at follow-up. The initial rotation was 15 degrees and 30 degrees at follow-up. Seven cases were treated with posterior spinal arthrodesis. The average initial curve magnitude was 44 degrees, preoperatively it was 51 degrees, and at follow-up it was 44 degrees. The average initial rotation was 0 degrees, preoperatively it was 6 degrees, and at follow-up it was 8 degrees. Two cases had the addition of Harrington rod instrumentation. The average initial curve in these two patients was 54 degrees, preoperatively it was 65 degrees, and at follow-up it was 29 degrees. Initially, neither patient had any measurable rotation. Prior to surgery, one of these patients had 15 degrees of rotation, which progressed to 45 degrees at the time of the last visit. The other patient had no rotation. The average age at follow-up was 19 years. Average follow-up in all patients with hemivertebrae was 8 years.

Wedged Vertebrae

There were eight cases of wedged vertebrae. The average follow-up was 10 years, at which time the average age of the patients was 22 years. Four of the patients were treated nonoperatively. The average initial curve magnitude was 31 degrees, and at follow-up it was 50 degrees. The average initial rotation was 4 degrees, and at follow-up it was 19 degrees. Two cases were treated with posterior spinal arthrodesis. The average initial curve magnitude was 58 degrees, preoperatively it was 67 degrees, and at follow-up it was 41 degrees. Both patients had no rotation at the time of the first visit. Preoperatively, one patient had 15 degrees of rotation, which progressed to 30 degrees at the time of the follow-up. The other patient never developed any rotation. Two cases had the addition of Harrington rod instrumentation. The average initial curve magnitude was 41 degrees, preoperatively it was 45 degrees, and at follow-up it was 28 degrees. The average initial rotation was 0 degrees, preoperatively it was 7 degrees, and at follow-up it was 23 degrees.

Complex Deformities

There were seven cases in which the congenital scoliosis consisted of an unclassifiable complex of multiple deformities. The average follow-up for these patients was 4 years, at which time their average age was 14 years. One case that was treated nonoperatively had an initial curve magnitude of 21 degrees that progressed to 31 degrees at follow-up. No measurable rotation was seen in this patient. Six cases were treated with posterior spinal arthrodesis. The average initial curve magnitude was 42 degrees, preoperatively it was 44 degrees, and at follow-up it was 38 degrees. In three patients, the rotation could not be measured. Two patients had no rotation, and one patient who had 0 degrees of rotation initially had 15 degrees of rotation at the time of the last visit.

Conclusions

Vertebral rotation in congenital scoliosis is a component of the spinal deformity. Asymmetric growth of congenitally deformed vertebrae make confirmation of the etiology of spinal rotation difficult. Vertebral rotation progressed prior to and after posterior spinal fusion in cases of unilateral bar, nonincarcerated hemivertebrae, or wedged vertebrae. This study advocates that posterior spinal fusion in congenital scoliosis halts lateral curve progression. The authors believe that progressive vertebral rotation in certain types of congenital scoliosis is part of the natural history. Our data show that progressive vertebral rotation continues after posterior spinal fusion of the congenital segment that demonstrated progressive rotation prior to the operation. Congenital scoliosis that had no vertebral rotation prior to posterior spinal fusion did not rotate postoperatively. The authors believe that anterior spinal fusion to prevent progressive vertebral rotation in immature patients (the crankshaft phenomenon) may not be necessary in certain types of congenital scoliosis that had no vertebral rotation prior to the operation.

Summary. We reviewed the embryology of the spine, the pathogenesis of congenital scoliosis, the natural history of lateral curvature, and discussed spinal rotation in congenital scoliosis. In a unilateral bar, rotation was progressive with or without posterior spinal fusion; however, the Cobb magnitude of scoliosis of the congenital component did not progress after posterior spinal fusion. In a hemivertebra, progression of curve magnitude and rotation varied. Posterior spinal fusion limited progression of the Cobb magnitude of the congenital components of this type of scoliosis. Rotation in the nonincarcerated vertebrae, however, increased from 15 to 26 degrees after spinal fusion and, in incarcerated vertebrae, rotation did not increase. In wedged vertebrae, a posterior spinal fusion stopped progression of the Cobb angle, but rotation continued to progress. In complex vertebral deformities, progression of rotation and scoliosis varied, and a posterior spinal fusion did not appear to significantly affect rotation. Vertebral rotation in congenital scoliosis is a major component of spinal deformity. Progressive rotation, which correlates with types of congenital curves, appears to be a major factor in the results of treatment; that is, vertebral rotation frequently continues to progress after a posterior spinal fusion of the congenital segments in congenital scoliosis caused by the unilateral bar, nonincarcerated hemivertebrae, or wedged vertebrae.

References

1. Ogden JA (1990) Development and maturation of the neuromusculoskeletal system. In: Morrissy RT (ed) Lovell and Winter's pediatric orthopaedics, vol I, 3rd edn. Lippincott, Philadelphia, pp 1–33
2. O'Rahilly R, Benson DR (1985) The development of the vertebral column. In: Bradford DS, Hensinger RN (eds) The pediatric spine. Thieme, New York, pp 3–17
3. Parke WW (1982) Development of the spine. In: Rothman RH, Simeone FA (eds) The spine, vol I, 2nd edn. Saunders, Philadelphia, pp 1–17
4. Winter RB (1987) Congenital spine deformity. In: Bradford DS, Lonstein JE, Moe JH, Ogilvie JW, Winter RB (eds) Moe's textbook of scoliosis and other spinal deformities. Saunders, Philadelphia, pp 233–270
5. Tsou PM, Yau A, Hodgson AR (1980) Embryogenesis and prenatal development of congenital vertebral anomalies and their classification. Clin Orthop 152:211–231
6. Watterson RL, Fowler I, Fowler BJ (1954) The role of the neural tube and notochord in development of axial skeleton of the chick. Am J Anat 95:337–339
7. Shapiro F, Eyre D (1981) Congenital scoliosis. A histopathologic study. Spine 6:107–117
8. Nogami H, Terashima Y, Tamaki K, Oohira A (1979) Congenital kyphoscoliosis and spinal cord lesion produced in the rat by β-aminoproprionitrile. Teratology 16:351–358
9. Tanaka T, Uhthoff HK (1981) The pathogenesis of congenital vertebral malformations. Acta Orthop Scand 52:413–425
10. Uden A, Nilsson IM, Willner S (1980) Collagen changes in congenital and idiopathic scoliosis. Acta Orthop Scand 51:271–274
11. Kuhns JG, Hormel RS (1952) Management of congenital scoliosis: Review of one hundred seventy cases. Arch Surg 65:250–263

12. MacEwen GD, Conway JJ, Miller WT (1968) Congenital scoliosis with unilateral bar. Radiology 90:711–715
13. MacEwen GD, Kumar SJ (1984) Congenital anomalies of the spine. In: Goldsmith HS (ed) Practice of surgery. Harper and Row, Philadelphia, pp 1–13
14. McMaster MJ, Ohtsuka K (1982) The natural history of congenital scoliosis. A study of two hundred and fifty-one patients. J Bone Joint Surg 64-A:1128–1147
15. McMaster MJ, David CV (1986) Hemivertebra as a cause of scoliosis. A study of 104 patients. J Bone Joint Surg 68-B:588–595
16. Nasca RJ, Stilling FH III, Stell HH (1975) Progression of congenital scoliosis due to hemivertebrae and hemivertebrae with bars. J Bone Joint Surg 57-A:456–466
17. Tanaka T (1988) A study of the progression of congenital scoliosis in non-operated cases. J Jpn Orthop Assoc 62:9–22
18. Winter RB, Moe JH, Eilers VE (1968) Congenital scoliosis. A study of 234 patients treated and untreated. Part I: Natural history. J Bone Joint Surg 50-A:1–15
19. Winter RB, Moe JH, Eilers VE (1968) Congenital scoliosis. A study of 234 patients treated and untreated. Part II: Treatment. J Bone Joint Surg 50-A:15–47
20. Winter RB (1971) The effects of early fusion on spine growth. In: Zorab PA (ed) Scoliosis and growth. Churchill, London, pp 98–104
21. Winter RB, Moe JH (1982) The results of spinal arthrodesis for congenital spinal deformity in patients younger than five years old. J Bone Joint Surg 64-A:419–432
22. Winter RB (1983) Congenital scoliosis. In: Winter RB (ed) Congenital deformities of the spine. Thieme-Stratton, New York, pp 177–227
23. Winter RB, Moe JH, Lonstein JE (1984) Posterior spinal arthrodesis for congenital scoliosis. An analysis of the cases of two hundred and ninety patients, five to nineteen years old. J Bone Joint Surg 66-A:1188–1197
24. Winter RB (1988) Congenital scoliosis. Orthop Clin North Am 19:395–408
25. Bernard TN Jr, Burke SW, Johnston CE III, Roberts JM (1985) Congenital spine deformities. A review of 47 cases. Orthopedics 8:777–783
26. Bunnell WP, MacEwen GD (1983) Congenital deformities of the spine. In: Evarts CM (ed) Surgery of the musculoskeletal system, vol 2. Churchill Livingstone, New York, pp 363–409
27. Hall JE, Herndon WA, Levine CR (1981) Surgical treatment of congenital scoliosis with or without Harrington instrumentation. J Bone Joint Surg 63-A:608–619
28. Andrew T, Piggott H (1985) Growth arrest for progressive scoliosis. Combined anterior and posterior fusion of the convexity. J Bone Joint Surg 67-B:193–197
29. Dubousset J, Herring JA, Shufflebarger H (1989) The crankshaft phenomenon. J Pediatr Orthop 9:541–550
30. Hefti FL, McMaster MJ (1983) The effect of the adolescent growth spurt on early posterior spinal fusion in infantile and juvenile idiopathic scoliosis. J Bone Joint Surg 65-B:247–254
31. Risser JC, Norquist DM, Cockrell BR Jr, Tateiwa M, Hoppenfeld S (1966) The effect of posterior spine fusion on the growing spine. Clin Orthop 46:127–139
32. Terek RM, Wehner J, Lubicky JP (1991) Crankshaft phenomenon in congenital scoliosis: A preliminary report. J Pediatr Orthop 11:527–532
33. Winter RB, Lonstein JE, Denis F, Sta-Ana de la Rosa H (1988) Convex growth arrest for progressive congenital scoliosis due to hemivertebrae. J Pediatr Orthop 8:633–638
34. Roaf R (1958) Rotation movements of the spine with special reference to scoliosis. J Bone Joint Surg 40-B:312–332

35. Roaf R (1963) The treatment of progressive scoliosis by unilateral growth-arrest. J Bone Joint Surg 45-B:637–651
36. Piggott H (1971) Posterior rib resection in scoliosis. J Bone Joint Surg 53-B:663–671
37. Lopez-Sosa F, Guille JT, Bowen JR (1992) Rotation of the spine in congenital scoliosis. Presented at the 58th annual meeting of the American Academy of Orthopaedic Surgeons
38. Winter RB (1990) Spinal problems in pediatric orthopaedics. In: Morrissy RT (ed) Lovell and Winter's pediatric orthopaedics, vol 2, 3rd edn. Lippincott, Philadelphia, pp 656–664
39. Cobb JR (1948) Outline for the study of scoliosis. AAOS Instructional course lectures. CV Mosby 5:261–275
40. Perdriolle R, Vidal J (1987) Morphology of scoliosis: Three-dimensional evolution. Orthopaedics 10:909–915
41. Moe JH (1958) A critical analysis of methods of fusion for scoliosis: An evaluation in two hundred and sixty-six patients. J Bone and Joint Surg 40-A:529–554

Diagnosis and Treatment of Tethered Spinal Cord Syndrome*

TAKAHIKO NAKAMURA, TAKAO HOMMA, SEIJI UCHIYAMA, and HIDEAKI E. TAKAHASHI[1]

Key Words. Tethered cord, diagnosis, treatment, spina bifida, spinal dysraphism

Introduction

Besides spina bifida aperta, there have been reports of an occult form of spina bifida, which was accompanied by bladder trouble, foot and toe deformities, gait disturbance, pain in the back and lower limbs, and a lumbosacral tumor. Recently, some authors have pointed out that in either aperta or the occult form of spina bifida, the essential pathology is a tethering state of the spinal cord. They reported this condition as tethered spinal cord syndrome. The purpose of this report is to relate our experiences in dealing with this syndrome.

Materials and Methods

Between 1976 and August 1983, there were 77 reported cases of tethered spinal cord syndrome in the department of Orthopedic Surgery at the Niigata University School of Medicine. Fifty-two cases were males and 25 were females. The patient's ages at the time of their initial visit to our hospital ranged from 5 months to 53 years. These patients were divided into two groups by the level of the conus. The first group was low-placed conus medullaris (LPCM), in which

[1] Department of Orthopedic Surgery, Niigata University School of Medicine, Asahimachi-dori 1-757, Niigata, 951 Japan

* This chapter was reproduced in part from an article in the *Journal of the Japanese Orthopedic Association* (58:1237–1251;1984), with permission.

Table 1. Signs and symptoms according to the type of tethered spinal cord syndrome.

Signs and symptoms	LPCM[a] (%)	TFT[a] (%)	Total[a] (%)
Incontinence or nocturia	30 (88)	32 (74)	77 (82)
Pain in back and lower limbs	1 (3)	9 (21)	10 (13)
Gait disturbance	8 (24)	1 (2)	9 (12)
Foot and toe deformities	28 (82)	7 (16)	35 (45)
Lumbosacral tumor	17 (50)	0 (0)	17 (22)
Sacral dimple	12 (35)	6 (14)	18 (23)

LPCM, Low-placed conus medularis; *TFT*, tight filum terminale
[a] Numbers of cases

the conus was below the L1 vertebral body, and the second was tight filum terminale (TFT) in which the conus was above the L2 vertebral body.

Of the 77 cases, the former (LPCM group) was comprised of 34 cases and the latter (TFT group) of 43 cases.

Results

Symptoms and Signs

Incontinence, gait disturbance, foot and toe deformities, lumbosacral tumor, and sacral dimple were seen more often in the LPCM group, whereas nocturia and pain in the back and lower limbs were seen more often in the TFT group (not shown).

In 54 cases, symptoms appeared before the age of 5 years but in 23 cases, symptoms appeared after the age of 5 years. Lasègue's sign was observed in 46% (LPCM: 24%, TFT: 23%).

As to neurological findings, abnormal sensation, motor weakness, and change of tendon reflex were seen in 38% (LPCM: 68%, TFT: 41%), 32% (LPCM: 62%, TFT: 9%), and 56% (LPCM: 76%, TFT: 40%), respectively. These findings were often seen in the LPCM group.

Diagnosis

Diagnosis was based on these symptoms and signs, and also through X-ray findings. Generally, authors have considered that this syndrome was accompanied by spina bifida, but in this series 9% (three cases) of the LPCM group and 23% (ten cases) of the TFT group exhibited no spina bifida on the plain X-ray film of the spine, indicating that cases affected by this syndrome did not always experience spina bifida at the same time.

Myelography was performed in 74 cases. In early cases, cisterna puncture was selected in 4 cases with pantopaque, but in the other 70 cases metrizamide myelography was carried out from a lumbar approach.

The A-P view in the supine position was most important in obtaining a correct diagnosis (Fig. 1). In the LPCM group, caudally tethered cord and ascending roots were found in all cases, and intraspinal lipoma was noted in 22 cases. In the TFT group, filum terminale was always visible in the myelogram. Computed tomography (CT) was carried out in 40 cases. Metrizamide CT clearly defined the three-dimensional anatomy of LPCM (Fig. 2), but it was not helpful for TFT since it visualized the filum terminale in only one case. Magnetic resonance imaging (MRI) is also a very useful procedure for diagnosis of this disease (Fig. 3).

Treatment

In the LPCM group, the operative procedure is a laminectomy (two or three lamina above the lipoma), careful dissection of intrathecal adhesion, resection of the lipoma and severance of the filum terminale (Fig. 4).

A release operation was performed in 58 cases (28 LPCM cases and 30 TFT cases). Forty-nine cases were examined 2 months or more after the surgery (27 LPCM cases and 22 TFT cases). Twenty-one cases (78%) in the LPCM group and 15 cases (68%) in the TFT group showed improvement of various degrees.

Conclusion

Spina bifida aperta and occulta, or neurospinal dysraphism, until now has always been evaluated from a horizontal plane of anatomy [1]. In many cases of the occult form with clinical symptoms and signs, abnormalities of the spinal

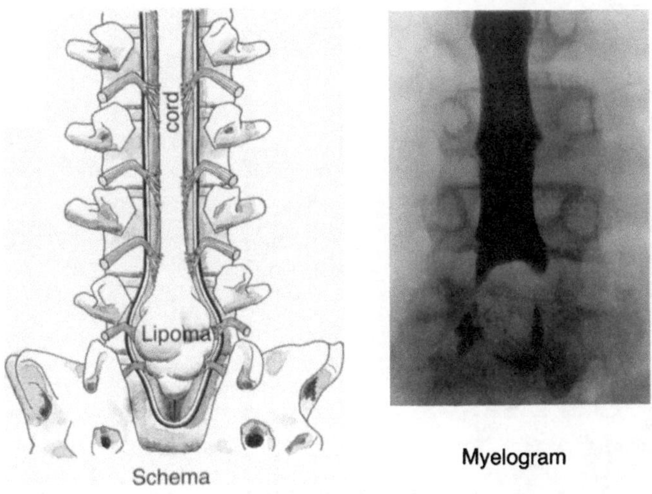

Fig. 1. Myelogram. Schematic illustration cord. Lipoma

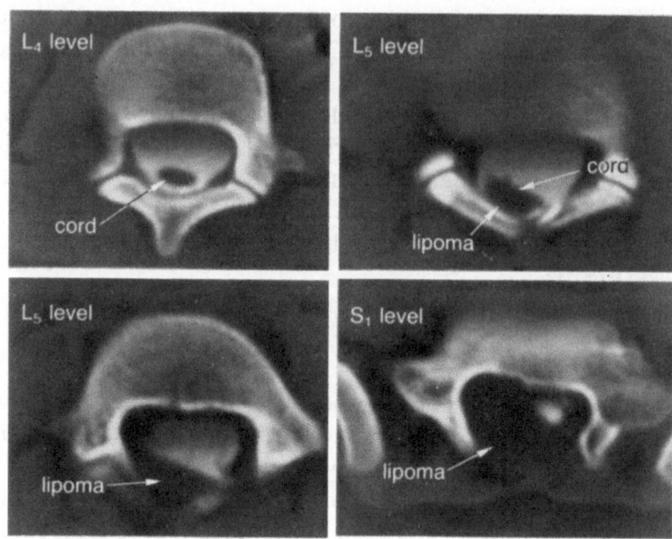

Fig. 2. Metrizamide computed tomography

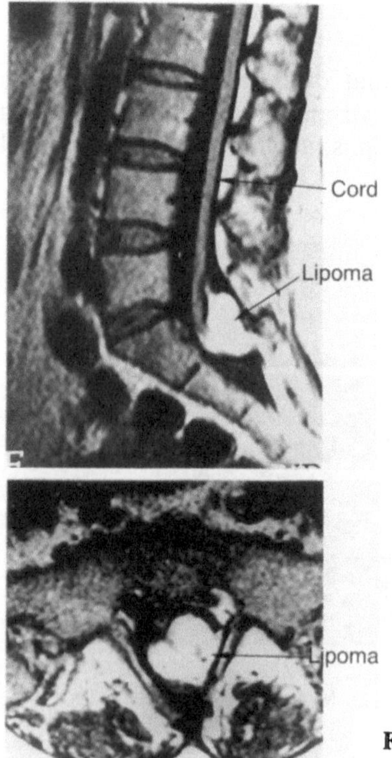

B

Fig. 3A,B. MRI **A** cord lipoma on T1-weighted sagittal view and **B** lipoma on T1-weighted axial view

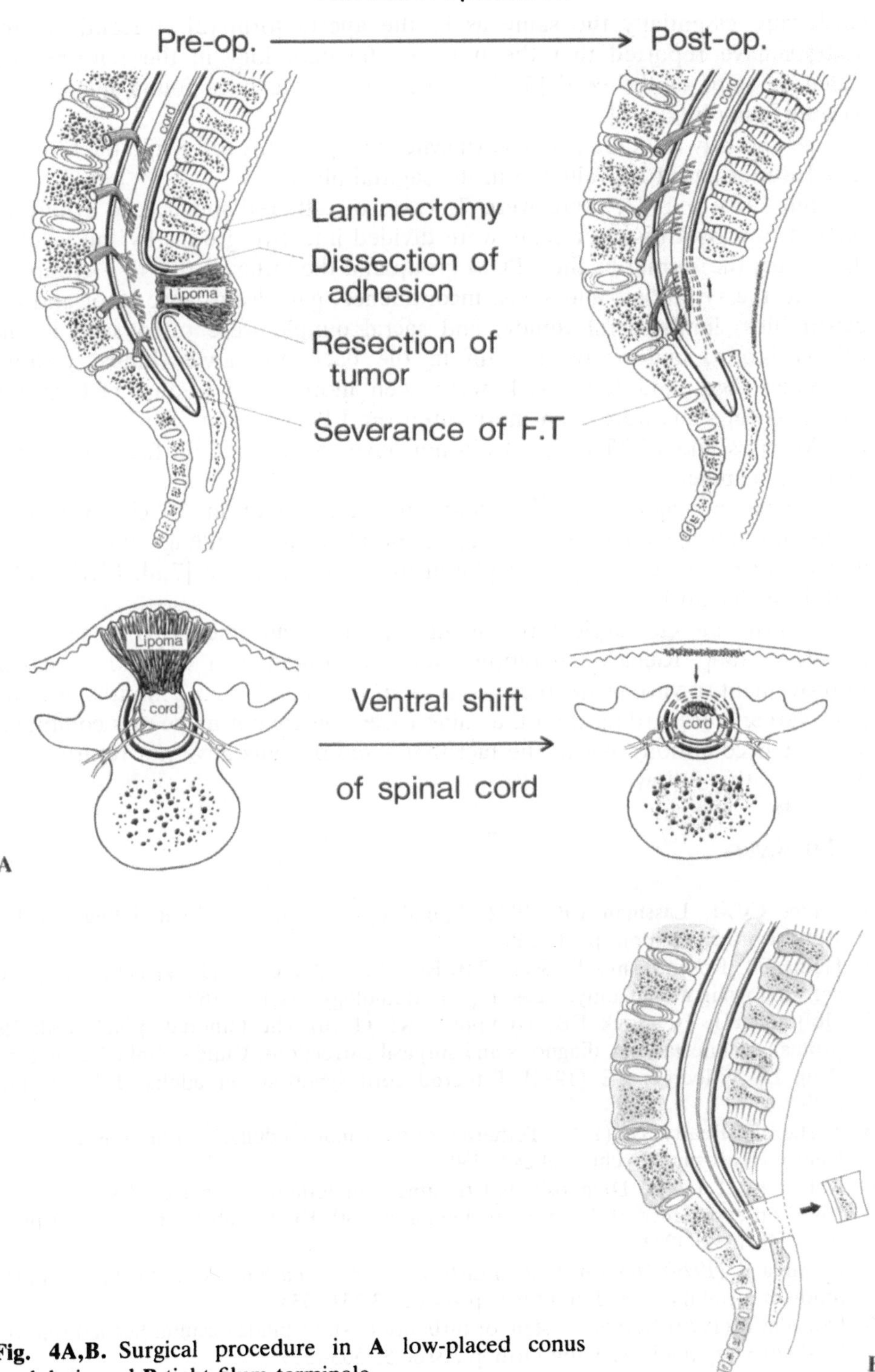

Fig. 4A,B. Surgical procedure in **A** low-placed conus medularis and **B** tight filum terminale

cord were essentially the same as in the aperta form [2]. Recently, some authors have reported that the fundamental pathology in these forms is a tethering state of the cord [3–5]. Furthermore, we have found many cases without spina bifida [6].

Consequently tethered spinal cord syndrome [6] is the most suitable term for this disorder and it is evaluated in the sagittal plane.

From 1976 to 1983, there were 77 cases of tethered spinal cord syndrome seen at our institution. Patients were divided into two groups by the level of the conus; the former as the LPCM group and the latter as the TFT group.

As to the symptoms and signs, incontinence, gait disturbance, foot and toe deformities, lumbosacral tumor, and sacral dimple were often seen in the LPCM group, and nocturia, pain in the back and lower limbs, positive Lasègue's sign, and tight back were seen more often in the TFT group. Neurological signs were seen more often the LPCM group. Thirteen cases (3 LPCM cases and 10 TFT cases) did not have spina bifida on the plain X-ray film of the spine.

To make a diagnosis of this syndrome, it is important to clarify clinical symptoms and signs, neurological signs, and plain X-ray findings, but a definite diagnosis was made by myelography in the supine position [7,8]. MRI is also useful for diagnosis.

The principle of surgical treatment for this syndrome is to release this tethering state. Release operations were performed in a total of 58 cases. Improvement of various degrees was seen in 73% of 49 cases 2 months or more after surgery. Regarding the other nine cases, we cannot make any comments as to their condition, due to the fact that some patients have not returned for post operative follow-up.

References

1. James CCM, Lassman LP (1972) Spinal dysraphism. In: Spina bifida occulta. Butterworths, London, pp 1–136
2. Heinz ER, Rosenbaum AE, Scarff TB, Reigel DH, Dryer BP (1979) Tethered spinal cord following meningomyelocele repair. Radiology 131:153–160
3. Hoffman HJ, Hendrick EB, Humphrey RP (1976) The tethered spinal cord: Its protean manifestations, diagnosis and surgical corrections. Child's Brain 2:145–155
4. Pang D, Wilberger JE (1982) Tethered cord syndrome in adults. J Neurosurg 57:32–47
5. Yashon D, Beatty RA (1966) Tethering of the conus medullaris within the sacrum. J Neurol Neurosurg Psychiat 29:244–250
6. Nakamura T (1984) Diagnosis and treatment of tethered spinal cord syndrome—based on experience of 77 cases (in Japanese, with English abstract). J Jpn Orthop Assoc 58:1237–1251
7. Ootsuka K (1979) Nervous system disturbance of spina bifida occulta. First report. Study of x-ray findings. J Jpn Orthop Assoc 53:331–334
8. Ootsuka K (1979) Nervous system disturbance of spina bifida occulta. Second report. Study of x-ray findings. J Jpn Orthop Assoc 53:505–519

Intermittent Claudication Due to Low Back Pain

SHINICHI KONNO and SHINICHI KIKUCHI[1]

Key Words. Intermittent claudication, lumbar compartment syndrome, intramuscular pressure, fasciotomy, low back pain

Introduction

Patients with chronic low back pain experience intermittent claudication [1]. This study examines the causal relationship between intermittent claudication and back pain in patients with lumbar compartment syndrome.

Intermittent claudication due to back pain has the following characteristics: (1) the patient is asymptomatic at rest, (2) back pain is induced by standing or walking, (3) the pain is dull, never sharp, (4) symptoms are relieved by lumbar extension, and (5) there are no neurologic deficits of the lower extremities.

Materials and Methods

Forty-five patients with intermittent claudication due to low back pain, including 20 males and 25 females between the ages of 51 and 78 years (mean, 61 years), were entered in the study. Twenty-seven patients had osteoporosis, 10 had spondylosis, and 6 had degenerative spondylolisthesis. Three patients became symptomatic following lumbar spine surgery. Patients were divided into two groups: those who could walk less, and those who could walk more than 10 min without stopping because of pain. The control group consisted of 20 normal adults without back pain (10 males and 10 females; mean age, 57).

Intramuscular pressure of lumbar back muscles was measured in patients with back pain and in the control group. Pressure was recorded with the

[1] Department of Orthopedic Surgery, Fukushima Medical College, 1 Hikarigaoka, Fukushima, 960-12 Japan

subject supine, prone, in the lateral decubitus position; standing with the spine in neutral position, in flexion, and in extension; sitting; and standing in 60° flexion holding a 5 kg weight. Measurements were obtained using a Microtip catheter transducer (Millar Houston, Texas) inserted at the level of the fifth lumbar spine, 2 to 3 cm lateral to the spinous process.

The angle of lumbar lordosis (from L1 to L5) was measured in patients with intermittent claudication to establish the radiographic characteristics of this syndrome and to determine the relationship between the severity of osteoporosis and the intramuscular pressure. The severity of osteoporosis was scored using the Jikei University scale [2].

Paraspinal fasciotomy was performed in 7 of 11 patients assessed as having severe disease, including 3 patients who had previously undergone surgery, 3 with osteoporosis, and 1 with spondylosis. These patients were re-evaluated postoperatively over 1–3 years, with a mean of 2 years and 2 months.

Results

Comparison of Intramuscular Pressure in Patients with Back Pain and Normal Controls

Back pain was rated as severe in 11 cases and as mild in 34 cases. Patients with severe pain had elevated intramuscular pressure in all positions, especially standing in the neutral and flexed positions (Fig. 1).

Radiographic Characteristics of Intermittent Claudication Due to Low Back Pain

The radiographic appearance of the spine in patients with intermittent claudication was characterized by osteoporosis in 32 cases and by decreased lumbar lordosis. The average angle of lordosis was −2.2° in severe cases, and 8.2° in mild cases. Both values were significantly less than in the control group ($P < 0.05$).

Furthermore, severe osteoporosis showed a positive correlation with the intramuscular pressure ($P < 0.05$).

The Effect of Fasciotomy on Intramuscular Pressure

Intramuscular pressure in the neutral and flexed positions while standing and with loading was significantly lower following fasciotomy. Postoperatively, intramuscular pressure was the same as in the control group (Fig. 2).

Operative Results

In all cases, intermittent claudication due to back pain was relieved completely or improved following fasciotomy, and all patients were satisfied with the

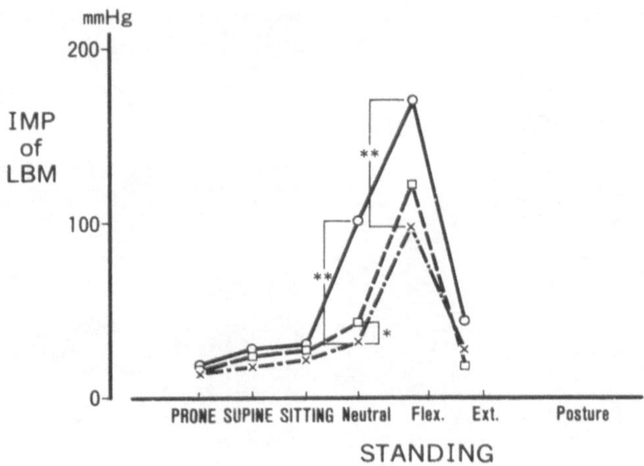

Fig. 1. Comparison of intramuscular pressure (*IMP*) in patients with back pain and normal controls. *LBM*, Lumbar back muscle; *open circle/solid line*, severe cases; *open square/dotted line*, mild cases; *"X"/chained line*, controls; *Flex*, flexion; *Ext*, extension. $*P < 0.05$, $**P < 0.01$

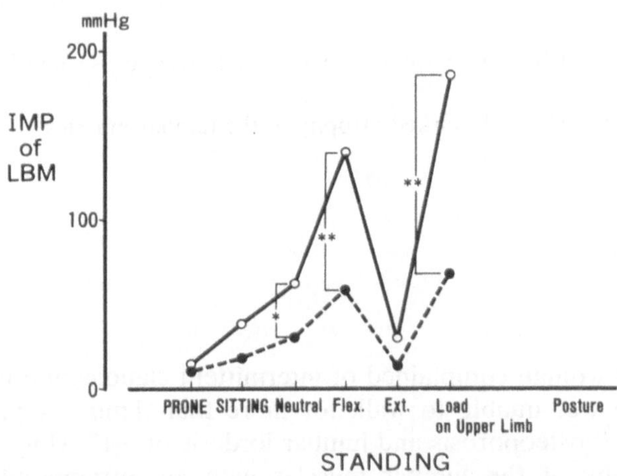

Fig. 2. The effect of fasciotomy in seven cases on intramuscular pressure (*IMP*). *Solid line*, before fasciotomy; *open circle*, after fasciotomy. $*P < 0.05$, $**P < 0.01$

outcome. One patient, who was severely symptomatic and was unable to perform routine activities of daily living without distress, was able to walk for 20 min without stopping following fasciotomy, though he could not walk for more than 10 s prior to it. However, his work as a farmer required prolonged spinal flexion, which still caused back pain. Three patients who had symptoms but no disability preoperatively were able to walk for more than 20 min following fasciotomy.

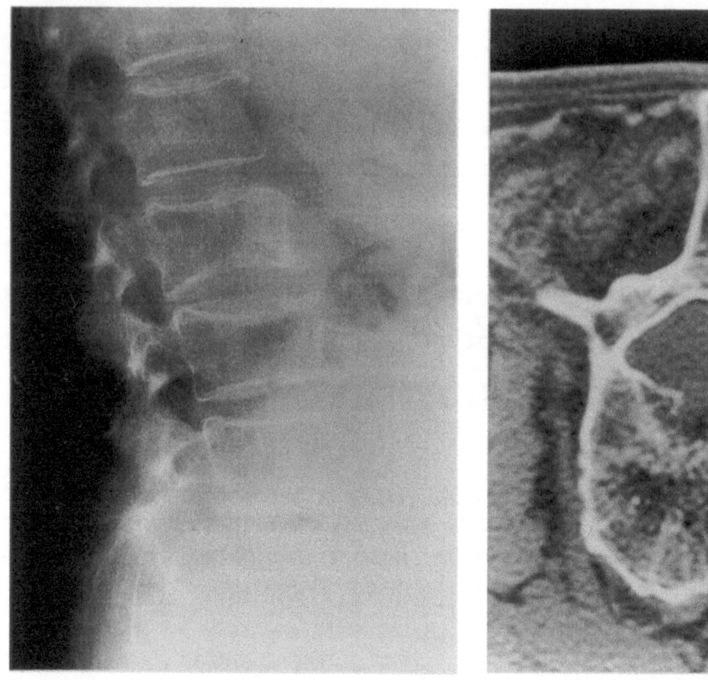

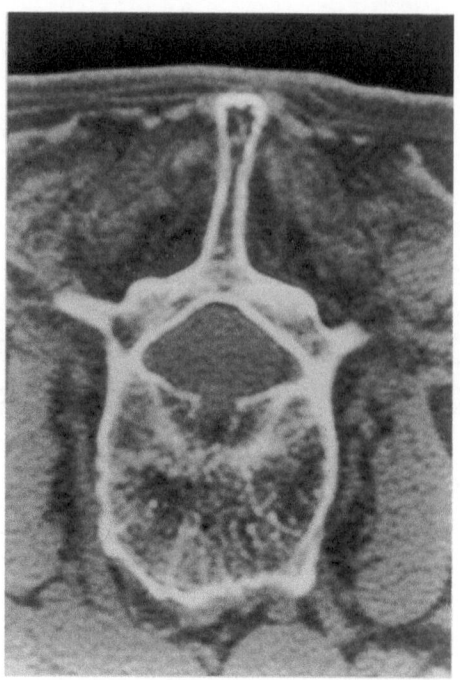

Fig. 3. Case 1: A plain radiograph revealed class 2 osteoporosis and lumbar lordosis of −12°

Fig. 4. Case 1: CT showed marked atrophy of the lumbar muscles

Case Report

Case 1

A 74-year-old woman complained of intermittent claudication because of back pain, and she was unable to walk for more than 1 min. A plain radiograph revealed class 2 osteoporosis and lumbar lordosis of −12° (Fig. 3). CT showed marked atrophy of the lumbar muscles with an intramuscular pressure of 200 mmHg (Fig. 4). Fasciotomy was performed, and the intramuscular pressure decreased to less than 50 mmHg with relief of the patient's back pain.

Case 2

A 65-year-old man underwent bilateral decompression of the L5 nerve roots. He began to experience intermittent claudication due to back pain about 3 months following surgery and could not walk for more than 4 min. Back pain was unilateral. Plain radiography revealed spondylotic change and lumbar lordosis of 10°. CT showed degeneration and atrophy of lumbar back muscles

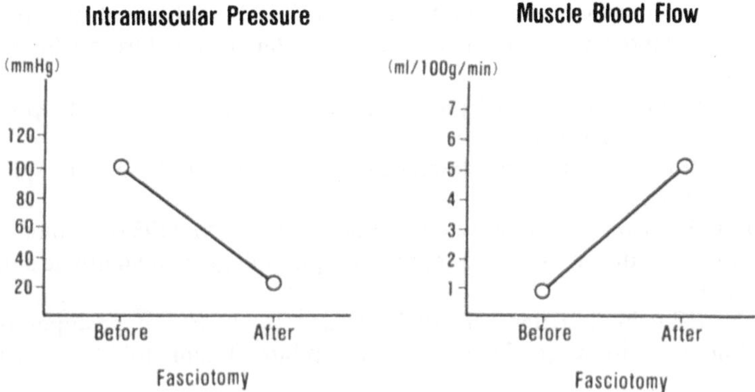

Fig. 5. Case 2: Fasciotomy was performed, and intramuscular pressure decreased and was equal bilaterally. Muscle blood flow also increased

with thickening of thoracolumbar fascia bilaterally. The intramuscular pressure was higher on the symptomatic side than on the asymptomatic side in all positions. Flexion and extension raised the pressure to 130 mmHg on the symptomatic side, while remaining 30 mmHg on the asymptomatic side and reproduced the back pain. Muscle blood flow was measured by using laser doppler. Muscle blood flow on the symptomatic side was one-fifth that on the asymptomatic side. Paraspinal fasciotomy was performed based on a diagnosis of compartment syndrome. Postoperatively, intramuscular pressure decreased and was equal bilaterally. Muscle blood flow also increased (Fig. 5).

Discussion

Most patients with intermittent claudication due to low back pain are elderly, have osteoporosis, and demonstrate a positive correlation between increased intramuscular pressure and the onset of pain. We perform lumbar fasciotomy in severe cases and have achieved dramatic relief of symptoms, with intramuscular pressure decreasing to normal. This observation strongly suggests a causal relation between intermittent claudication and low back pain in patients with lumbar compartment syndrome.

Only one acute and one chronic case of compartment syndrome of lumbar muscles has been reported apart from our series [3–5]. We believe that lumbar compartment syndrome develops most often in elderly patients who have a decreased angle of lumbar lordosis, osteoporosis, or who have previously undergone lumbar surgery. Lumbar compartment syndrome should be ruled out in all elderly patients complaining of intermittent claudication due to low back pain.

References

1. Nagaosa Y, Kikuchi S, Konno S (1992) Clinical analysis of the patients with intermittent claudication due to backache (in Japanese). Orthop Surg Traumatol 35:683–688
2. Itami Y, Inushima Y (1964) Epidemical and clinical study of osteoporosis. J Jpn Orthop Assoc 38:487–489
3. Styf J, Lysell E (1987) Chronic compartment syndrome in the erector spinae muscle. Spine 12:680–682
4. Carr D, Gilbertson L, Frymoyer J, Krag M, Pope M (1985) Lumbar paraspinal compartment syndrome—A case report with physiologic and anatomic studies. Spine 10:816–820
5. Tajino T, Kikuchi S, Konno S (1992) Two case reports of postoperative lumbar compartment syndrome (in Japanese). Orthop Surg Traumatol 35:695–700

Posterior Lumbar Interbody Fusion with Pedicle Screws in the Treatment of Lytic and Degenerative Spondylolisthesis

SAKAE SATO[1], KUNIO IBARAKI[1], HIROAKI TAKARA[1], FUMINORI KANAYA[1], SATOSHI MORI[1], and TAKAHIKO NAKAMURA[2]

Key Words. Posterior lumbar interbody fusion, pedicle screw, lytic spondylolisthesis, degenerative spondylolisthesis, surgical outcome

Introduction

Three fusion techniques—posterolateral fusion, posterior lumbar interbody fusion (PLIF), and anterior spinal fusion—have been used for the treatment of spondylolisthesis. In general, it seems more desirable to combine instrumentation with fusion when the slipping vertebra is unstable. The instrument not only provides rigid stability immediately after surgery, but also decreases the late correction loss.

Pedicle screws and plating can be used in the posterior approach. We prefer PLIF to posterolateral fusion because only a little room is left for the bone graft after plating and the rates of screw breakage and correction loss are higher following posterolateral fusion than after PLIF [1,2]. PLIF is now widely accepted for the treatment of spondylolisthesis. However, there are few reports in the literature comparing the surgical results of PLIF for lytic spondylolisthesis (LS) with those for degenerative spondylolisthesis (DS) [3].

The purpose of this study is to compare the outcome of PLIF with pedicle screws in cases of LS and DS.

[1] Department of Orthopedic Surgery, University of the Ryukyus, 207 Uehara, Nishihara, Okinawa, 903-01 Japan
[2] Nakamura Orthopedic Clinic, 779-1 Kawasaki, Nagaoka, Niigata, 940 Japan

Patients and Methods

Patients

Eighteen patients (12 females and 6 males) were operated upon between 1989 and 1992 at our institutions. LS was found in 8 patients (2 females and 6 males) and DS in 10 females (Tables 1 and 2). The age at operation ranged from 24 to 63 years (average 45.1 years) for LS and from 54 to 70 years (average 60.4 years) for DS patients. DS patients were significantly older than LS patients ($P < 0.005$).

Eight patients had only leg symptoms such as intermittent claudication and radicular pain, two patients had low back pain alone, and eight patients had both.

Single-level fusion was performed in 16 cases (L4–5 in 11 cases, L5–S1 in 3 cases, L4–S1 in 1 case of sacralization, and L5–6 in 1 case of lumbarizaton). Two-level fusion for slippage was performed in 1 LS patient (L4–5 + L5–S) and 1 DS patient (L3–4 and L4–5).

Table 1. Radiological results in patients with lytic spondylolisthesis.

Case No.	Age	Sex	Fusion sites	Union results	Correction loss (%)	Collapse of grafts (%)
1	48	Female	L4/5	Union	0	0
2	63	Male	L4/5	Nonunion	0	23.1
			L5/S1	Nonunion	4.7	33.3
3	40	Male	L4/5	Union	0	0
4	57	Male	L4/5	Collapsed union	0	14.3
5	37	Male	L4/S1	Union	0	0
6	24	Female	L5/S1	Union	0	0
7	48	Male	L5/S1	Union	0	0
8	44	Male	L5/S1	Union	0	0

Table 2. Radiological results in patients with degenerative spondylolisthesis.

Case No.	Age	Sex	Fusion sites	Union results	Correction loss (%)	Collapse of grafts (%)
1	60	Female	L4/5	Union	0	0
2	70	Female	L4/5	Collapsed union	0	30
3	69	Female	L4/5	Union	0	0
4	62	Female	L4/5	Union	0	0
5	58	Female	L4/5	Union	0	0
6	55	Female	L5/6	Union	4.8	0
7	56	Female	L3/4	Union	0	0
			L4/5	Union	0	0
8	59	Female	L4/5	Nonunion	0	50
9	54	Female	L4/5	Union	0	0
10	61	Female	L4/5	Union	2.4	0

The follow-up ranged from 5 months to 2 years 7 months (average 1 year 5 months).

Indication for PLIF with Pedicle Screws

Our indication for LS is intervertebral instability regardless of leg symptoms, since it was reported that the rate of union after anterior spinal fusion without instrumentation in LS was not as high as that in spondylolysis without spondylolisthesis [4].

Our indications for DS are: (1) leg symptoms at rest, (2) the complete block of contrast medium on myelogram even at lumbar flexion, and (3) osteophyte formation in the superior articular processes of the lower vertebra on computed tomography (CT) scan.

Surgical Techniques

The patient is first placed in the prone position, then a midline skin incision is made. Laminae are exposed from one above to one below the slipping vertebra.

In LS, the separate posterior arch is resected and the medial part of the superior articular facets is excised. The fibrocartilagenous masses at isthmus, which compress nerve roots, are completely removed.

In DS, the inferior two-thirds of the slipping lamina and the superior one-third of the lower lamina are resected. The intervertebral disc material is removed, and the osseous end-plates of recipient beds are shaved off using rasps. Three blocks of corticocancellous bone, as large as possible, are inserted into the disc space.

Pedicle screws are inserted and plates are applied. All instruments we used are the products of the variable screw placement (VSP) system [5]. The plates were not aggressively bent for reduction of the deformity, nor was the persuader technique [5] used.

Free fat harvested under the lumbodorsal fascia is grafted over neural tissue in order to prevent adhesion. The wound is then closed layer by layer.

Postoperative management consists of bed rest for 3 weeks and then external immobilization with a hard corset for 2–3 months.

Radiological Evaluation

The percent of slip was measured in lateral X-ray films before operation, just after operation, and at follow-up. Correction loss was determined by subtracting the percent slip at follow-up from that just after operation.

The percent of collapse in the height of grafted bones was calculated from the formula, [(height just after operation) – (height at follow-up)]/(height just after operation)] multiplied by 100.

We considered that bony union was completed when the border lines between grafts and vertebral body disappeared.

Clinical Evaluation

The JOA (Japanese Orthopedic Association) score [6] for assessment of low back pain was used (Table 3). This score includes subjective symptoms, clinical signs, restriction of activities of daily living (ADL), and urinary bladder function. The maximum score is 29 points. Improvement rate was calculated as [(Postoperative score) − (Preoperative score)] divided by [(29 points) − (Preoperative score)] multiplied by 100.

We divide the JOA score into three subscores: leg score (12 points), low back score (3 points), and ADL score (14 points). Leg score is used for the evaluation of the effectiveness of decompression because it consists of radicular symptoms (I-B), gait (I-C), and clinical signs (II). The low back score is used to evaluate the effectiveness of fusion based on the level of low back pain (I-A). The ADL score consists of restriction of ADL (III).

Results

Operation Time and Bleeding

The average operation time was 291 and 257 min and the average blood loss was 523 ml and 662 ml in LS and DS, respectively.

Radiological Results

The slipping deformities were corrected in most cases even though no effort had been made to do so. The preoperative percent of slip in LS ranged from 4.7% to 22.7% (average 16.3%); at follow-up, the values were 0% to 15.6% (average 5.7%). In DS, the preoperative values were 6.7% to 32.5% (average 22.2%) and at follow-up, 0% to 15.0% (average 5.5%) (Tables 1 and 2).

Postoperative correction loss occurred in one LS case and two DS cases. The degrees of loss were 4.7%, 4.8%, and 2.4%, respectively.

Union was achived in 16 of 18 cases, union without collapse of the graft in 14, and union with more than 2 mm collapse, in 2 cases (1 LS and 1 DS patient). Nonunion was seen in one LS and one DS patient each. As a result the union rate was 88.9%.

The cases with the collapsed grafts showed higher incidences of nonunion than those with the correction loss. The collapsed grafts were clearly discernible in four cases, two of which (LS case no. 2 and DS case no. 8) developed into nonunion. The other 14 cases had no collapse at all.

Clinical Results

In comparing LS with DS, the preoperative total score and subscores were not significantly different (Table 4). The postoperative scores of LS patients,

Table 3. Assessment of Treatment for Low Back Pain (Japanese Orthopedic Association).

I. Subjective symptoms	
A. Low Back Pain	(9 points)
a. None	3
b. Occasional mild pain	2
c. Frequent mild or occasional severe pain	1
d. Frequent or continuous severe pain	0
B. Leg Pain and/or Tingling	
a. None	3
b. Occasional mild symptoms	2
c. Frequent mild or occasional severe symptoms	1
d. Frequent or continuous severe symptoms	0
C. Gait	
a. Normal	3
b. Able to walk farther than 500 m, even muscle weakness	2
c. Unable to walk farther than 500 m, owing to leg pain, tingling, and/or muscle weakness	1
d. Unable to walk farther than 100 m, owing to leg pain, tingling, and/or muscle weakness	0
II. Clinical signs	(6 points)
A. Straight leg raising test (including tight hamstrings)	
a. Normal	2
b. 30–70 degrees	1
c. Less than 30 degrees	0
B. Sensory disturbance	
a. None	2
b. Slight disturbance (not subjective)	1
c. Marked disturbance	0
C. Motor disturbance (MMT)	
a. Normal (Grade 5)	2
b. Slight weakness (Grade 4)	1
Marked weakness (Grade 3–0)	0

III. Restriction of activities of daily living (ADL) (14 points)

ADL	Severe restriction	Moderate restriction	No restriction
a. Turn over while lying	0	1	2
b. Standing	0	1	2
c. Washing	0	1	2
d. Leaning forwards	0	1	2
e. Sitting (about 1 hour)	0	1	2
f. Lifting or holding heavy objects	0	1	2
g. Walking	0	1	2

IV. Urinary bladder function	(−6 points)
a. Normal	0
b. Mild dysuria	−3
c. Severe dysuria*	−6
* Incontinence	
* Urinary retention	

Table 4. Changes of score and improvement rate.

	Preoperative (Points)	Postoperative (Points)	Improvement rate (%)
Total score	LS 17.5 ± 3.7 N.S.	LS 28.3 ± 1.0*	LS 94.5 ± 7.9**
	DS 16.0 ± 3.3	DS 24.4 ± 2.6	DS 61.5 ± 23.3
Leg score	LS 8.6 ± 2.1 N.S.	LS 11.8 ± 0.7*	LS 95.0 ± 14.1**
	DS 7.5 ± 1.9	DS 10.0 ± 1.6	DS 50.9 ± 40.3
Low back score	LS 1.1 ± 0.6 N.S.	LS 2.9 ± 0.4*	LS 95.8 ± 11.8*
	DS 1.6 ± 0.7	DS 2.2 ± 0.8	DS 40.0 ± 65.8
ADL score	LS 7.8 ± 2.6 N.S.	LS 13.6 ± 0.7 N.S.	LS 95.9 ± 7.6*
	DS 7.0 ± 2.4	DS 11.8 ± 2.4	DS 62.9 ± 37.6

* $P < 0.05$; ** $P < 0.01$ (between LS and DS)
N.S., Not significant; *LS*, lytic spondylolisthesis; *DS*, degenerative spondylolisthesis; *ADL*, activities of daily living

however, were significantly higher than those of DS patients in terms of the total score ($P < 0.05$), leg score ($P < 0.05$), and low back score ($P < 0.05$).

The improvement rate of JOA score among LS patients was significantly higher than that DS in the total score ($P < 0.01$), leg score ($P < 0.01$), low back score ($P < 0.05$), and ADL score ($P < 0.05$).

Actually, all symptoms disappeared in seven LS patients with leg symptoms and in five patients with low back pain. In two of nine DS patients with leg symptoms and one of five DS patients with low back pain, these symptoms improved but did not resolve.

LS differed very much from DS especially in the improvement rate of the leg score. This suggests that the leg symptoms of LS responded very well to decompression, and those of DS responded moderately well.

Clinical and Radiological Results of Nonunion Cases

Nonunion did not necessarily indicate a poor clinical result: Both nonunion cases showed improvement of low back pain. There was no intervertebral movement in functional lateral roentgenograms at follow-up. The plates and screws might fix the vertebrae under fibrous union.

Complications

There were no cases with metal breakage or infection. Transient paresthesia in the legs was observed in two DS and two LS patients. The paresthesia disappeared after 2 weeks and 1 month in the LS patients, and after 2 weeks and 6 months in the DS patients. No motor paresis was observed.

Discussion

Surgical Procedures

We have been making efforts to reduce bleeding, especially from epidural veins and the recipient beds, which disturbs and limits the field of vision during surgery. One of our techniques to reduce bleeding is to use rasps instead of using osteotomes for the removal of osseous end-plates.

As much disc material is removed as possible, paying attention to the anterior margin of the disc, and large grafts are inserted into the rasped

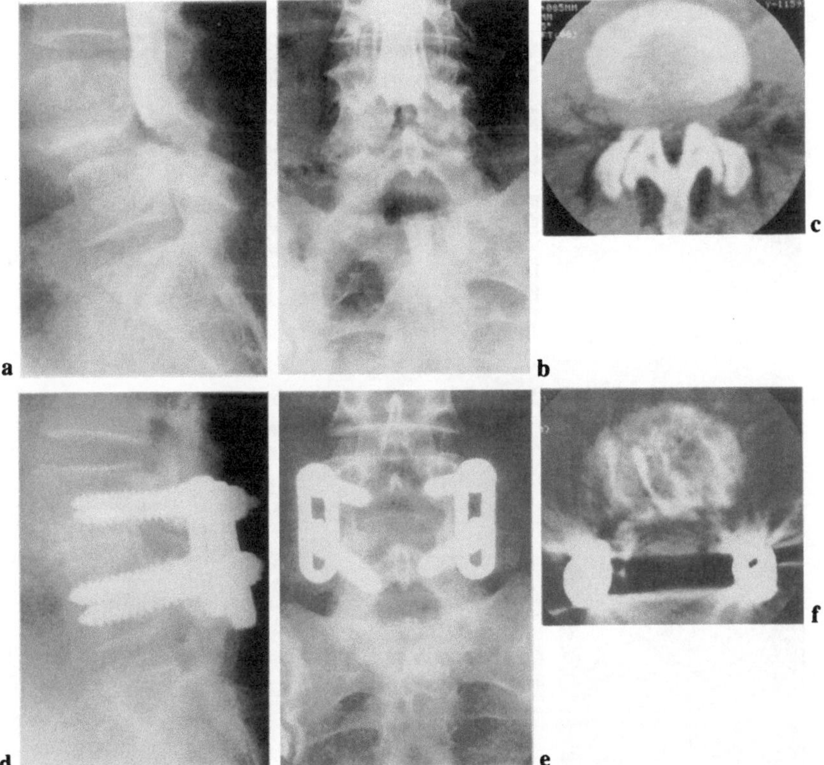

Fig. 1. A 54-year-old woman with intermittent claudication due to bilateral leg numbness. **a,b** Myelograms show complete block at the L4–5 level due to degenerative spondylolisthesis with 27.0% slip (grade 3 in Satomi's classification). **c** Computed tomography (CT) myelogram reveals that the anteriorly displaced inferior facets and the bulged L4–5 disc completely obstruct the dural sac as well as the nerve root sleeves (stage 3 in Satomi's classification). **d** The slipping is realigned into 10.5% on postoperative lateral roentgenogram. **e** Anterolateral roentgenogram shows the remaining upper one-third of the L4 spinous process. **f** CT illustrates large grafts placed at intervertebral space

intervertebral space. The total lateral diameter of the grafted bones is equal to the distance between the medial margin of the pedicles. Large grafts increase mechanical strength and seem to prevent both metal breakage and correction loss of slipping.

Difference of Clinical Results Between LS and DS

The severity of DS was classified by Satomi et al. in 1990 [7]. Myelogram grade 3 showing complete block is equal to CT Myelogram stage 3 or 4, in which the dura is markedly compressed by the bulged disc and slipping articular

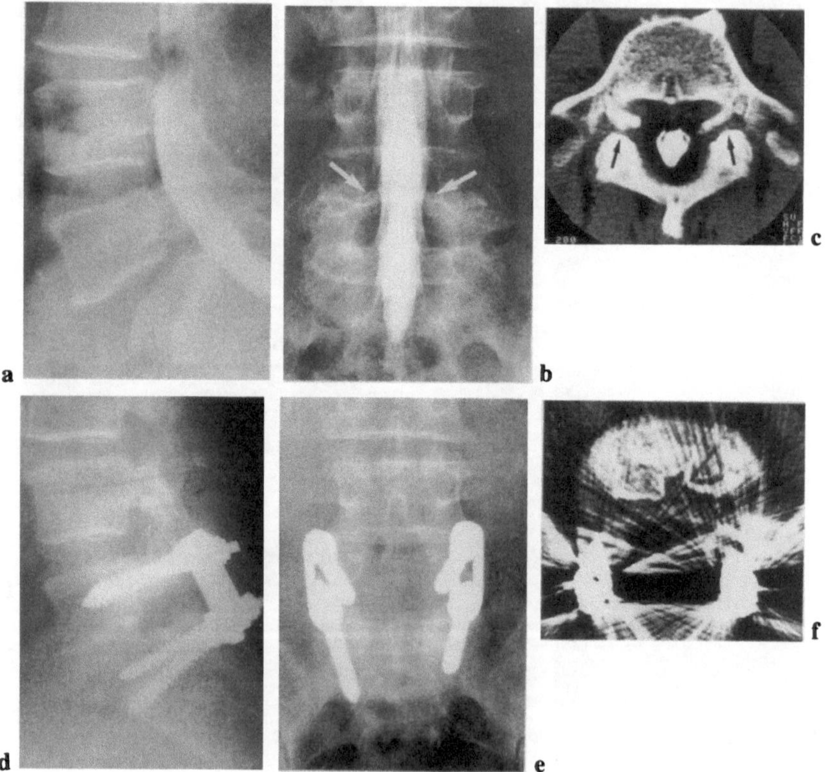

Fig. 2. A 44-year-old man with low back pain and painful intermittent claudication in both legs. **a** Preoperative lateral myelogram demonstrates 20.5% displacement of L5 due to lytic spondylolisthesis (LS). **b** Anteroposterior myelogram shows obliteration of the bilateral L5 nerve root sleeves and the intact dural sac. **c** CT myelogram reveals the cracked pars interarticularis and the intact dural sac. **d,e** in roentogenograms following PLIF with pedicle screws, the slipping is reduced into 15.6% and the separate posterior arch is resected. **f** CT illustrates three corticocancellous grafts incorporated in the disc space. All of the patient's symptoms disappeared

processes. In our series, there were nine cases in stage 3 and one in stage 4. There were no cases in either stage 1 or stage 2. All our cases were classified in the advanced stages (Fig. 1). Some cauda equina fibers might have deteriorated before operation, which may lead to the lower degree of neurological improvement seen in DS than in LS.

On the other hand, leg symptoms in LS are generally caused only by the compression of bilateral nerve roots, which are located beneath the fibrocartilagenous masses at the pars interarticularis (Fig. 2). The compressed neural tissue in LS is markedly smaller than that of DS in which the cauda equina is compressed. That is one reason why LS patients could achive better results than DS patients.

DS patients were significantly older than LS patients in our series, and it is very likely that the advanced age of DS patients worsened the neurological recovery after surgical decompression (Fig. 3).

Advantages and Complications of PLIF with Pedicle Screws

No surgical intervention in the area of the anterior great vessels, which lie anterior to the lumbar spine, is necessary. This point is clearly advantageous for elderly patients with DS who also have arteriosclerosis.

Four patients complained of paresthesia in the legs. Abumi et al. reported neurological complications after excessive reduction of slipping deformity in transpedicular screw instrumentation [8]. In this series, however, the reduction of slipping deformity might be caused solely by plating after thorough removal of disc material, rather than by intentional reduction. Furthermore, because all paresthesia was transient, it might not be caused by entrapment of nerve roots but rather by the retraction of neural tissue during operation. The paresthesia was a minor complication.

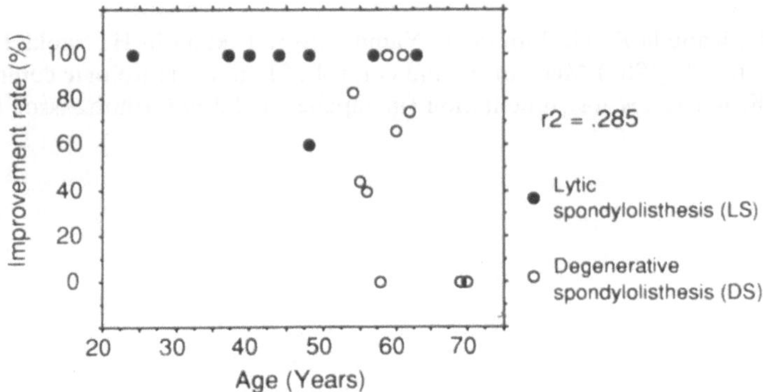

Fig. 3. Scattergram—Improvement rate of leg score *vs* age at operation

Conclusions

Overall, LS demonstrated better improvement than DS, which might be caused by the amount and degree of compressed neural tissue, and the age at operation. Additionally, our experience showed that reduced bleeding increases the surgical field of view and facilitates the insertion of large grafts in order to achieve better mechanical strength.

Bony union was achieved in 88.9%, and nonunion seemed to be related to the collapse of grafts. There was no metal breakage and little correction loss. Posterior lumbar interbody fusion with pedicle screws is the eminent surgical procedure for both LS and DS.

References

1. Whitecloud TS, Butler JC, Cohen JL, Candelora PD (1989) Complications with the variable spinal plating system. Spine 14:472–476
2. Matsuzaki H, Tokuhashi Y, Matsumoto F, Hoshino M, Kiuchi T, Toriyama S (1990) Problematical factors in pedicle screw fixation (in Japanese). Rinsho Seikei Geka 25:563–570
3. Yamamoto T, Kadowaki T, Owada T (1992) Posterior lumbar interbody fusion (PLIF) combined with pedicle screw fixation for degenerative and spondylolytic spondylolisthesis (in Japanese). Spine and Spinal Cord 5:355–362
4. Matsui N, Inoue S, Miyasaka H, Watanabe T, Saegusa O, Tanaka T, Yamagata M, Otsuka Y (1982) Selection in surgical methods after clinical results of spondylosis and spondylolisthesis (in Japanese). Rinsho Seikei Geka 17:357–366
5. Steffee AD (1989) The variable screw placement system with posterior lumbar interbody fusion. In: Lin PM, Gill K (eds) Lumbar interbody fusion: Principles and techniques in spine surgery. Aspen, Rockville, pp 81–93
6. Japanese Orthopedic Association (1986) Assessment of treatment for low back pain (in Japanese). J Jpn Orthop Assoc 60:391–394
7. Satomi K, Hirabayashi K, Toyama Y, Fujimura Y (1992) A clinical study of degenerative spondylolisthesis. Radiographic analysis and choice of treatment. Spine 17: 1329–1336
8. Abumi K, Kaneda K, Hashimoto T, Yamamoto I, Takahashi H, Naoki T, Narita Y, Hatakeyama A (1989) Mechanism and control of lumbar neurologic complication by transpedicular screw instrumentation (in Japanese). J Jpn Orthop Assoc 63:S64

Cotrel-Dubousset Instrumentation in Trauma, Metastatic Tumor, and Degenerative Spine Disease

Kazunori Yagi, Naoshi Hayashi, Toshiaki Seki, Kazuo Takahashi, and Tomoo Yamada[1]

Key Words. Cotrel-Dubousset instrumentation, spine injury, metastatic spinal tumor, spondylolisthesis, degenerative spine

Introduction

Initially conceived for the correction of scoliosis, Cotrel-Dubousset instrumentation (C-D-I) is now used for various spine pathologies. After the experience of Harrington and Luque instrumentation, we introduced C-D-I in 1988 to our hospital with expectation of its rigid stability and wide applicability. On the other hand we had been anxious about the burden of the operative procedure which would increase operating time, increase blood loss, and cause more complications. The purpose of this report is to assess the utility of C-D-I in various pathologies, except scoliosis, from the viewpoint of operating stress and complication.

Material Method

Sixteen males and 18 females from 15 to 78 years of age (mean of 50) had undergone operative procedures utilizing C-D-I between December 1988 and August 1992. The diagnoses were trauma in 6 cases, tumor metastasis in 12, spondylolisthesis in 14, degenerative scoliosis in 1, and postoperative instability in 1. Our indications for C-D-I in cases of spinal trauma were dislocation-fracture of the lumbar spine (4 cases) and burst fracture of fifth lumbar vertebra (2 cases). Three cases sustained traffic accident, two fell from heights and one fell down on the back.

[1] Department of Orthopedic Surgery, Niigata City General Hospital, 2-6-1 Shitikuyama, Niigata, 950 Japan

The origin of malignant tumors were the lung in four cases, prostate in three, gastrointestinal tract in two, and the uterus, bladder, and breast in one each. Localization of metastasis was lumbar in five, thoracic in three, thoracolumbar in three, and cervicothoracic in one. Seven cases out of 12 had multiple lesions. Fourteen cases of spondylolisthesis were classified into isthumus spondylolisthesis (n = 7), degenerative spondylolisthesis (n = 6), and dysplastic spondylolisthesis (n = 1).

Localization of spondylolisthesis was at L4 in seven cases, L5 in four, and multiple in three. Nine cases suffered from Meyerding grade I, four from grade II, and one from grade IV. Clinical outcome, operating time, blood loss, and complications were compared to those of conventional methods.

Operative Technique

The lesions located in the cervical and thoracic spines were fixated with rods and hooks. The lesions from the lumbar spine to the sacrum were treated by transpedicular screws combined with various hooks. Bone graft was not done in a patient who sustained an osteoporotic L5 burst fracture and all cases of metastatic tumors. Transpedicular screwing was performed in all cases of spondylolisthesis, which were usually combined with posterior interbody fusion (PLIF) with or without posterolateral fusion (PLF). We made it routine to fixate the neighbor motion segment of spondylolisthesis of which discs were considered to be the origin of low back pain. Hard corsets were applied postoperatively at least for 6 months in the patients who underwent bone graft, and through life in the cases without bone graft.

Results

The follow-up of 34 cases was 2–42 months (mean 18 months). The mean number of fixated motor segments was mean 2.3 in traumatized patients, 5.9 in the cases of metastatic tumors, 2.0 in the cases of spondylolisthesis, and 4 in all others. All six cases with spine injuries maintained anatomic reduction. Solid fusion was achieved in all five cases who underwent bone graft. The other case treated without bone graft had no instrument failure (example 1).

Nine out of 12 cases (75%) suffering from metastatic tumor were able to walk and maintain walking ability for 2–33 months (mean 8.3 months). Spondylolisthesis was corrected completely in five cases and improved up to Meyerding grade 1 in nine cases. The average of operating time was 240 min for spine injuries 258 min for metastasis, and 312 min for spondylolisthesis. Mean blood loss was 1695 g for spine injuries, 1346 g for metastasis, and 1415 g for spondylolisthesis.

Complications

Transient root irritation was observed in six cases of spondylolisthesis. There was no correlation between irritated root and PLIF: Irritation occured at the same level as PLIF in three cases and at a lower level in two cases. One screw breakage occured in a case of spondylolisthesis which led to removal of the instrument and additional PLF. The instrument was removed 2 years after the operation in another patient who complained of skin irritation above one of the hooks. One case of deep methicillin-resistant *S. aureus* (MRSA) infection was treated by closed irrigation. Appropriate administration of antibiotics could suppress the infection but complete cure was not achieved until removal of the instrument.

Example 1

Severe low back pain with cauda equina syndrome disappered after laminectomy at L5 and C-D-I in a 78-year-old woman (Fig. 1). Bone graft was not done because we considered that the grafted bone would not survive in such an osteoporotic patient. She had maintained walking ability until 82 years of age, nearly for 3 years, in spite of the successive osteoporotic vertebral

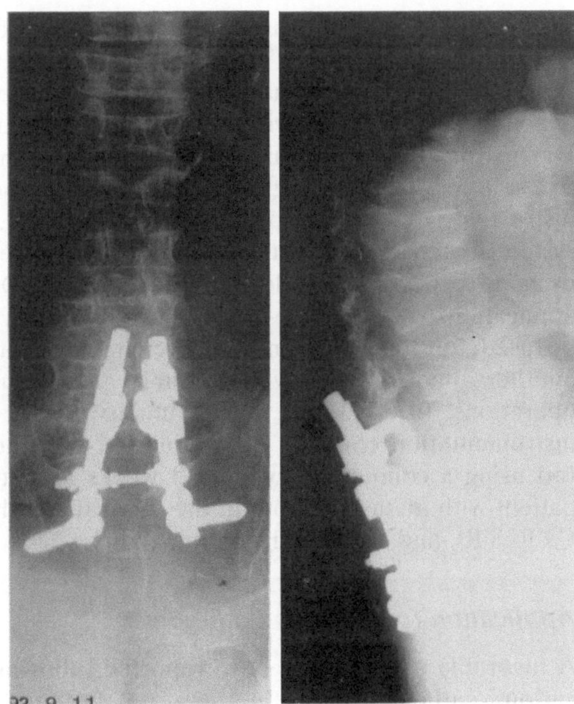

Fig. 1. Example 1: A 78-year-old woman with osteoporotic burst fracture (3 years postop.)

fracture at other levels. No loosening of the instrument was observed. C-D-I showed satisfactory stability over a long period of time even though osteoporosis was relatively advanced and though no bone graft was done.

Example 2

C-D-I from 11th thoracic vertebra to the sacrum, combined with laminectomy at L4, was done in a 53-year-old man (Fig. 2). He began to walk 2 weeks after the operation and continued for 6 months until 3 weeks before his death.

Example 3

This 56-year-old woman had lumbago, intermittent claudication, and vesicorectal disturbance. Myelogram demonstrated complete block at the L4/5 disk level. C-D-I combined with L4/5 PLIF and PLF from L4 to the sacrum was carried out, and her symptoms disappeared completely.

Discussion

Biomechanical Considerations

C-D-I is a system fundamentally composed of two rods and several hooks and/or screws. A frame is constructed using two rods combined with two depositif de traction transversale (DTT). The combination of these elements depends neither on a wire binding as with Luque nor on a hitch as with Harrington, but rather on a metal crush [1]. These structual components give C-D-I remarkable strength in all directions, not only to axial compressive-distractive stress but also to rotatory force [2]. Only C-D-I and the Steffee system match the strength of the normal spine model, according to a study using a corpectomy model [3]. Moreover, C-D-I has such a wide variety of applications owing to the availability of various hooks and screws, that it can be used for fixation from the occipital bone to the sacrum [4]. C-D-I has another unique capacity for cranial and caudal extension in subsequent operations. In this series, a case underwent the second operation to elongate instrumentation cranially by uniting a 7-mm thoracic rod to a 5-mm cervical rod using a connection cylinder 3 weeks after the first operation. Finally the patient with metastasis both in the cervical and thoracic spines was fixated from C3 to T10, and recovered walking ability.

Application for Various Pathologies

A favorable outcome has been reported following the application of C-D-I for various pathologies [5]. In the pre-C-D-I era, "two above two below" or

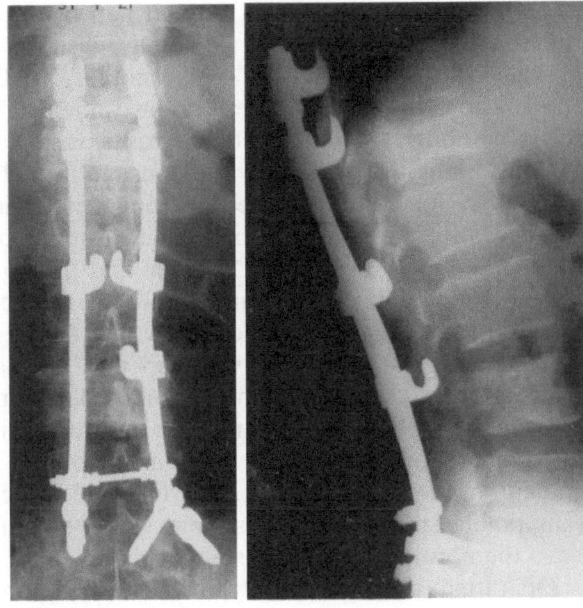

Fig. 2. Example 2: A 53-year-old man with cancer metastasis of bile duct origin in L1 and L4

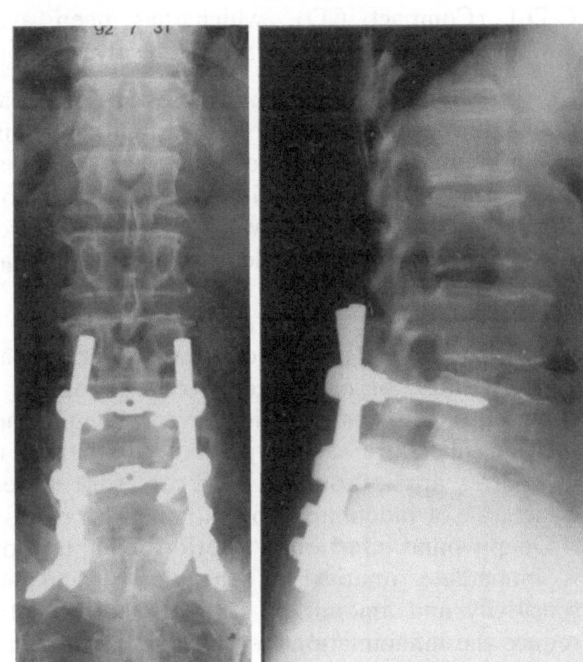

Fig. 3. Example 3: A 56-year-old woman with L4 degenerative spondylolisthesis

"Three above three below" fixation had been advocated in the treatment of spinal injury [6], but short fusion is desirable for traumatized patients to prevent concomitant loss of spinal mobility. C-D-I had sufficient strength for short fusion. In fact there were no instrument failures or correction loss in our series, although the number of the cases was small.

Considering the possibility of extension of the bone lesion, short fusion is not mandatory for patients suffering from metastatic tumor. On the other hand, the operative stress should be kept to a minimum. The average of operating time and blood loss were 258 min and 1346 g, which exceeded or Luque instrumentation by 90 min and by 400 g, respectively, on the comparison of data of our hospital. On the contrary, the recovery rate of walking in the cases treated with C-D-I (75%) was superior to that of the cases treated with Harrington or Luque instrumentation (45%). Patients who had severe collapse of a vertebral body tended to have residual pain after Harrington or Luque instrumentation and could not stand upright probably due to insufficient stability of the spinal column. The favorable outcome of C-D-I depends on the remarkable strength of the system which does not need a vertebral body to have the normal strength of spinal column.

Operating time in spondylolisthesis was long beyond the fusion length especially before introduction of the tulip screw. Previously, it was not easy to pass the rods through the screws located close together. The new system of C-D-I (Compact CD), which has been available recently of facilitate lumbosacral instrumentation, may resolve this problem.

Complications. New pain and dysesthesia appeared after the operation is not apt to be complained in the seriously ill with spinal trauma or metastasis. This is why root irritaion occurred exclusively in cases of spondylolisthesis. In these cases, postoperative CT did not demonstrate root injury caused by malposition of the pedicular screws. Therefore, streching with correction of spondylolisthesis or irritation during root release was considered to be the cause in most instances.

An instrument failure can be caused by PLIF failure resulting from insufficient grafted bone. Considering that the patients with a low daily activity level, because of either advanced age or the presence of cancer, did not experience this complication even when bone graft was not performed, mechanical failure can be prevented either by reducing the patients' activity level or by application of a hard corset for no less than 6 months in cases with bone graft or indefinitely for patients with metastasis.

Deep wound infection is a serious complication. The most common remedy is immediate removal of the device and administration of appropriate sensitivity and amount of antibiotics. Alternatively, if the antibiotics could reduce the inflammation, removal of instrument might be postponed until the goal of surgery could be achieved. In this series, a removal had been postponed for 3 months until the grafted bone was considered solid in the case of severe spondylolisthesis.

Conclusion

Not only the rigid stability but also the flexibility of surgical procedure make C-D-I useful in treatment of various spine pathologies.

References

1. Dubousset J, Cotrel Y (1989) Die CD-Instrumentation in der Behandlung von Wirbelseulendeformitäten. Orthopaede 18:118–127
2. Farcy J, Weidenbaum M, Midheksen C (1987) A Comparative biomechanical study of spinal fixation using Cotrel-Dubousset instrumentation. Spine 12:877–881
3. Gurr KR, McAfee PC, Shin C (1988) Biomechanical analysis of anterior and posterior instrumentation system after corpectomy. J Bone Joint Surg 70-A:1182–1190
4. Hopf C, Grimm J, Arai Y (1991) Ergebnisse der operativen Behandlung bei Spondylolisthesen sowie bei lumbalen und sakralen Wirbelseuleneingriffen. Z Orthop 129:365–373
5. Gurr KR, McAfee PC (1988) Cotrel-Dubousset instrumentation in adults. Spine 13:510–520
6. Willen J, Lindahl S, Nordwal A (1985) Unstable thoracolumbar fractures, a comparative clinical study for conservative treatment and Harrington instrumentation. Spine 10:111–112

Surgical Indication, Procedure, and Method of Postoperative Evaluation for Spinal Metastasis

Yoshio Ota, Yoshihiko Oshima, Taro Nagashima, Masahiro Hayashi, and Toshiaki Samoto[1]

Key Words. Spinal metastasis, surgical treatment, spinal instrumentation

Introduction

Owing to recent progress in the multidisciplinary approach for malignant tumors, patients now survive longer. However, the incidence of metastasis to the skeletal system increases with longevity. Of all osseous metastasis, the spinal column is most frequently involved, accounting for one-half of all osseous metastasis because of anatomical and pathophysiological features. Spinal metastasis may cause significant bone destruction resulting in spinal instability which may develop into pain and paralysis.

Based on these situations, spinal surgeons have been responsible for the treatment of spinal metastasis and have developed a variety of innovative methods of treatment, especially surgical treatment. Today, surgical treatment for spinal metastasis has become accepted as one of the best modalities of treatment. This article reports the authors' experience with the surgical treatment of spinal metastasis, surgical indications, surgical procedures, methods of postoperative evaluation, and results.

Methods and Materials

Methods

Surgical Indications. When clinical instability is present or at risk, surgical intervention is indicated. Clinical instability consists of two elements: Mech-

[1]Department of Orthopaedic Surgery, Yamagata University School of Medicine, Iida Nishi 2-2-2, Yamagata, 990-23 Japan

anical and neurologic [1]. These principally reflect pain and paralysis, respectively. However when more than one of following three contraindications were present, operation was not indicated: (1) The general condition of the patient was so poor that the patient could not tolerate the surgery or could not long survive the surgical outcome; (2) the extent of metastasis was so wide with either longitudinal spread or metastasis to the pelvis that effective stabilization could not be obtained and the patient could not become ambulatory; and (3) a more effective conservative method was available.

Surgical Procedure. The main factors to be considered in the selection of the surgical procedure were tumor location and tumor malignancy. Elements of procedure were spinal stabilization and neural decompression. Spinal stabilization was chiefly for the purpose of mechanical stabilization but also partly for neurological stabilization. Neural decompression was effective only for neurologic stabilization, with possibly compromised mechanical stabilization. When a low grade metastasis was localized within the anterior and middle column, and was limited within two contiguous vertebrae, anterior decompression and reconstruction was performed incorporating autogenous bone graft, methylmethacrylate and other instrumenting devices. However, these cases were rare. In the majority of cases, metastasis was multifocal and extirpation was impossible. Besides, relentless growth of the remnant tumor and occult metastasis could result in clinical instability. Consequently, multifocal metastasis, three-column involvement, or distant metastasis were treated by posterior spinal stabilization through multi-segmental instrumentation with many supporting anchor points. For this purpose, Luque segmental spinal instrumentation (SSI) was used widely. However, that has little resistance against axial load, and reinforcing by methylmethacrylate was sometimes necessary. In 1984, the authors developed a modified Luque rod named "grooved rod" (G-rod) because a helical groove is carved on an original Luque rod into which sublaminar wires are placed snugly to hold the rod in place (Fig. 1a) [2]. With this modification, posterior segmental instrumentation became mechanically more resistant, especially against axial loading.

Our standard procedure consisted of the following four elements [2,3]: (1) Posterior instrumentation with a grooved rod and sublaminar wiring spreading usually as far as three spinal segments above and below the metastasis was performed; (2) if necessary, decompression was done through a posterolateral approach (Fig. 1a–d); (3) for patients with an anticipated survival of over 6 months, autogenous bone grafting was added; and (4) anterior reconstruction was combined for cases with a longer anticipated survival with low malignancy growth.

Postoperative Evaluation. Since malignant tumor with remote metastasis is still an uncurable and progressive disease, the aim of surgical treatment should be to improve the quality of life and postoperative evaluation should reveal the duration of improvement until the death of a patient. Postoperative pain relief was evaluated by the duration of effective pain relief. In order to measure this,

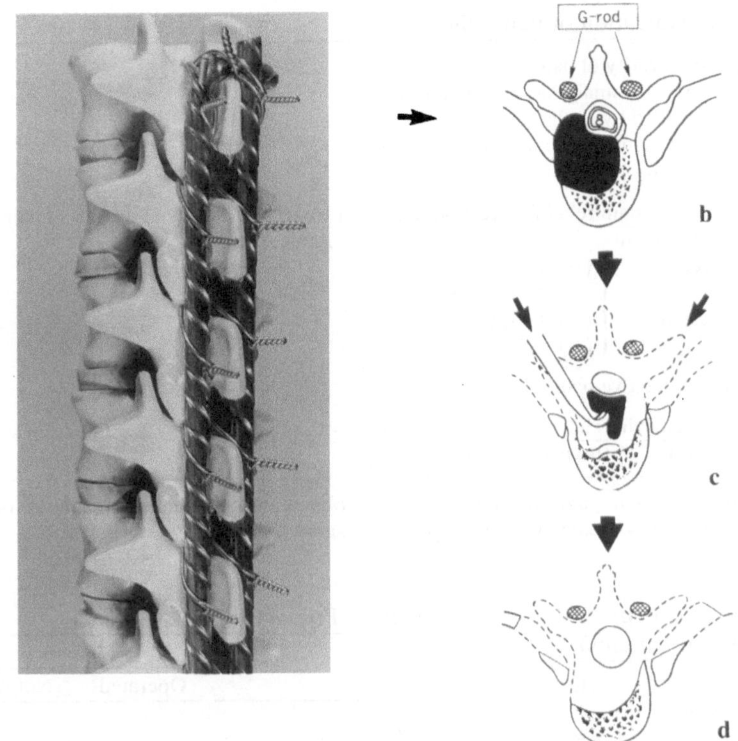

Fig. 1. **a** Photograph shows the Grooved rod (G-rod) sublaminar wiring system used on a spine model. Wires placed in the groove hold the rod tightly. **b** Diagram showing transverse section of the spine stabilized with a G-rod. **c** Diagram showing decompression through a posterolateral approach. **d** Diagram shows completion of decompression (**b**,**c**,**d** with permission, from [3])

we first graded the severity of pain and then defined the effectiveness of pain relief. The former was graded into four stages according to medication or nerve blocks used to control the pain. The latter was defined as the concept that through effective pain relief, patients should be helped to lead a meaningful life either without pain [grade(−)] or with pain controlled by analgesics [grade(+)]. In those cases where the severity of pain became (−) or (+) at a certain time after treatment, pain relief was evaluated as "effective". However, in those cases without preoperative pain [grade(−)] which became painful [grade(+)], the pain relief was evaluated as "not effective" [4] (Table 1).

Neurologic-improvement was evaluated by comparing motor function of the patient just before surgery and 1 month after surgery. Because of insufficient patient records, it was impossible to determine the duration of neurologic improvement.

Table 1. Evaluation of pain relief.

Grading for severity of pain
- (−): no pain, or analgesics not required
- (+): controlled by analgesics
- (2+): controlled by narcotics or nerve blocks
- (3+): uncontrolled

Effectiveness of pain relief at a certain time after treatment based on severity of pain

	Before treatment		After treatment
Effective:	(−), (+), (2+), (3+)	→	(−)
	(+), (2+), (3+)	→	(+)
Not effective:	(−), (+), (2+), (3+)	→	(2+), (3+)
	(−)	→	(+)

Duration of effective pain relief

$$\frac{\text{period when pain relief was assessed as “effective”}}{\text{period of survival after treatment}^{a}} \times 100\ (\%)$$

[a] The period when pain was no longer a problem due to deteriorated level of consciousness was excluded from the period of survival

Table 2. Operative procedure (number of patients).

Stabilization	110
Posterior approach	
G-SSI*	46
L-SSI*	2
HI, H-SSI*	40
Others	8
Anterior approach	11
Combined approach	3
Non-stabilization	17
Laminectomy	12
Others	4

L, Luque rod; *G*, grooved Rod (modified Luque Rod); *HI*, Harrington instrumentation; *SSI*, segmental spinal instrumentation

Table 3. Primary tumor.

Origin	Number: Operated	Number: Not operated
Lung	35	4
Breast	16	8
Gastrointestinal	8	3
Prostata	10	0
Kidney	7	2
Myeloma/Lymphoma	10	0
Liver	6	1
Thyroid	2	1
Unknown	19	7
Total	113	26

Materials

From 1977 to 1991, 113 patients underwent a total of 127 operations in which 110 were stabilizations and 17 were non-stabilizations. During this period, 26 patients were treated non-surgically (Table 2).

Stabilization was achieved mostly through the posterior approach in which G-rod spinal instrumentation was most frequently used because of greater stability. Operative procedures represent an evolution of our experience over a 14-year interval, beginning from laminectomy through the Harrington system to the G-rod system. Besides surgery, irradiation or hormonal therapy were combined when the tumor was sensitive to treatment. The most frequent primary tumor was lung cancer, followed by breast and gastro-intestinal cancer (Table 3).

Results

Pain Relief

Duration of effective pain relief and the period of survival was significantly longer in surgical cases (70.7%) than in non-surgical cases (36.1%). In those cases with higher malignancy, effective pain relief was a little shorter than those with lower malignancy but still quite longer than non-surgical cases. Among surgical cases, the stabilization group (72.4%) was longer than the laminectomy group (57.3%). G-rod SSI showed the longest duration of effective pain relief (77.5%).

Neurologic Improvement

Neurologic deficits were improved or unchanged in 84% in the stabilization group and 44% in the laminectomy group, and were worsened in 16% in the stabilization group and 23% in the laminectomy group.

Case Reports

Patient 1

A 51-year-old man with lung cancer developed resting and motion pain in his back as well as neurologic deficits in his legs due to metastasis to T7,8,9 spine. He underwent decompressive laminectomy and posterior stabilization ranging from T3 to L1 using G-rod SSI system (Fig. 2). Preoperative back pain of grade (2+) was improved to grade (−) throughout the 8 months before death, which means the duration of effective pain relief was 100%.

Patient 2

A 75-year-old woman with stomach cancer developed low back pain due to L2 metastasis. She underwent posterior stabilization using Harrington system with segmental sublaminar wiring (Fig. 3). Postoperative low back pain of grade (2+) was relieved to grade (−) until the rod became dislodged. After this accident, pain recurred and the duration of effective pain relief was 12%.

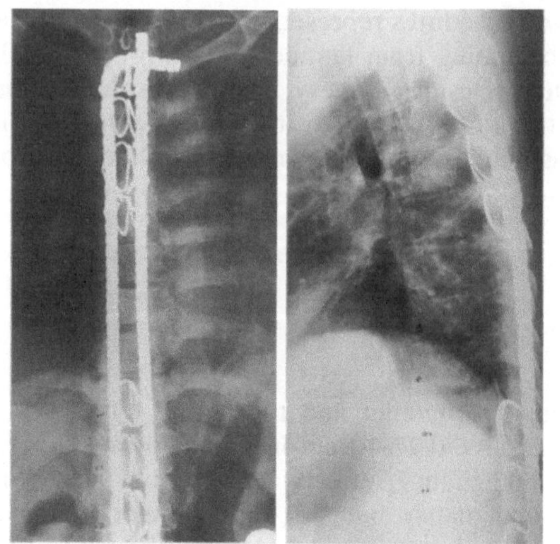

Fig. 2a,b. Patient 1. A-51-year-old man with lung cancer metastasis to T7,8,9 underwent decompressive laminectomy and posterior stabilization using G-rod SSI ranging from T3 to L1. **a** Postoperative anteroposterior radiograph of the spine. **b** Postoperative lateral radiograph of the spine

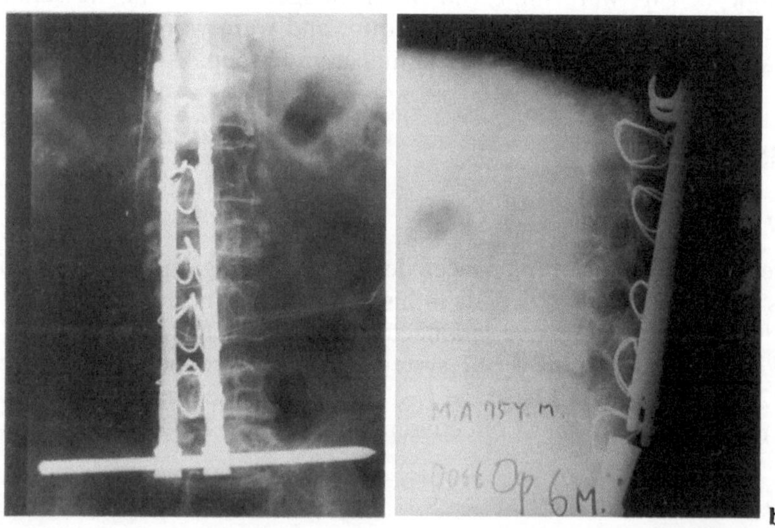

Fig. 3. Patient 2. A 75-year-old woman with stomach cancer metastasis to L2 underwent stabilization using Harrington system with segmental sublaminar wiring. **a** Postoperative anteroposterior radiograph of the spine. **b** Postoperative lateral radiograph of the spine. Dislodging of the rod occurred

Discussion

The basic problem arising from spinal metastasis is clinical instability of the spine. Treatment of spinal metastasis should be re-stabilization or prevention of clinical instability, including mechanical and neurologic instability, to eliminate or prevent pain and neural deficit. Stabilization procedures of the metastatic spine for clinical instability have been proven to be successful by other authors [5–7]. From our results, surgery was more effective than other therapeutic modalities. However, there were contraindications for surgery such as poor general condition of the patient, diffuse metastasis, and alternative, effective non-surgical methods. Concerning surgical procedures, when metastasis was located anteriorly and limited to one or two vertebrae, the anterior approach was reasonable. However, the remnant tumor and occult metastasis could jeopardize the stability obtained after anterior surgery. Posterior surgery, using instrumentations, especially the G-rod system, were more appropriate. It is a fundamental requirement in choosing procedures to predict the stability of the diseased spine, which decreases until death. Based on this prediction, we can decide how much stability needs to be given to the spine. Postoperative evaluation should reveal the duration of the improvement until the death of the patient, because malignant tumors with remote metastasis are an uncurable and progressive disease. The duration of effective pain relief newly devised by us gave a reasonable indicator for evaluation.

Summary

The authors' experience in the surgical treatment of spinal metastasis concerning surgical indication, procedure, method of postoperative evaluation, and results were reported. Surgery should be an integral part of the overall treatment for improvement of the quality of life of patients with spinal metastasis.

Acknowledgments. The authors thank Professor Yoshihiro Watanabe for reviewing and revising the manuscript.

References

1. Denis F (1984) Spinal instability defined by the three-column spine concept in acute spinal trauma. Clin Orthop 65–76
2. Samoto T (1989) Experimental study and clinical application of the modified Luque rod (Grooved rod) (in Japanese). Yamagata Medical Journal 7:47–58
3. Hayashi M, Oshima Y, Samoto T (1990) Surgical indication and technique of metastatic spinal tumor (in Japanese). Spine and Spinal Cord 3:291–299

4. Nagashima T, Oshima Y, Ota Y, Sato H, Hayashi M, Yokota M, Hiramoto N, Mori M, Ito T, Owashi K, Takei H (to be published) Pain relief through surgical treatment for spinal metastases—evaluation of pain and pain relief (in Japanese). Rinsho Seikei Geka
5. Hammerburg KW (1992) Surgical treatment of metastatic spine disease. Spine 17:1148–1153
6. Onimus M, Schraub S, Bertin D, Bosset JF, Guidet M (1986) Surgical treatment of vertebral metastasis. Spine 11:883–891
7. Kostuik JP, Errico TJ, Gleason TF, Errico CC (1988) Spinal stabilization of vertebral column tumors. Spine 13:250–256

Follow-Up Study of Modified Luque Instrument (G-Rod) for Spinal Trauma

MASAHIRO HAYASHI, YOSHIHIKO OHSHIMA, YOSHIO OHTA, HIROSHI SATOH, NORITOSHI HIRAMOTO, MINORU YOKOTA, TOMOKAZU ITOH, HIROSHI TAKEI, YOUNOSUKE ARII, and YOSHIHIRO WATANABE[1]

Key Words. Modified Luque instrument, G-rod, spinal trauma, segmental spinal instrumentation, follow-up study

Introduction

Luque sublaminar wiring is one of the most rigid spine stabilization techniques, with the advantages of being easy to apply, technically simple, and low in cost [1]. However, its stabilizing capabilities are not perfect, especially against axial loads. The authors have an adaptation of the Luque instrument, called a grooved rod (G-rod), which has a helical groove carved into an original Luque rod (L-rod), with a 2-mm width, an 0.8-mm depth, and a 19-mm pitch. Both rods are shown in Fig. 1.

We have already reported the results of our biomechanical studies [2], in which we used a normal spine model consisting of nine plastic vertebrae in which discs were simulated by polyethylene slices. The vertebrae were fixed with original Luque rods or with G-rods used in conjunction with sublaminar wiring. The results of this test showed that deformity with use of G-rods was less than with L-rods, as shown in Fig. 2. Models of injured spines were made by removal of the central spine section from the normal model. In tests of such models, L-rods provided little resistance to axial compression, but the G-rods were able to resist such axial loads (Fig. 3).

At first G-rods were indicated for metastatic spinal tumors, and we obtained good clinical results of rigid fixation and a high percentage of pain relief [3]. Later on, we used the G-rods not only for metastatic spinal tumors, but also spinal trauma, as well. The purpose of this paper is to evaluate the use of the G-rod for spinal traumas.

[1] Department of Orthopaedic Surgery, Yamagata University School of Medicine, Iida Nishi 2-2-2, Yamagata, 990-23 Japan

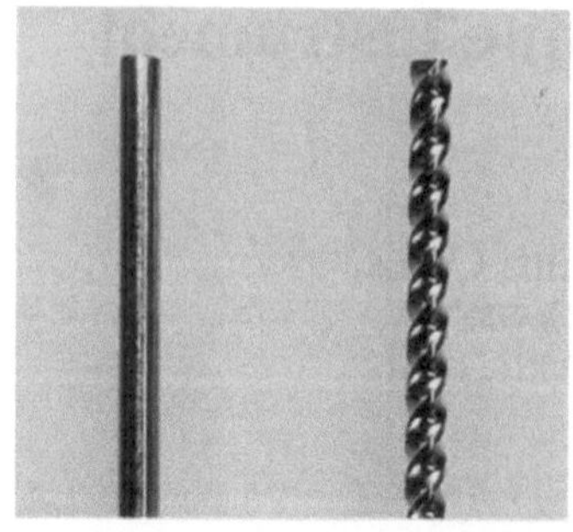

Fig. 1. Presentation of rods. *Left side* is original Luque rod and *right side* is newly developed modified Luque rod (*G-rod*)

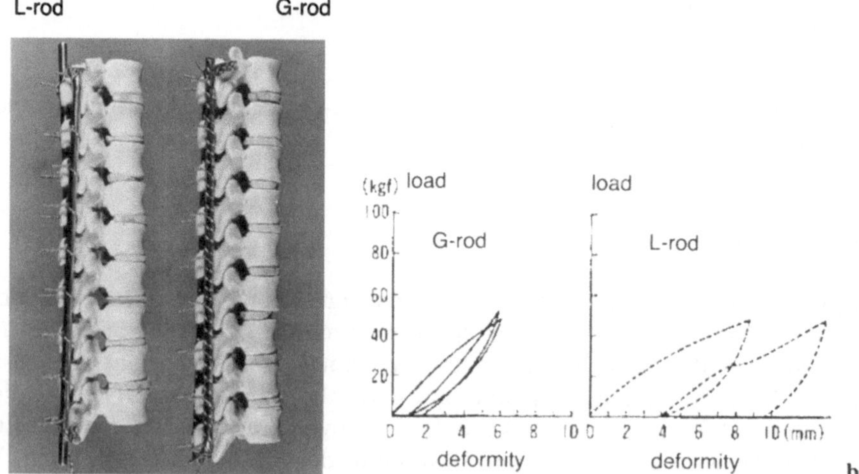

Fig. 2a,b. Biomechanical study 1. **a** Normal spine model was fixed with original Luque rod or G-rod associated with sublaminar wiring. **b** Result was that deformity of G-rod was less than that of L-rod by one-fourth

Patients

From 1985 to 1992, we operated on 50 patients, using G-rods for spinal fractures and dislocations. The follow-up period was 2 years and 9 months on average, with a range of 6 months to 7 years.

Twenty-nine cases were male and 21 were female. Classifying the injuries by Denis three-column theory [4], 28 cases were burst fractures, 2 were seat-belt injuries, and 20 were fracture dislocations. None were compression fractures.

The average age of these patients was 49.9 years, ranging from 16 to 80 at the time of surgery. There were two age peaks, one in their 20s and one in their 50s to 70s. Many cases in their 20s peak had fracture dislocations caused by motor vehicle accidents. Many cases in the 50s to 70s peak had burst fractures caused by falls (Fig. 4).

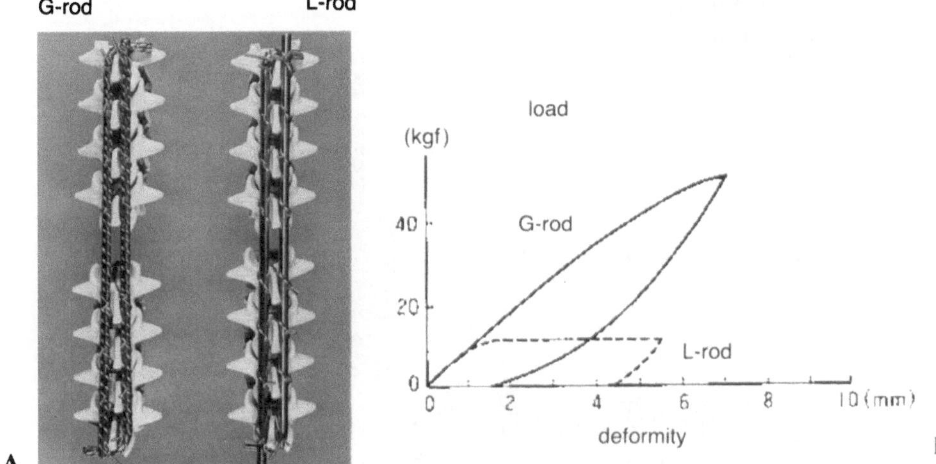

Fig. 3A,B. Biomechanical study 2. **A** Injured spine model was fixed with original Luque rod or G-rod. **B** The result was that the model using L-rod revealed little resistance to axial compression, whereas G-rod could resist axial loading

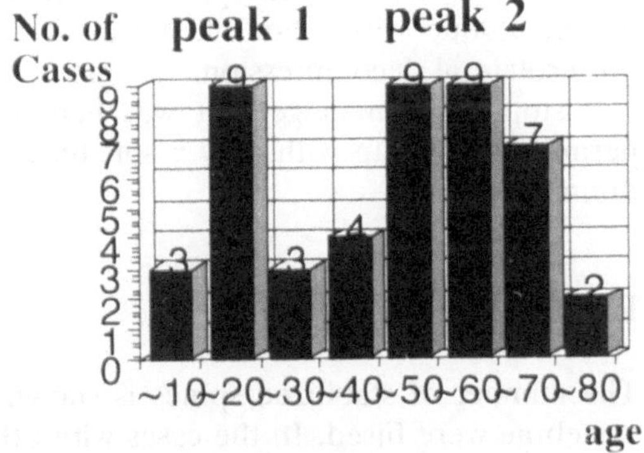

Fig. 4. There were two peaks in the 20s and from the 50s to the 70s in the incidence of burst fractures

The most frequent location of fracture was the thoracolumbar junction (Fig. 5).

Methods

In principal, the area of instrumentation was two or three vertebrae above, and two vertebrae below, the injured area of the spine. The prone position with Hall's frame was somewhat helpful, but reduction was mainly achieved using Harrington's outrigger. After achieving displacement reduction and

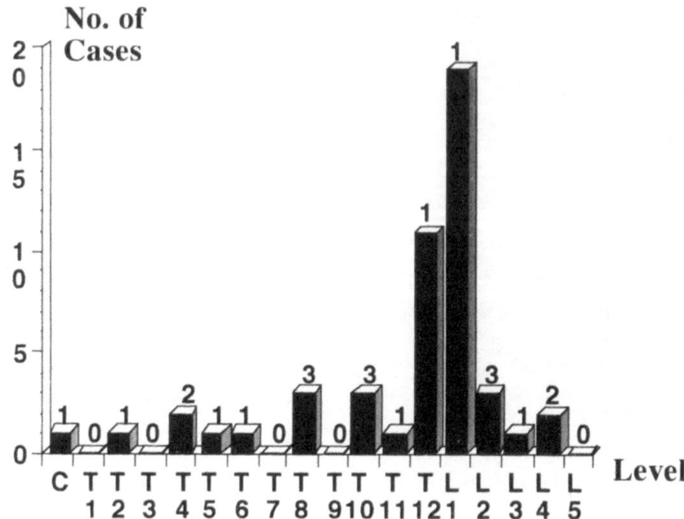

Fig. 5. The injured spinal level. Thoracolumbar junction was the most frequently injured. *C*, Cervical; *T*, thoracic; *L*, lumbar

realignment, the injured spine was stabilized with a rectangular G-rod and double Luque wires. For burst fractures, this treatment was combined with posterolateral decompression.

Postoperative management was handled on the principle that patients be permitted to sit up with only a soft brace soon after the removal of a suction drain.

Results

The number of stabilized spines is shown in Fig. 6. In principle, four or five vertebrae were fused. In the cases with other spinal body or laminar fractures, longer segments (five or six) were fused. In cases of fracture dislocations, we tried shorter fusion, stabilizing only two or three vertebrae.

Before surgery, the average kyphosis was 22.3 degrees, with a range of 50 degrees kyphosis to 5 degrees lordosis. After surgery, on average, the kyphosis was reduced to 8.3 degrees, with a range from 32 degrees kyphosis to 21 degrees lordosis. However, at the follow-up, the average kyphosis was 17.1 degrees, with a range 37 degrees kyphosis to 8 degrees lordosis. There was an average 8.8 degrees correction loss, but no occurrence of psuedoarthrosis (Fig. 7).

Neurologic status was evaluated using Frankel's classification [5]. In 13 cases, there was a complete lesion, none of which recovered. In 31 cases, there was an incomplete lesion, and 6 had absolutely no neurologic deficiency.

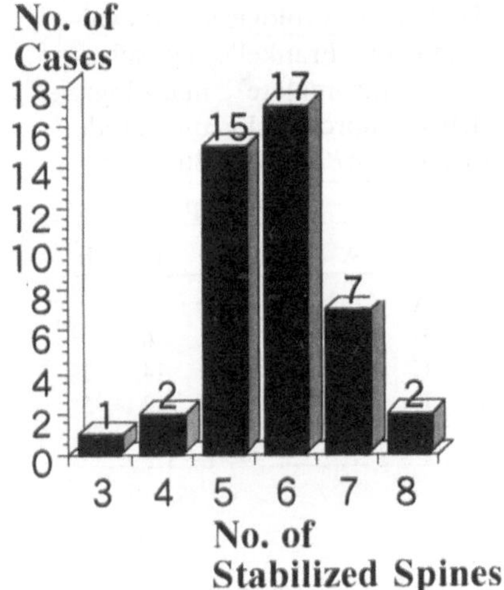

Fig. 6. The numbar of stabilized spine. Four or five vertebral segments were fused in most cases

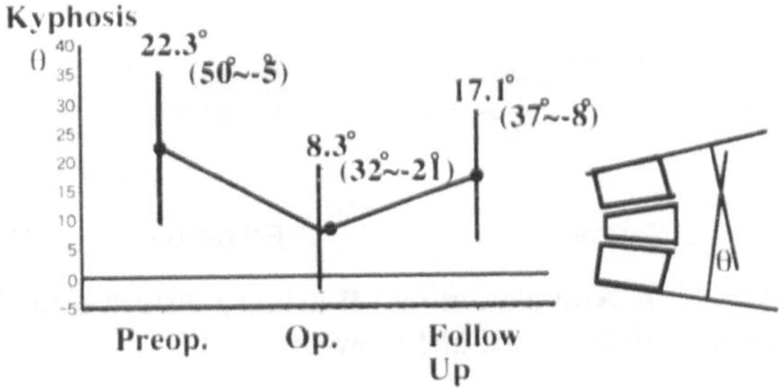

Kyphosis (°)
22.3° (50°~-5°)
8.3° (32°~-21°)
17.1° (37°~-8°)
Preop. Op. Follow Up
θ

Fig. 7. Changes of alignment. The average kyphosis preoperatively was 22.3 degrees, at the time of surgery 8.3, at follow-up 17.1

Postoperatively, of the 31 cases with an incomplete lesion, 27 improved one grade or more (87%). We did not find any cases of neurologic deterioration (Table 1).

Gait and urinary disturbance were evaluated (Fig. 8). Preoperatively, 43 cases were unable to walk, but only 15 cases postoperatively. Preoperatively, 26 cases (of 38) had urinary disturbance, but this number was reduced to 12 postoperatively.

Complications during and after surgery are shown in Table 2. There was no infection, no neurologic deterioration, and no broken rods. Broken wires were observed in 12 cases (of 50), representing 3% of the total of 800 wires used.

Case Presentation

Case

A 17-year-old male with T8 fracture dislocation caused by traffic accident was given emergency treatment at another hospital and then transferred the same

Table 1. Neurologic status evaluated on Frankel's classification. Incomplete neurologic deficit improved by one grade or more (87%) in 27/30 cases.

		Postop.				
		A	B	C	D	E
Preop.	A	13				
	B		1		6	
	C			1	14	2
	D				2	5
	E					6

Table 2. Complications during and after surgery. Only breakage of wire was seen in 12 cases.

1. Infection	0
2. Neurologic deterioration	0
3. Breakage of rod	0
4. Breakage of wire	12/50 cases
	24/800 wires (3%)

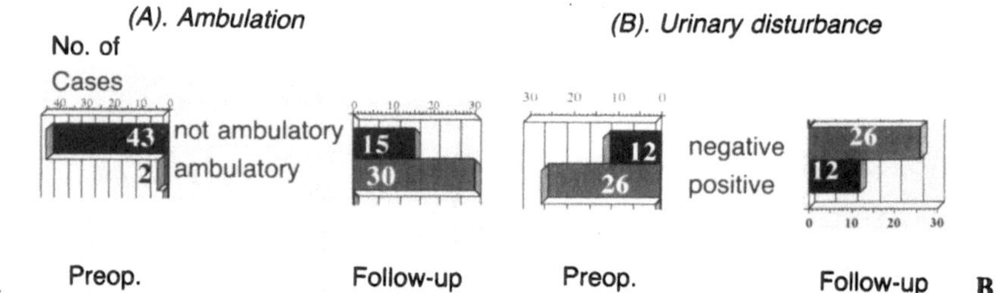

Fig. 8. **A** Ambulation and **B** urinary disturbance: 30 patients could walk and 26 had no urinary disturbance at follow-up

day to our institution. At the time of arrival, neurologic status was Frankel B (Fig. 9). The spinal injury was accompanied by crush injury of lung and diaphragm, with fractures of mandible and clavicle. The operation was performed without delay on the same day as the accident.

preoperatively, there was 37 degrees kyphosis between T8 and T9, with anterior displacement of 16 mm. Surgery reduced the kyphosis to 10 degrees and anterior displacement to zero.

At follow-up, 1 year later, neurologic status had recovered to Frankel D, and he was able to run as well as others in his age. He had suffered a loss of correction of only four degrees.

Discussion

We see following four points as advantages of the original Luque instrument, as compared with other posterior instruments:

1. Rigid fixation is achieved which enabled more rigid stabilization for osteoporotic spines than any other posterior instruments.

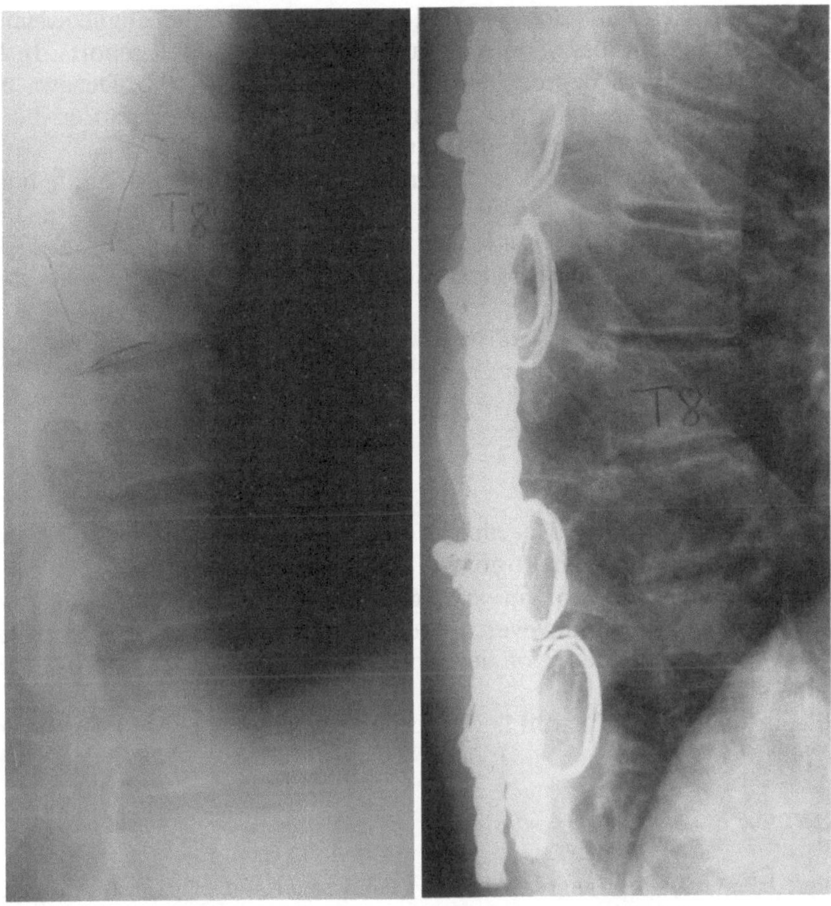

Fig. 9. This case was 17-years-old high school student. T8 fracture dislocation caused by traffic accident. Preoperative kyphosis was 37 degrees, but at the time of follow-up kyphosis reduced to 10 degrees

2. The Luque instrument can be used at any level. The Harrington device can not be used on the cervical spine. Pedicle screwing can not be used on the level of narrow pedicles, such as the cervical spine.
3. Luque SSI offers an easy operative procedure without difficult preparation, and can be performed without the need of an image intensifier.
4. The hardware is inexpensive compared to other posterior instruments.

However, the Luque system also has some disadvantages:

1. The Luque system may not provide adequate protection against axial loads postoperatively. The G-rod, however, offers adequate protection against axial loads.

2. In many cases, some loss of correction was seen in the Luque system. In our cases, subsequent loss of correction was less than in other reports. In 1985, Nasca reported an 18 degree loss of correction [6]; in 1985 Dezawa et al. reported that kyphosis had been reduced at the time of operation, but had regressed to preoperative levels at the time of follow-up. [7]

3. Neurologic complications had been reported previously [8], but in none of our 50 cases were there neurologic complications.

4. The Luque system needs a longer fusion than the P.S. system. The G-rod still has the disadvantage of long fusion, but it is more stable than shorter fusion.

5. In some cases, breakage of wire was seen. For that problem, the authors have recently used cable wire, as reported by Songer et al. [9].

Conclusion

In this paper we presented a clinical study of the use of a modified Luque instrument (G-rod) for spinal trauma.

Kyphosis improved from an average 22.3 degrees preoperatively to 8.3 degrees postoperatively; however, there was an 8.8-degrees loss of correction.

Twenty-seven of 31 cases of incomplete neurologic lesion improved by at least one grade (87%).

We conclude that the G-rod is very useful for thoracolumbar trauma repair.

References

1. Luque ER, Cassis N, Ramirez-Wiella G (1982) Segmental spinal instrumentation in the treatment of the thoraco-lumbar spine. Spine 7:312–317
2. Hayashi M, Ohshima Y, Samoto T, Satoh H, Yokota M, Togashi K, Itoh T, Nagashima T (1991) Experimental and clinical study of modified Luque segmental spinal instrument (in Japanese). Bessatu Seikei Geka 20:45–49
3. Hayashi M, Ohshima Y, Samoto T (1990) Surgical indication and technique of metastatic spinal tumors. Spine and Spinal Cord 3:291–299
4. Denis F (1983) The three-column spine and its significance in the classification of acute thoracolumbar spinal injuries. Spine 8:817–831
5. Frankel HL (1969) The value of postural reduction in the initial management of closed injuries of the spine with paraplegia and tetraplegia. Paraplegia 7:172–192
6. Nasca RJ (1985) Segmental spinal instrumentation. South Med J 78:303–309
7. Dezawa A, Inoue S, Kitahara H, Nagase J, Murakami M, Yamasaki M (1985) Clinical study of spinal instrumentation in the treatment of fracture of thoracic and lumbar spine (in Japanese). Rinsho Seikei 20:442–453
8. Herring JA (1982) Early complications of segmental spinal instrumentation. Orthop Trans 6:22
9. Songer MN, Spencer DL, Myer PR, Jayaraman G (1991) The use of sublaminar cables to replace Luque wires. Spine 16:S418–S421

Hyperthermia and Spinal Cord —An Experimental Study

Seiji Uchiyama, Hideaki E. Takahashi, and Takao Homma[1]

Key Words. Hyperthermia, spinal cord, evoked potentials, temperature, spinal cord injury

Introduction

Hyperthermia is one of the recent topics in cancer treatment and is being applied to tumors in many locations [1]. When hyperthermia is used to treat a tumor, the surrounding tissue is heated as well. With any technique available, it is extremely difficult to heat only the tumor. Extra care should be taken whenever the spinal cord is involved in the heating region because of possible injury to the spinal cord. In some cases, paraplegia occurred following hyperthermia [2]. Under these circumstances it is vital that the effects of hyperthermia on the spinal cord be understood. Unfortunately, there are very few reports on this subject. This study was done to obtain basic information about thermal damage to the spinal cord to make the hyperthermia treatment safer, and to explore the possibility of applying it to the spine or spinal cord tumors. Part of this study has already been reported [3]. In the present study, we did radio frequency (RF) local heating of canine spines and studied spinal cord evoked potentials (SCEP) and histological changes following spinal cord heating, then estimated the tolerable temperature of spinal cord.

Experiment 1: Temperature Disrtibution in the Spinal Canal

The relation between the intramedullary and epidural temperatures was studied to see if the intramedullary temperature could be estimated from the

[1]Department of Orthopedic Surgery, Niigata University School of Medicine, Asahimachidori 1-757, Niigata, 951 Japan

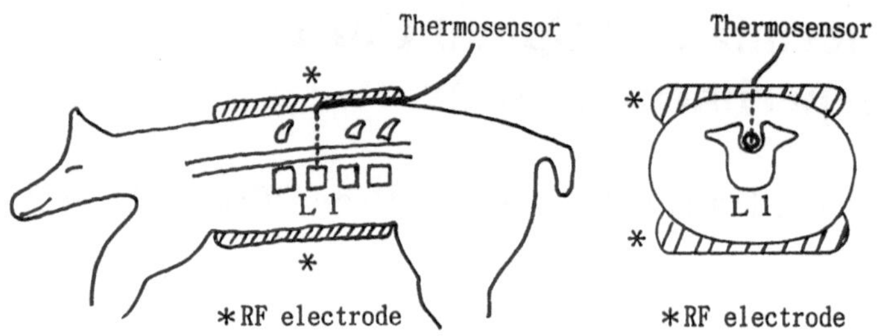

Fig. 1. Radio frequency (*RF*) heating of canine spine

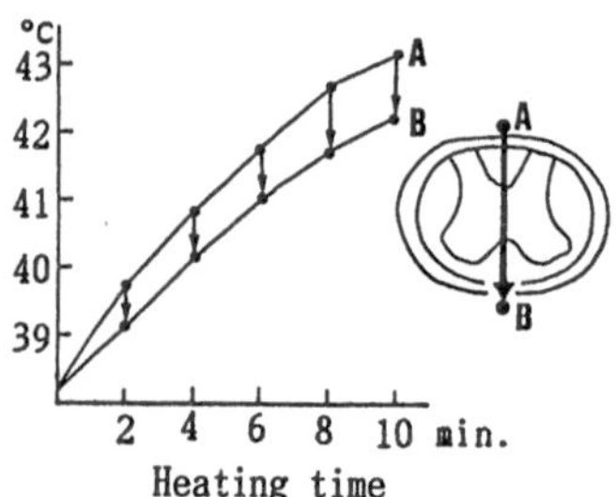

Fig. 2. Temperature in spinal canal in the dorsal epidural space (*A*) and the ventral epidural space (*B*) (with permission, from [3])

epidural temperature, because using on invasive instrument such as a thermal sensor will cause injury to the spinal cord and should be avoided whenever possible.

Materials and Methods

Five adult mongrel dogs weighing 10–15 kg were used and anesthetized with katamine hydrochloride, pentobarbital, and placed under controlled ventilation with pancronium bromide. After laminectomy of L1, an indwelling catheter 1.1 mm in diameter was inserted from the dorsal side of the dura, passing through the spinal cord to ventral epidural space, to guide the flexible thermosensor. The catheter was then secured to the dorsal fascia and the wound was closed. Disc-shaped RF electrodes with a diameter of 15 or 20 cm were placed in close contact on back and abdomen (Fig. 1) [4]. Heating was done by RF capacitive heating, a technique widely used in Japan for hyperthermia [1]. The output power and heating time were adjusted to raise the temperature about 45°C, and were between 200 and 400 W, and between 10 and 20 min, respectively. During heating, the temperature was recorded at 1-mm intervals by moving the thermosensor in the catheter.

Results

Temperature in the dorsal epidural space was same as, or 1°C to 2°C higher than, that in the ventral epidural space, and the temperature changed linearly between the two points including the spinal cord. The results of one dog are shown in Fig. 2. These results showed that the intramedullary temperature could be estimated from epidural temperature monitors.

Experiment 2: Spinal Cord Evoked Potentials and Histological Changes Following Heating

Materials and Methods

Spinal cord was heated in 29 other adult mongrel dogs in the same way as in experiment 1. Thermosensors were placed only in the epidural space to avoid injury due to sensor insertion, and the intramedullary termperature was estimated from the results of experiment 1. This time, the temperature in the dorsal side of spinal cord was about 1°C higher than that in the ventral side in some animals. Under these conditions, intramedullary temperature was taken to be that of the higher, dorsal side. Estimated temperature of spinal cord was raised to a target level between 43°C and 47°C, and it was maintained for 30 min by adjusting RF output, then heating was finished. The stimulus and recording site of SCEP were L4 and T4 or T5 respectively, and flexible bipolar electrodes placed in the dorsal epidural space were used for both stimulation and recording. Stimulation was done by rectangular waves of 0.2 msec in duration with the supramaximal intensity to the recording potentials. The filter range was 10–1500 Hz and 25 to 50 responses were averaged with the analysis time of 10 msec. During RF irradiation, monitoring of SCEP was impossible so that SCEP were recorded before heating, at the end of 30 min heating, and after the return of the spinal cord temperature to preheating level which took 1–2 h after the end of heating. For histological study, spinal cord was taken out immediately after the last SCEP recording in 26 dogs and 1 week later in 2. Evans-Blue vital staining and Hematoxilyn and eosin (H&E) staining were employed.

Results

Spinal Cord Temperature and Evoked Potentials. The basic pattern of SCEP was divided into three components: The initial potential with a high amplitude, second potential with a little smaller amplitude, and small polyphasic potentials (Fig. 3). The initial and second potentials were stable and recorded in all animals, but polyphasic potentials had large interanimal variations. With a rise in temperature, shortening of the latency of all components was observed. After 30 min heating up to the intramedullary temperature of 44°C, the amplitude was unchanged or changed less than 20%. At 45°C, reduction in the amplitude of the second potential by 20% to 40% in addition to shortenting of the latency took place, but the amplitude of initial potential was maintained (Fig. 3). At 46°C, the amplitude of second potential decreased by about 50%, and that of initial potential decreased by 20% to 30%. At 47°C, changes

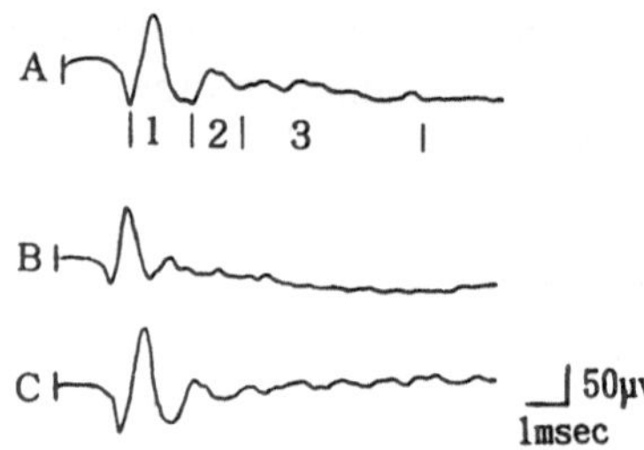

Fig. 3. Spinal cord evoked potential following heating. Preheating control (*A*): *1*, initial potential; *2*, second potential; *3*, polyphasic potentials. At the end of 30 min heating at 45°C (*B*), latency shortened and amplitude decreased. After return of spinal cord temperature (*C*), complete recovery of latency and amplitude was observed

observed at 46°C became more remarkable. Throughout this experiment, reduction in amplitude accompanied a shortening of the latency, and prolongation of latency was not observed (Table 1).

After heating up to 45°C, both the latency and the amplitude returned to preheating levels in all 17 aminals with the return of spinal cord temperature. After heating at 46°C, complete recovery took place in one and incomplete recovery of amplitude in two out of three dogs. At 47°C, incomplete recovery of amplitude occurred in three and no recovery was seen in two out of five dogs. Yet the latency was restored after the return of temperature even though the amplitude remained decreased (Table 1).

Thermal Injury of Spinal Cord. Heating up to 44°C revealed no detectable histological change. After heating at 45°C, despite full recovery of SCEP in all five animals, histological changes were found in five out of seven animals in both the white and the gray matter of the posterior portion of spinal cord. H&E staining revealed spongy destruction with many tiny vacuolations and hemorrhagic spots, and Evans-Blue staining showed pigment exudation and hemorrhage. These changes appeared first around the border between the dorsal column and the dorsal horn (Figs. 4,5). Heating at 46°C or above caused

Table 1. Spinal cord evoked potentials following spinal cord heating [3].

Estimated temperature in spinal cord	At 30 min. heating		Recovery after heating	
	Latency	Amplitude	Latency	Amplitude
43 C (7)	↓	→	Full	No change
44 C (5)	↓	→	Full	No change
45 C (5)	↓	↓ *1	Full	Full
46 C (3)	↓	↓ *2	Full	Full (1) Incomplete (2)
47 C (5)	↓	↓ *2	Full	Incomplete (3) No recovery (2)

( ) = No. of dogs
↓ Decreased; → unchanged
*1 = Second potential
*2 = Initial and second potential

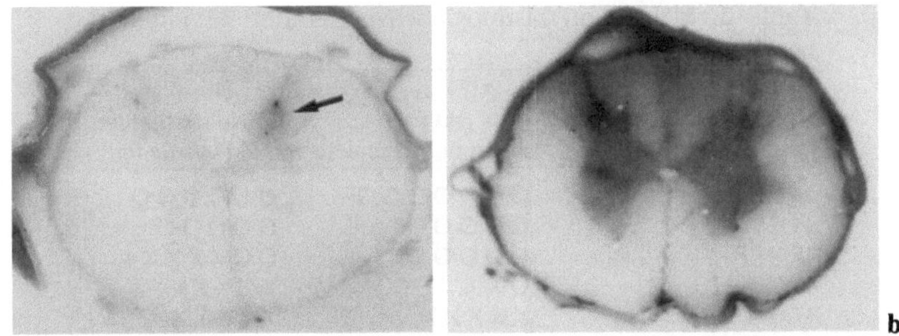

Fig. 4. Thermal injury of spinal cord (Evans-Blue vital staining). At 45°C (**a**), pigment exudation can be seen around the border between dorsal column and dorsal horn. At 46°C (**b**), marked exudation in the dorsal portion of spinal cord was seen

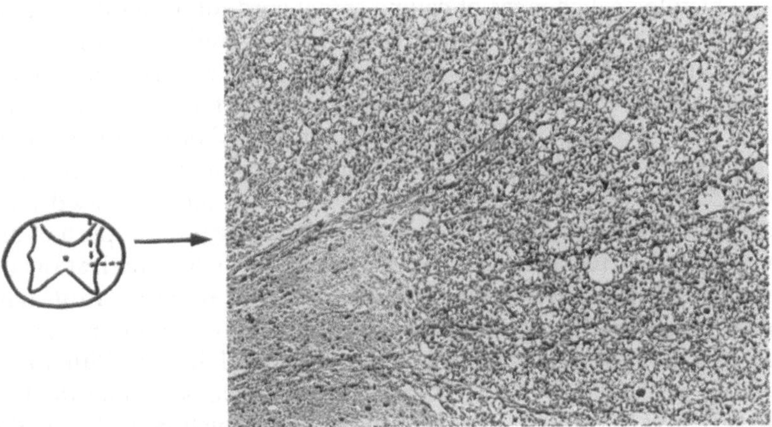

Fig. 5. Thermal injury after heating at 45°C in the same animal as in Fig. 3. Hemorrhage and vacuolation can be seen in spite of full recovery of SCEP. (H&E, ×20)

injury in all animals. Two dogs were observed for a week after the experiment: In one dog heated to 44°C no motor paralysis was seen; in the other, heated to 46°C, paresis occurred so that the animal could hardly stand up from a lying poition. From these results the torelable spinal cord temperature of 30 min heating was estimated to be 44°C (Table 2).

Discussion

Hyperthermia requires knowledge of the thermal effects on tissues or organs involved in the heating area since normal tissue is heated simultaneously during the treatment, and this is especially true of the spinal cord. Paraplegia after

Table 2. SCEP and histologic changes after 30 minutes' hearting [3].

Estimated temperature in spinal cord	SCEP recovery O Full X No or incomplete	Histology O No destruction X Destruction
43 C	OOOOOOO	OOOOOO
44 C	OOOOO	OOOOO
45 C	OOOOO	OOXXXXX
46 C	OXX	XXXXX
47 C	XXXXX	XXXXX

hyperthermia of lung cancer has been reported [2], however few studies have been reported so far on the effects of heat on the spinal cord. We studied SCEP and histological changes of canine spinal cord following RF local heating to see the thermal effects on spinal cord. In this study, we found a strange pattern in the SCEP hitherto unreported, and a torelable spinal cord temperature which has not been mentioned in any leterature was estimated.

In SCEP, the increase of spinal cord temperature shortened latency, but the amplitude did not change up to an estimated intramedullary temperature of 44°C. At 45°C or higher, shortening of the latency and decreased amplitude were observed together. This combination has not been reported hitherto. Yokota et al. reported on the effects of heat from polymerization of bone cement on SCEP [5]. The result of their study was different from ours, and heat caused prolongation of latency with reduction of amplitude. The bizarre pattern observed in our experiment may arise as follows: With the rise of temperature, conduction velocity in spinal cord increases, so that the latency is shortened. Below a certain temperarture, nerve conduction itself is maintained and amplitude does not decrease. When the intramedullary temperature exceeds the critical level, conduction block occurs without passing the stage of latency prolongation. Theoretically, this would lead to the strange phenomenon observed of shortening of latency in combination with reduction of amplitude.

In the present study, small thermal injury could not be detected by SCEP. After heating to 45°C, histological examinations revealed tissue damage in the spinal cord in five of seven animals, yet SCEP showed full recovery of latency and amplitude in all five animals studied. Some experiments of spinal cord compression have indicated that not all spinal cord injuries could be detected by SCEP, and Yasukawa reported that it was difficult to detect degeneration near the central canal or unilateral destruction of spinal cord [6]. In the present study, histological changes after heating at 45°C were hemorrhage, vacuolation, and exudation of pigment. Even with these changes, conduction pathways of SCEP may have remained preserved. SCEP is very important for intraoperative spinal cord monitoring [7]. Our experiment, which is a very special one and the mechanism of spinal cord injury, is much different from other experiments or operations, so the results of this study never diminish the significance of SCEP in spinal cord monitoring.

This study suggests the highest tolerable temperature for normal spinal cord for a 30-min heating is approximately 44°C. The results should be kept in mind whenever hyperthermia is applied in an area which involves the spinal cord.

References

1. Abe M, Hiraoka M, Takahashi M, Egawa S, Matsuda C, Onoyama Y, Morita K, Kakehi M, Sugahara T (1986) Multi-institution studies on hyperthermia using an 8-MHz radio frequency capacitive heating device (Thermotron RF-8) in combination with radiation for cancer therapy. Cancer 58:1589–1595
2. Douglas MA, Parks LC, Bebin J (1981) Sudden myelopathy secondary to therapeutic total body hyperthermia after spinal cord irradiation. N Engl J Med 304:583–585
3. Uchiyama S, Yashiro K, Takahashi H, Homma T (1989) An experimental study of spinal cord evoked potentials and histologic changes following spinal cord heating. Spine 14:1215–1219
4. Uchiyama S, Takahashi H, Homma T, Yashiro K, Sato S, Saitoh Y (1989) Bone and spine heating by radio frequency wave (RF): An experimental study. In: Onoyama Y (ed) Proceedings of the 3rd annual meeting of the Japanese Society of Hyperthermic Oncology. Mag Bros, Tokyo, pp 85–86
5. Yokota H, Masuhara K, Iwasaki H, Kanbara K, Ishii K, Fujii S (1982) A study of thermal effect for spinal cord. Cent Jpn J Orthop Traumatol 24:1235–1237
6. Yasukawa K (1980) Experimental and clinical studies of the evoked electrospinogram for monitoring spinal cord function. J Jpn Orthop Assoc 54:1661–1677
7. Tamaki T, Noguti T, Takano H, Tsuji H, Nakagawa T, Imai K, Inoue S (1984) Spinal cord monitoring as a clinical utilization of the spinal evoked potential. Clin Orthop 184:58–64

Part II.

Biomechanics of Spine in Growth and Aging

An Overview: Spinal Tissue Vital Biomechanics for Clinicians

H.M. Frost[1]

Key Words. Spine, bone, ligament, cartilage, intervertebral disc, modeling, remodeling, joint, arthrosis, internal fixation, biomechanics

Introduction

This article summarizes some physiology learned after 1964 about bone, cartilage, and fibrous tissues. It complements other cellular, molecular-biologic, and physiologic knowledge and by the next decade should be essential to the work of clinicians concerned with spinal problems. It belongs in a new paradigm of skeletal biology [1–30]. Its complexity requires *extreme* brevity and selectivity. If some find new ideas here, skeletal science's poor interdisciplinary communication explains that. For simplicity, a *single asterisk* identifies facts, no matter how arcane they may seem. *Double asterisks* identify hypotheses considered true by most who are qualified to judge them. *Triple asterisks* identify clinicopathologic facts not yet studied systematically by basic scientists.

The text reviews some basic mechanics and bone biology, and some properties of bone, bones, fibrous tissues, ligament, cartilage and joints. The discussion focuses on the human spine and what happens after birth (some structural tissue properties differ in other animals). Table 1 lists and defines the symbols used in this article.

---

[1] Department of Orthopedic Surgery, Southern Colorado Clinic, 41 Montebello, Pueblo, CO 81001, USA

The asterisk system used throughout this chapter classifies the indicated text passages into the following categories:

* Facts.

** Hypotheses generally considered valid.

*** Clinicopathologic facts that have not yet been studied systematically.

Table 1. Abbreviations and acronyms in the text.

BMU:	Basic multicellular unit
CGFRC:	The chondral growth-force response curve that can describe how cartilage growth responds to mechanical forces
MDx:	Microdamage, meaning microscopic and submicroscopic mechanical fatigue damage
MES:	A general term for the minimum effective signal that begins to turn an adaptive, protective or healing skeletal activity ON
MESm:	The minimum effective strain range that can turn adaptive modeling drifts ON
MU:	Mechanical usage, in the sense of the typical peak mechanical loads on skeletal structures instead of their frequency. Weight lifting has a greater effect on them than walking or running
RAP:	Regional acceleratory phenomenon
μE:	Microstrain
MESr:	Minimum effective strain range that begins depressing BMU creations and equalizing their resorption and formations
MLA:	Momentarily loaded area

Basic Mechanics

Strain

Mechanical loads always deform or strain tissues. Expressed as microstrain (μE), 2000 μE in tension stretches a bone or ligament 0.2%, or from 100% to 99.8% of its original length. Compression of 25 000 μE can shorten a bone 2.5%, or from 100% to 97.5% of its original length. Special gauges can measure the three principal strains (tension, compression and shear) in vivo. A tissue's fracture or rupture strain can provide a yardstick to compare with other strains [31,32].

Stress

Straining a tissue stretches its intermolecular bonds, which resist with a force called stress. Three principal stresses correspond to the principal strains, and can be expressed as the force per unit area. How much stress a given strain causes depends on a material's *stiffness*. For equal strains, stiffer materials generate larger stresses than less stiff or "compliant" materials. The stiffness of skeletal tissues decreases in this order: Enamel > lamellar bone > woven bone > mature tendon and ligament > cartilage > scar.

Total and Unit Loads

As examples, kilograms, Newtons, or pounds can express an external mechanical force or *load* on a given structure. For a 20-kg *total load* on a whole intervertebral disc, if the disc's cross section area equals 15 cm^2, each cm^2 would carry 1/15th the total load (20/15 = 1.33 kg/cm^2). That defines the disc's *unit loading*, and also its compression stress (Fig. 1).

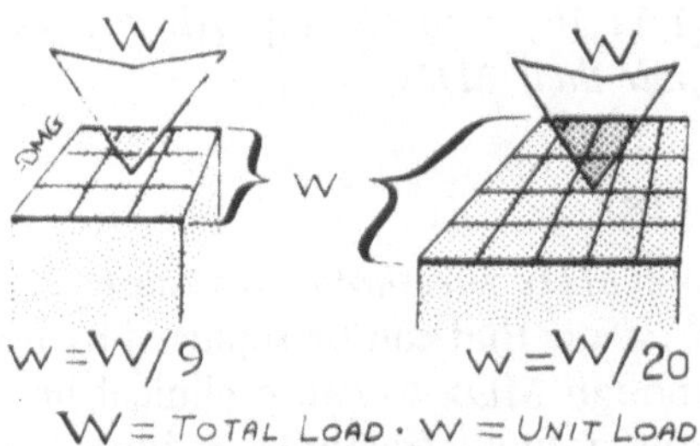

Fig. 1. The meaning of unit loads. Total load (*W*), and unit load (*w*): A basic concept in vital biomechanics. Each surface shown here carries the same total load. Yet each unit area of the *left* surface carries one-ninth the total load, while each unit area of the larger surface on the *right* carries 1/20th of the same total load

Strength

The load or corresponding strain or stress that breaks or ruptures a tissue can define its strength, and this article is concerned with three kinds of strain [18]. First, the load, strain or stress that causes a fracture or rupture when applied only once defines the *ultimate strength*. The ultimate or "fracture strain" of normal bone is roughly 25 000 ± 5000 μE, which corresponds to a stress of about 130 MPa or 16 000 psi. The ultimate strain of normal ligament is roughly 70 000 μE in tension. Second, the strain at which permanent deformation (also called plastic flow) of a material begins to occur defines its *yield point*. It is equal to about one-third of a structural tissue's ultimate strain. A third kind of strength concerns fatigue (see below).

Elasticity

Elasticity is defined as a material's ability to return to its original shape and dimensions after deloading, whether quickly as with springs (which shows *resilience*), or slowly as with oranges and cartilage (which shows *viscoelasticity*). The viscoelasticity of structural tissues decreases in this order: Scar > cartilage > mature fibrous tissues > woven bone > lamellar bone > enamel.

Fatigue and Microdamage

Repeatedly straining and destraining (or loading and deloading) a tissue even well below its yield point can eventually cause a sudden fracture or rupture due to accumulated microscopic, physical fatigue damage called microdamage (MDx). *All structural tissues can develop MDx under cyclic loading*. It increases with the size of the loads and number of loading cycles. The number of cycles of a given strain that cause a fatigue failure defines a third kind of strength known as *fatigue life* [1,11,16,17,30,33–41]. *All structural tissues have mechanisms to detect and repair their MDx.*

Microdamage Thresholds

All skeletal tissues have *MDx thresholds*, meaning strain (or stress) ranges below which little MDx occurs that can be repaired by normal mechanisms, but above which there is enough MDx to cause clinical harm.*** Increased MDx can cause bone pain and fatigue fractures in bone,* pain and spontaneous ruptures in fibrous tissues,* and chondromalacia and arthroses in cartilage.* Under equal loads the fatigue life of bone loaded parallel to its grain exceeds that when loaded across the grain, so "parallel-grain" and "across-grain" thresholds exist*** (an analog probably exists for cartilage) [15–17]. The MDx thresholds of structural tissues tend to lie well below their fracture or rupture strains, and somewhat below their yield points.** The strains or unit loads associated with the above features would rank as follows: Rupture strength > yield point > fatigue life > MESm (the MESm is defined below).

Basic Biology

Certain spinal features are established at birth, and later several basic biologic activities combine to control the spine's architecture, adapt it to various challenges, keep it healthy throughout life, and affect its healing and reactions to disease and other challenges.

Growth

Both general body growth and longitudinal bone growth have the basic function of increasing size by increasing the total numbers of cells and the total amounts of intercellular materials.* However, "pure" growth not otherwise guided tends to produce disorganized masses of tissue, as in anaplastic neoplasms. All tissues can grow in this sense [19,31,41–43], but that tends to stop after skeletal maturity.

Macromodeling

During growth, many circulating and local agents can retard growth in some places and increase it in others.* This control normally shapes (hence "modeling", as in modeling statues in clay) growing structures such as joints, bones, ligaments, livers, and kidneys. *In skeletons it creates functionally and biomechanically purposeful architecture.* Since this process usually occurs during growth, it tends to be less effective in adults [1,19,31,41]. Modeling activities can either act or be ON, or lie dormant and OFF. By 1990, a related, important fundamental concept evolved: *The biologic activities probably "model" a growing skeleton's architecture to keep the typical peak strains of* *each structural tissue below its MDx threshold.*** This idea should apply to whole bones, joints, ligaments, tendons, and their parts [16,17].

Micromodeling

While any new tissue is forming, a special activity determines the organization and "grain" of its cells and intercellular materials. This "micromodeling" helps to determine what *kind* of tissue forms;*** macromodeling controls *where and when* it forms.* As examples, micromodeling helps to make scar different from tendon, meniscus different from growth plate cartilage, and fracture callus and woven bone different from lamellar bone.* In mature tendon, ligament, fibrocartilage, and bone, micromodeling *always* makes the tissue's grain parallel to the major tension or compression loads on it *during the time it was forming* [7,31].

Remodeling

Bone and fibrous tissues can undergo turnover in small packets. A multicellular unit or BMU (basic multicellular unit) can do that by removing a bit of tissue and then replacing it with newly formed tissue, either of the same or different kind.* An "activation event" is required for a new BMU to begin, so it functions in an activation-resorption-formation sequence that usually takes several months to finish. The responses of BMU-based remodeling to an agent can also act or be ON, or lie dormant and OFF [1,6,12,19,31,44]. Many have studied BMU-based bone remodeling but not the comparable fibrous tissue activity. Cartilage lacks such BMUs.

Macrohealing

All structural tissues can heal gross injuries but they do it differently. The healing process usually involves creating an original healing tissue ("callus"), and then replacing it piecemeal with the "mature" type of tissue. This usually takes months. The callus has worse mechanical properties than the mature tissue. Normally OFF, gross injuries can turn macrohealing ON [4,43,45].* "Macrohealing" is distinguished from the biologically different "microrepair" of MDx.

Mechanical Usage and Loading Histories

The skeleton's biologic activities respond to some time-averaged value of many loads instead of to single ones, and the largest or "typical peak loads" (or strains) have far greater effects than smaller ones no matter how frequent.* "Loading history" refers to these properties (D.H. Carter coined the term) [31,46–50]. While evidence suggests that the skeleton's MDx and biologic activities can respond somewhat differently to *intermittent and continuous* *loads*, this has not yet been studied.*** The human spine does carry significant continuous loads, unlike the extremities [14–18].

Creep

This slow, irreversible deformation under a load can happen in tension, compression, shear, or any combination thereof. It is always abnormal when it occurs in bone, but not always in fibrous tissues and articular cartilage [30,31,34,51,52].***

Regional Acceleratory Phenomenon

An injury or other noxious stimulus normally accelerates all ongoing regional biologic activities.*** Effective stimuli can include any operation, fracture, or local infection. The affected activities can include healing, perfusion, growth, modeling, remodeling, MDx repair, creep compensation, and combatting infections. Failure to develop a normal regional acceleratory phenomenon (RAP) after an injury or operation can delay or prevent healing and promote infection.*** It can cause a biologic failure of bone healing after osteotomy, bone grafting, arthrodesis, or fracture.* Such failures happen much more often in adults than children, and more often where sensory denervation exists.* Excessive RAPs can also happen, as in causalgia minor and algodystrophy in the spine and extremities [20,28,31,41;53–55].***

Mechanoreceptors

Bone and fibrous tissues have nerves that can signal pain when overstrained or injured.* Cartilage lacks such nerves. These mechanoreceptors explain some of the bone pain associated with osteoporoses, osteomalacias, and arthroses, and in the presence of some internal fixation devices and artificial joints. They explain some of the pain in fibrous tissue structures in some athletes (shin splints, tendonitis, charley horse), and in back pain arising in the annulus fibrosis or longitudinal ligament of the spine [17,56–59].*

Table 2 lists a few diseases that involve malfunctions of the above features to give some idea of how widespread they are in skeletal pathophysiology. Attention now turns to some properties of specific tissues.

Bone and Bones

Bone Types

As D.B. Burr, W.S.S. Jee and R.B. Martin note, the healthy human skeleton contains mostly *lamellar bone*. It has a "grain" or long-range order, and more strength, stiffness and fatigue resistance than other bone types [15,16,60]. It forms relatively slowly, its formation cannot exceed a maximal rate, and it

Table 2. Some skeletal diseases in which altered perception and adaptation to mechanical usage play major causative roles.

Osteoporoses, adult-acquired	Osteoporoses, in children
Osteopenias in disuse	Osteopenias in chronic disease
Osteogenesis imperfecta	Arthroses
Spinal stenosis	Increased bone fragility
Spontaneous tendon ruptures	Spontaneous fractures
Osteochondritis dissecans	Aseptic necroses
Hernias	Varices
Aneurysms	Keloid
Joint contractures	Osteochondromas
Retarded bone healing	Retarded tendon healing
Dwarfisms	Frozen shoulder
Hallux rigidus	Genu varum and valgum
Congenital hip dysplasia	Club foot
Dentinogenesis imperfecta	Prognathism
Ehlers-Danlos syndrome	Chondromalacia

carries the loads on bones throughout life.* *Woven bone* lacks the grain, stiffness, strength, and fatigue resistance of lamellar bone.*** It can form faster than lamellar bone but it takes more intense stimuli to induce its formation than does lamellar bone.*** It usually lasts only a few months in the body.* If it carries loads, less lamellar bone usually replaces it.*** Fibroareolar tissue usually replaces it if it carries no loads [4,19,26,31,43,61,62].***

Bone Modeling Drifts

When osteoblasts deposit new bone on broad bone surfaces without local coupling to osteoclasts, this constitutes a *formation drift*. When osteoclasts resorb bone from other surfaces without local coupling to osteoblasts, this constitutes a *resorption drift*. As Fig. 2 suggests, patterns of these drifts can move bone surfaces in tissue space to shape and size cortical bone and trabeculae. During growth, drifts usually maintain a bone's shape and increase its outside diameter and cortical thickness.* These "modeling drifts" become inefficient on cortical bone in adults but can continue on trabeculae throughout life [2,3,19,20,26,31,44,49,50,52,63].***

*Global modeling can increase bone size and mass but apparently does not reduce them.*** *It becomes inefficient in cortical bone in adults.** "Global" means all the drifts in a whole bone combined (obviously a single resorption drift can remove local bone). As used below, the term modeling means via these drifts.

Mechanical Usage and Modeling Drifts

Beginning with C.E. Lanyon in 1974, bone strains measured in many normally functioning, intact animals revealed the following [7,26,41,46,64–66]. The

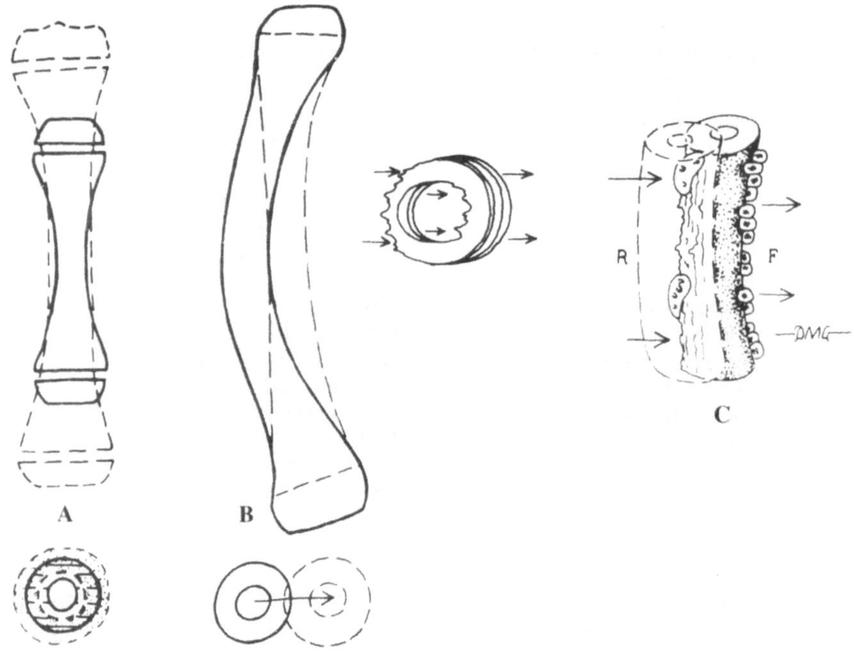

Fig. 2A–C. Modeling drifts. **A** An infant's long bone, its original size and shape shown by the *solid line*. To keep that shape as it grows, its surfaces must move in tissue space as suggested by the *dotted line*. Formation drifts build some surfaces up, resorption drifts remove material from others. **B** A different drift pattern corrects the bowed bone (due to a fracture malunion) shown by the *solid line*. The cross section view on the *right* shows the cortical-endosteal and periosteal drifts. The segment at **C** shows how the drifts in **B** would move the whole segment to the right in tissue space (from [63], with permission)

largest range of bone strain which animals can cause by a deliberate effort may center on about 12% of the fracture strain during growth, and on about 6% in adults. When and where typical peak strains stay below those ranges, mechanically controlled modeling drifts tend to stay OFF.* When strains equal or exceed those ranges, drifts usually turn ON and begin changing bone architecture and mass in ways that lower the subsequent strains toward the bottoms of those ranges, which can be defined as the *minimum effective signals* for turning modeling ON (hence, MESm). When and where strains stay below the MESm range, adaptive and mechanically controlled modeling drifts usually go OFF and stay OFF [7].**

*Global modeling drifts can adapt bones to overloads but apparently not to underloads.** By the "MESm criterion", loads that cause strains smaller than the MESm represent underloads; higher loads represent overloads.*

When and where typical peak bone strains enter a higher threshold, around 12% to 16% of the fracture strain, woven bone formation can begin;* when it

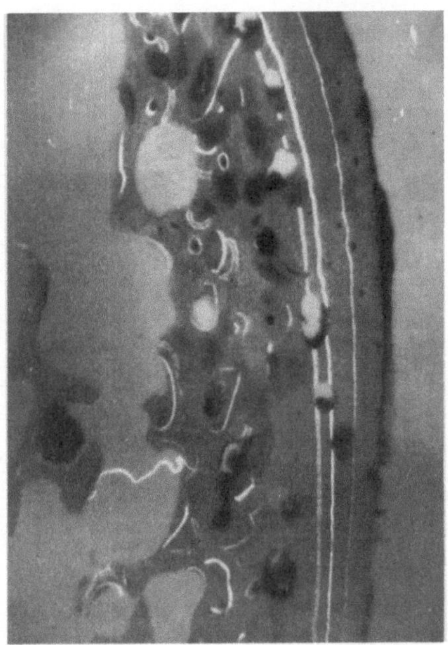

Fig. 3. Modeling drifts. Undecalcified cross-section of the cutaneous cortex of the middle third of a young girl's 7th rib, obtained at the time of thoracotomy for cardiac surgery. About 10 X in blue-light, transmitted, fluorescence microscopy. The *long white, vertical lines* are tetracyclines deposited by lamellar bone formation drifts during growth. The *smaller, semicircular white lines* in the cortex are secondary osteons that were forming at the same time as the drifts. This whole cortex was drifting toward the *right* (which is the normal pattern) (from [38], whith permission)

does, it always suppresses local lamellar bone drifts [15,31].* Figure 3 illustrates these drifts, and also the BSUs described below.

Bone Remodeling and the Basic Multicellular Unit

A BMU can turn bone over in packets in an activation-resorption-formation sequence,* as Fig. 4 suggests. In humans a typical packet can turn over about $0.05\,mm^3$ of bone in about 4 months; several million of them can arise in the skeleton annually. A BMU's resorption is coupled to its formation so both occur in the same place.* BMUs can turn bone over on periosteal, haversian, cortical-endosteal, and trabecular surfaces (E. Sedlin's "envelopes") throughout life. Inside cortical bone they form secondary osteons. Where bone touches marrow, BMUs usually form slightly less than they resorb.* That causes a negative local bone balance and the resultant marrow cavity expansion and trabecular thinning and losses that normally happen throughout life, which L.C. Johnson first reported and R.R. Smith, H. Takahashi and R.R. Walker

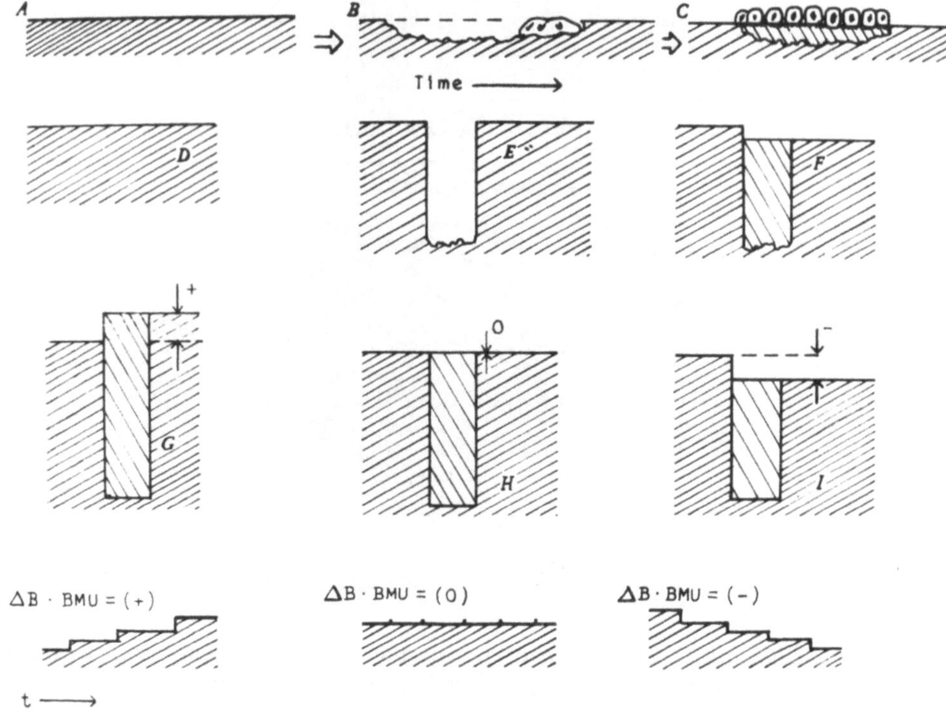

Fig. 4. The bone remodeling basic multicellular unit (BMU). *Top row*: An activation event on a bone surface at (*A*) creates a pocket of resorption (*B*) followed by replacement of the resorbed bone (*C*). *Second row*: Idealize these events to show the bone resorbed (*E*) and formed (*F*) by completed BMUs. *Third row*: In these "BMU graphs" (after the author) (*G*) shows a small excess of formation over resorption as on periosteal surfaces. (*H*) Shows equalized resorption and formation as on haversian surfaces. (*I*) Shows a net deficit of formation, as on cortical-endosteal and trabecular surfaces. *Bottom row*: These "stair graphs" (after P.J. Meunier) show effects on the local bone balance and mass of a series of BMUs of the kind immediately above. The ΔB.BMU in this figure is the same thing as Greek rho in the text (from [63], with permission)

documented [65,67–69]. Increasing both BMU creations (called "mu" by histomorphometrists) and the deficit of bone in completed BMUs (called "rho", shown in Fig. 5) increases the net loss of bone and tends to cause osteopenia, as Fig. 6 suggests.* Reducing BMU creations and equalizing their resorption and formation tends to conserve bone and prevent osteopenia [1,8,19,20, 26,29,31,41,70–75].*

Mechanical Usage and Basic Multicellular Units

In acute disuse, bone strains would fall and stay below about 1/500th the fracture strain. BMU creations increase everywhere in such bone, while next to

Fig. 5. The rho fractions. These drawings show the meanings assigned in the text to Greek rho, rho-sub-r and rho-sub-f. A negative value of rho means completed BMUs resorb more bone than they make

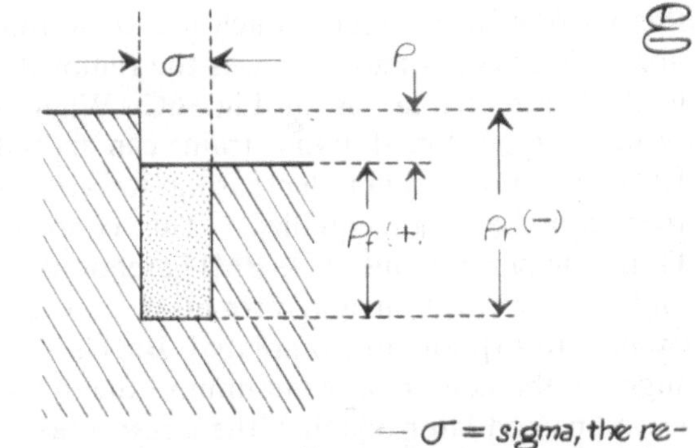

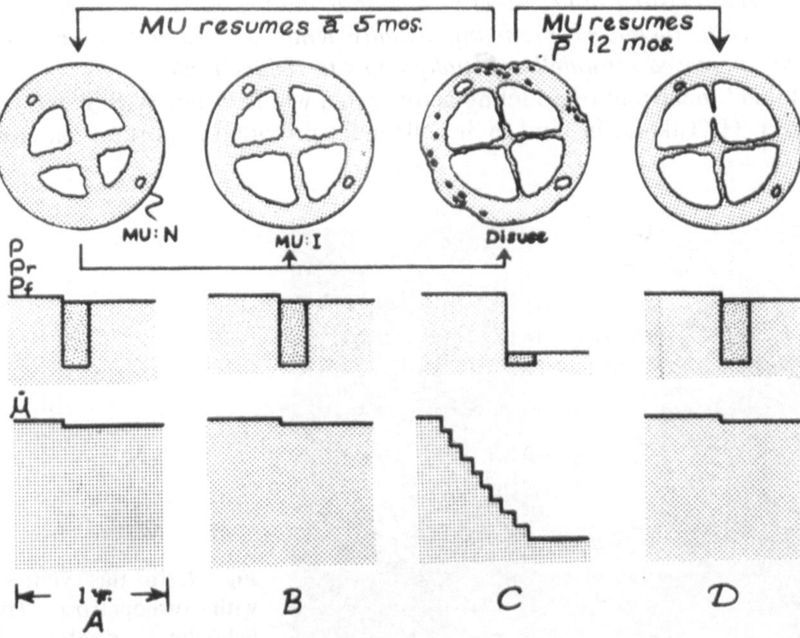

Fig. 6. Some mechanical usage effects on remodeling. *Top row*: Bone cross sections to illustrate effects of normal and increased mechanical usage (MU) and disuse. *Second row*: The rho fraction values for the MU cases above. *Third row*: These "stair graphs" show the changes in BMU creations associated with the MU states above. Column (*A*) applies to normal MU, column (*B*) to hypervigorous MU, column (*C*) to acute disuse, and column (*D*) to the return to normal MU. When the disuse lasts a short time, most of the losses shown in (*C*) can be restored. When it lasts for a long time, some permanent trabecular and cortical thinning and marrow cavity expansion exist (from [14], with permission)

the marrow BMUs make much less bone than they resorb, and in some cases none.* This combination causes the removal of bone touching marrow and can lead to osteopenia, as in Fig. 6C. When normal mechanical usage (MU) resumes, typical peak bone strains can exceed the MESr. Where that happens, BMU creations begin decreasing towards normal and their resorption and formation begin to equalize.* This conserves existing bone, as in Fig. 6B. During hypervigorous MU, BMU creations remain normal or may even decline and their resorption and formation stay equalized; formation still does not exceed resorption in completed BMUs, as in Fig. 6D.* The above strain suggests the center of a minimum effective range that can first depress BMU creations and later equalize their resorption and formation. Hence, the MESr for BMU-based remodeling [8,20,23,24,26,28,68,74,76–78]. In sum:

Global remodeling can remove or conserve bone but cannot add to it, at least not without pharmacologic assistance [41,70,79]. Global remodeling can adapt bone to disuse and underloads, but not to overloads.

Loads that cause strains equal to or above the MESr can reduce remodeling and conserve existing bone; otherwise remodeling begins removing it.

Also, while increased modeling usually tends to increase bone mass and strength, increased remodeling usually tends to reduce both.

"Global" means all remodeling activity in a whole bone. W.S.S. Jee, Z.F.G. Jaworski, H. Takahashi, and their colleagues provided important experimental

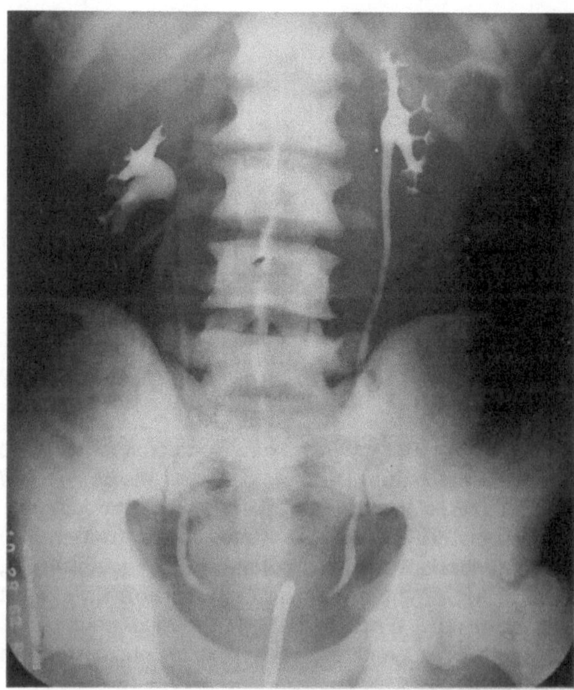

Fig. 7. In this young adult with osteopetrosis (Albers-Schönberg disease) BMU-based remodeling is impaired, usually from birth. As a result, bones tend to keep the spongiosa formed even years before. That limits "medullarization" of bone as shown here. It can also lead to fatigue fractures and impaired fracture healing

data about these features. Figure 7 shows one effect on an adult's bone density of a lifelong decrease in remodeling.

Microdamage Thresholds and Repair

Bone's parallel-grain MDx threshold range (hypothesized by Martin et al. in 1983 [27]) may center on about 12% of its fracture strain, since its fatigue life can fall below 20000 cycles above 16%, while below 8% its fatigue life can exceed 10 million cycles.* Normal living bone can detect MDx in its early stages and create a local BMU to remove and replace the damaged bone with new bone. As R.B. Martin and D.B. Burr note, that effectively repairs the MDx.* If MDx accumulates faster than normal BMUs can repair it, or if something impairs that repair mechanism, MDx can accumulate and cause fatigue fractures of whole bones or loosening of internal fixation devices and artificial joints.* MDx repair is impaired in dead bone, in all osteomalacias, in many osteoporoses, and in an occasional apparently healthy person as well.* Bone's across-grain MDx threshold has yet to be studied systematically.*** The closeness of the MESm to the somewhat higher MDx threshold suggested to D.H. Carter and the author that the adaptation of normal bone to its MU may aim to minimize MDx rather than to provide great momentary strength. If so, the latter became a secondary benefit [1,11,16,18,26,30,33–39,80–83].

Fibrous Tissues

This discussion focuses on ligament and the annulus fibrosis. Other texts discuss analogous problems of other ligaments, tendon, fascia, and joint capsule [10,17,36,42,57,58,61,84–91].

Longitudinal Growth

The spine's ligaments grow in length by end-growth and creep-growth [17].

End-Growth. During general body growth, ligaments attach to bones across a layer of cartilage. Growth of that cartilage parallel to the tension which the ligament puts on it explains the normal migration of bony ligament attachments between birth and maturity.* Increasing tension on the attachments can slightly increase this end-growth.***

Creep-Growth. Under *intermittent loading*, fibrous tissues normally do not creep significantly in tension (they do not stretch irreversibly).* However, as L.E. Dahners, C. Frank, and clinical observations (wedging casts or constant traction on contracted joints or muscles for example) show, enough *constant tension* can stretch them in creep.* In growing subjects who have not reached maturity, many ligaments span steadily growing epiphyses (as in the knee, hip

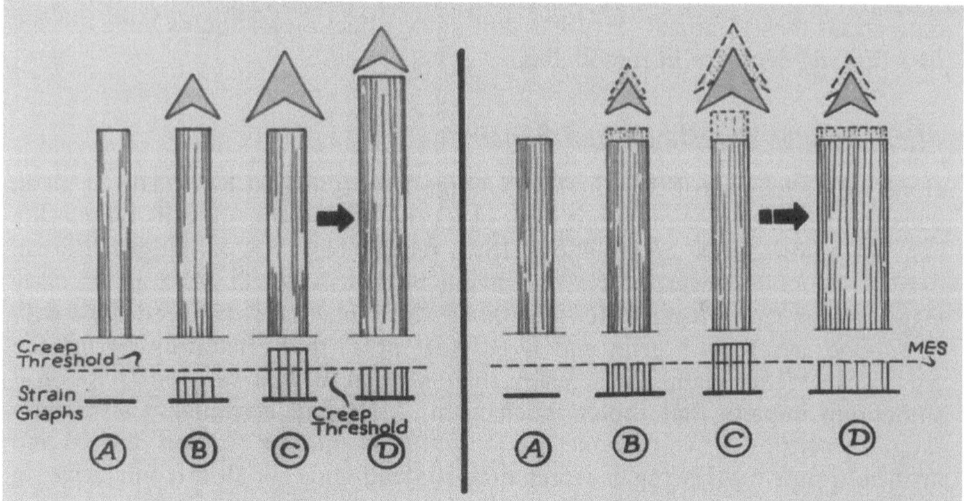

Fig. 8. *Left*: Creep-growth. Most ligament growth in length comes from stretching in the middle, meaning creep growth. It happens under continuous tension strain above some kind of threshold value. As the strain graphs suggest, at (*B*) that value is not exceeded. At (*C*) it is, which leads to (*D*): A longer ligament. Growth in ligament length is usually directly proportional to growth in height of the epiphysis which it spans. *Right*: Diametric modeling. These drawings suggest how diametric growth or modeling of ligament responds to intermittent tension strains. Strains above the minimum effective signal (*MES*) for diametric modeling would make the tissue's cells begin adding new collagen to increase its diameter, stiffness, and strength, as at (*D*). When those increases lower tension strains back to the bottom of the MES (note the strain graphs at the *bottom*), the addition of further collagen would stop. Fascia and tendon can also increase in thickness by this mechanism

capsule, or longitudinal ligament). The resulting constant tension on the ligaments can stretch them in creep, and most increases in ligament length during general growth are believed to occur by this mechanism (Fig. 8) [17].* That may also explain why creep usually stops after skeletal maturity. These results imply that there is a minimum range of continuous tension that can induce creep.*** If so, an MES for creep exists.

Diametric Modeling

As proposed in 1973, when the intermittent loads on a fibrous tissue structure repeatedly exceed some minimum value, its cells begin to synthesize collagen to increase the structure's thickness and cross sectional area [49].* This synthesis continues until the increased stiffness reduces the tension strains to within a minimum value or range. Referred to as diametric modeling (Fig. 8), the strain range that controls collagen synthesis appears to have its own MES which is centered on about 20% of the rupture strain.*** This may explain why intermittent stretching of contracted joint capsules and scars can make them worse instead of better. In sum:

Intermittent tension strains above a threshold can thicken ligaments but not lengthen them. Continuous tension above a different but lower threshold can make them stretch without thickening.

Creep and Creep Compensation

Living fibrous tissues tend to shorten if not periodically stretched, which reveals a vital mechanism(s) that would tend to correct or prevent excessive creep.*** This mechanism may depend on the protein actin [90]; it can cause muscle and capsular contractures in joints immobilized for long periods of time, especially after an injury or when for some other reason a local RAP accelerates the process.*** It could explain why intermittently loaded structures like tendons do not stretch appreciably throughout life, but continuously tensioned ligaments (and fascia?) can. While the latter happens during normal growth, it can happen sometimes in adults too (as in the intervertebral ligaments in spondylolisthesis) [17].*** Overactive creep compensation activity happens in Dupuytren's contracture, frozen shoulder (pericapsulitis), during a RAP, and in "arthrofibrosis" of fingers and some other joints after injury [17].***

Microdamage

This can happen in all fibrous tissues including the annulus and longitudinal ligament [17,31,49].* It likely begins at the molecular level and progresses upwards from there in steps, from the rupture of a few collagen fibers, to bundles of them, to a complete rupture. Normal fibrous tissues detect and repair their MDx before it becomes excessive. Dead fibrous tissue cannot repair MDx.* Therefore, there seems to be a minimum amount of MDx required to activate the biologic repair system.*** If so, there would also be an MES for turning MDx repair ("microhealing") ON. Most intervertebral disc herniations result from fatigue failures of the overlying annulus.

Microdamage Threshold

Fibrous tissues must have an MDx threshold as well.*** That is, below a certain range of cyclic tension strains, the healthy tissue develops little MDx and can repair it to prevent accumulated fatigue. Above that range, new MDx occurs faster than it can be repaired. In the annulus, the problems include "bulging" discs and frank herniations. This threshold has yet to be systematically studied.

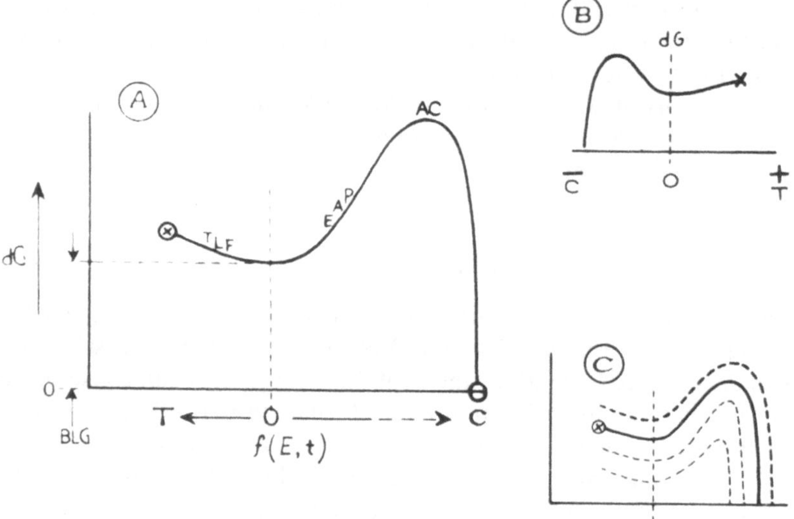

Fig. 9. The chondral growth-force response curve (CGFRC). (*A*) shows this curve. The horizontal axis plots tension (*T*) and compression (*C*) loads on a cartilage plate. (*B*) shows another way to plot the CGFRC, with positive values to the *right* (tension) and negative ones (compression) to the *left*. The family of curves in (*C*) shows how different inherent growth potentials of different chondral planes might cause different amounts of modeling without necessarily changing the kind of responses to mechanics. This might partly explain why chondral planes grow slower in fingers than in knees, and slower in mice than giraffes. *TLF*, tendon, ligament, fascial bony attachments; *EAP*, epiphyseal and apophyseal plates; *AC*, articular cartilage

Cartilage and Joints

Chondral Growth-Force Response Curve

Figure 9 shows some responses of growing hyaline cartilage to mechanical forces. During growth and in the absence of normal mechanical loads, there is a "baseline growth" in the growth plates and articular cartilage.*** Increasing the compression loads can increase growth, but only to a point,*** beyond which further increases in compression decrease growth, and large enough loads can arrest growth altogether. On the concave side of a scoliosis, this can retard vertical growth of the centrae, which leads to wedging when growth continues on the convex side.* Growth plates normally load on the curve's growth-ascending limb, so increases in loading would increase growth, and decreases would do the opposite. Articular cartilage (and likely the cartilaginous end plates of vertebral centrae) normally loads near the curve's peak so both increases and decreases in loading could retard growth.*** However, increases should have the greater effect. These responses to mechanics may explain the alignment of normal growing limbs, spines and their facets, many of their malalignments (including scoliosis), and why joints tend to retain their birth shapes during subsequent growth [9,17,31,49,92].***

Microdamage. Cartilage—which probably has an MDx threshold also, although this, too, awaits systematic study—can develop MDx (chondromalacia is one result) which vital mechanisms normally repair while the damage is still microscopic or ultramicroscopic,*** thus preventing harmful amounts of damage from accumulating. Excessive MDx in articular cartilage plays a causative role in most arthroses (osteoarthritis),*** and in many inflammatory arthritides, too.* In the ring epiphyses, it may play a causal role in Scheuermann's disease.

The "Conductor". In determining skeletal architecture, including the joints, cartilage conducts and bone only plays violin [19,31,52]. In other words, cartilage determines the gross outer shape and size. By replacing its deeper layers with bone, the endochondral ossification process copies that shape and size. An enlarged, osteoarthritic facet stems from reactivated local cartilage growth at the joint margins, which bone then begins replacing. Large vertebral osteophytes reflect resumption of chondral growth at ligament attachments or at the remnant of the centrum's perichondral ring in response to "pathologic overload window" stimuli. The bony osteophytes seen in X-rays (Fig. 10) merely replaced some of that cartilage [17,43,62].

Joints

A recent vital biomechanical model explains the design of normal joints and the pathogenesis of arthroses, including the spine. It has considerable predictive and explanatory power but it takes two monographs to describe it, so only a partial abstract follows here [16,17].

The model makes this basic proposal: *A joint's design keeps each of its tissue's* unit *loads and strains—and their gradients—below its MDx threshold.* That would apply to articular cartilage, subchondral spongiosa, ligament, and meniscus. Between birth and maturity the *total* loads on joints can increase by a factor of 25,* so, in the absence of changes in shape, size, and stiffness, the unit loads on the joint's tissues would increase similarly and far exceed their MDx thresholds. That would cause early arthroses of affected joints.

Articular Cartilage and the Momentarily Loaded Area. A joint has no control over the size of the *total* loads on it. It must either adapt to them by increasing its load-bearing area (called here the "momentarily loaded area" or MLA) to reduce its *unit* loads to acceptable levels, or break down (i.e., develop an arthrosis). To keep unit loads below the MDx thresholds of its load-bearing tissues, a growing joint's bearing area can enlarge by increasing its diameter (Fig. 11), changing its shape (including reducing the curvature of its surfaces), and adjusting the stiffness of its articular cartilage and the subchondral

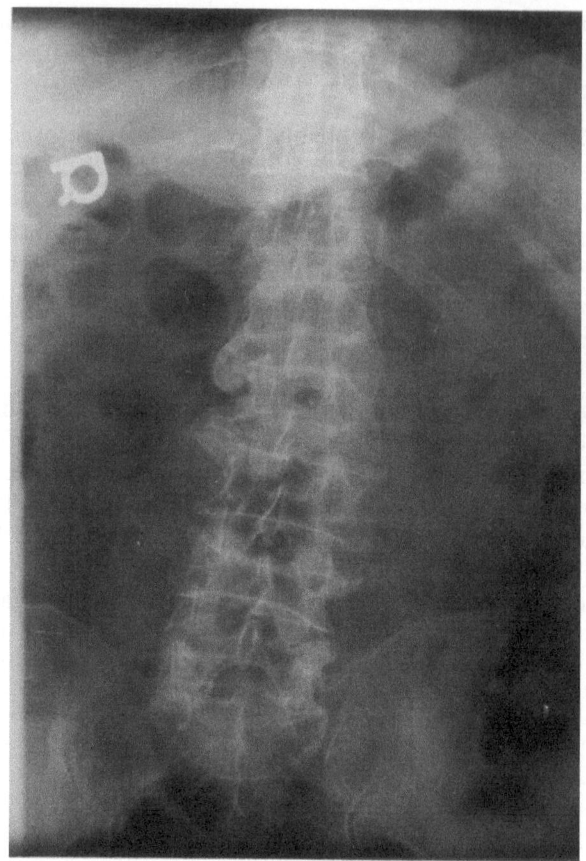

Fig. 10. Vertebral osteophytes. Here bone replaces cartilage at the bony attachments of ligaments, and/or at the remnant of the perichondral ring. That cartilage resumed growing in adult life when it should not have. In principle, that could stem from the stimulus of too much microdamage (MDx) in the ligament attachment or in the disc. In turn, that could stem from increased setpoints for MDx repair, or underadaptation of skeletal architecture during growth (so that in adult life it was mildly overloaded), or from tissues made abnormal in a way that caused more MDx than normal from normal MU. Or it could come from increased loading in adult lift due to adult-acquired obesity. Rheumatologists are just beginning to think about these vital biomechanical features

spongiosa supporting it. Growth at the perichondral ring can increase a joint's diameter. Chondral modeling in ways the chondral growth-force response curve (CGFRC) predicts can change its shape and surface curvature. Bigger joints with less sharply curved surfaces, as in Fig. 12, would have larger MLA's and thus reduced unit loads and gradients on both the articular cartilage and supporting bone. Presumably, these adaptations can be controlled within

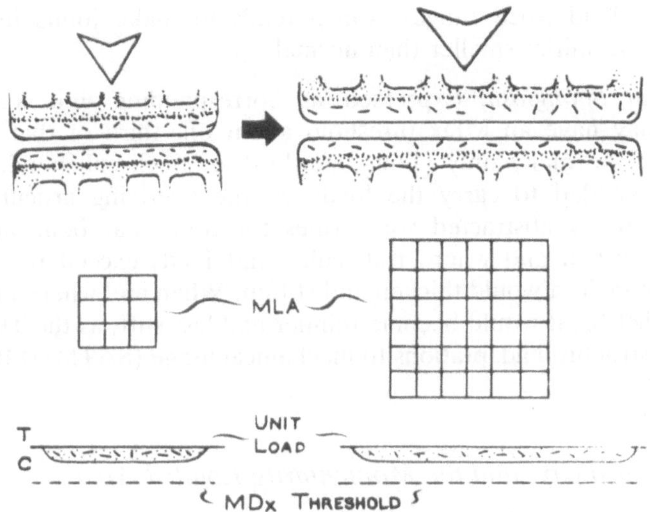

Fig. 11. Effect of joint diameter on the momentarily loaded area (MLA). When the diameter of the joint surface on the left doubles, as on the *right*, four times more unit areas could carry the joint's total load. That would tend to keep typical peak unit loads (and gradients) below the microdamage threshold of the tissues supporting its surface (from [92a] with permission)

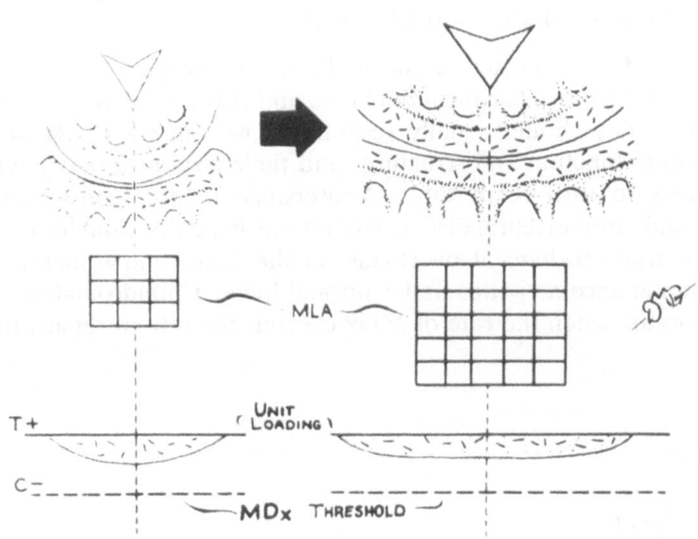

Fig. 12. Effect of curvature and size on the MLA. As the joint on the left grows the curvature of its surfaces decreases, which permits a larger MLA separately from the effect of increased diameter (from [92a] with permission)

certain unit load MES ranges, which tends to make joints in congenitally paralyzed extremities smaller than normal.

Subchondral Spongiosa. Expressed as corresponding unit loads, articular cartilage may have an MDx threshold about one-third of that of trabecular bone. If so, normally only about one-third as much subchondral bone area should be needed to carry the loads on the overlying articular cartilage.* The text already abstracted some rules for trabecular bone adaptations to mechanics. When and where trabecular unit loads exceed the MESm, subchondral spongiosa would thicken and stiffen. When and where those loads fall below the MESr, it would become thinner and less stiff, as the Three-Way and Four-Way structural adaptations to mechanical usage (SATMU) Rules describe [7,8].

Stiffness, Elasticity, and the Momentarily Loaded Area

Joint tissues are elastic and always deform (strain) under loads in ways that tend to increase the area or MLA carrying a load at any given moment. The effectiveness of this mechanism depends on the stiffness of the tissues. Chondrocytes can control articular cartilage stiffness, while modeling drifts and BMU-based remodeling control the stiffness of the subchondral spongiosa. For these reasons, the MLA of a joint under large loads usually exceeds that under small ones. This tends to lower the unit loads and their gradients on these tissues under large loads, as in Fig. 13. Reducing a growing joint's curvature should make this mechanism more effective and may partly explain why these curvatures decrease during normal growth.

Maintenance. Chondrocytes can normally repair cartilage MDx, prevent excessive creep, and control cartilage thickness and stiffness, partly by controlling its hydration.* They should usually respond to MU in ways that promote continued normal function and structure, and their responses may have their own MES ranges to turn them ON. Maintenance failures cause most acquired arthroses and intervertebral disc degenerations in adults. Sometimes the failures stem from true mechanical overloads on the joint, and sometimes from impaired maintenance activities under normal loads. Chondromalacia of articular cartilage occurs when the rate of MDx exceeds the rate of repair, for whatever reason.

Comment

Setpoint Effects

For modeling and remodeling, the genome must partly determine the MES values or "setpoints" in life. Certain hormones, drugs, cytokines, and other agents might modify those setpoints and circumstantial evidence suggests that

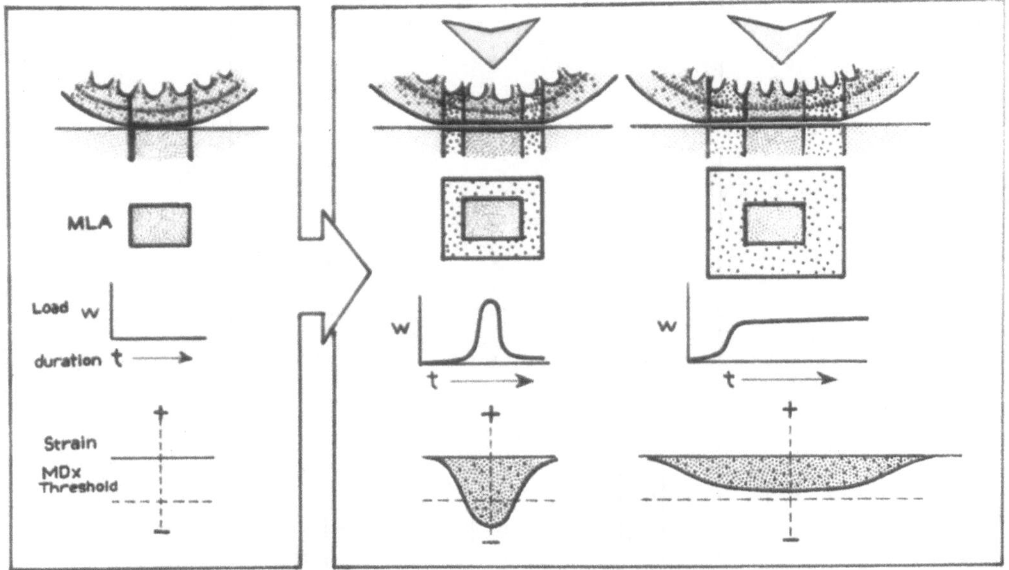

Fig. 13. Effect of elasticity on the MLA. *Left*: How a joint surface could deform under a load to increase its deloaded contact area (which under a load becomes the MLA). That would tend to reduce peak unit loads and their gradients. The graphs below show the total loads (*W*), their duration (*t*) and the microdamage thresholds. *Middle* and *right*: A brief load can deform the joint tissues somewhat to increase the MLA, but the same size load applied continuously as on the right will cause more deformation, and thus a larger MLA with smaller unit loads. This stems from the viscoelasticity of the cartilage and supporting bone. The size of these effects awaits systematic study (from [92b] with permission)

this is the case [3,14–17,31,41].*** *Raised setpoints* for bone, cartilage and ligament modeling are thought to have the same effects as disuse.** During growth, the structures may become subnormal in size, stiffness, and strength which would make them more susceptible to injury. Congenital spinal stenosis probably reflects such increased setpoints. *Lowered setpoints* should make growing skeletal structures become stiffer and stronger than normal during growth.** It has also been suggested by authorities on metabolic bone disease that the osteopenias in many osteoporoses may stem from increased setpoints for bone's MESr and MESm ranges [14];** they would cause smaller accumulations of bone during growth and greater losses in adults than the subject's MU justified. In the annulus a lowered MES for diametric modeling should make the ligament become thicker and stronger than normal.** An elevated MES should make it become thinner and weaker than normal.** A lowered setpoint in a scar could cause keloids. Figure 14 shows some setpoint effects on the bone configuration in children and adults. Figure 15 shows the result of increased modeling and remodeling setpoints in osteogenesis imperfecta.

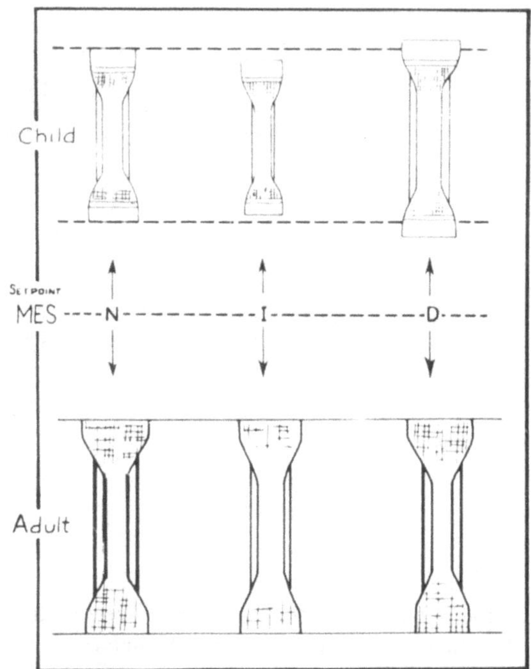

Fig. 14. *Top*: What a long bone would look like if it grew with normal (*N*), increased (*I*), or decreased (*D*) setpoints for longitudinal growth and bone modeling and remodeling. *Bottom*: Given the normal adult bone on the left, years later it would look as in the *middle* if the bone modeling and remodeling setpoints became increased, and as on the *right* if they were decreased. The right drawing shows good conservation of the original bone but no real additions to it

Joint Architecture. During growth, increased setpoints for chondral modeling may cause joints to become too small for their typical loads.** The joint tissues could be normal but their increased unit loads (and local gradients) could increase their MDx enough to eventually cause arthrosis.** Lowered setpoints should make growing joints become somewhat larger than normal, which would reduce their peak unit loads and theoretically should make them less prone to arthroses.**

Here four facts seem important: (1) Chondral modeling depends on chondral growth;* (2) that growth stops after skeletal maturity so an adult's joint must accept the architecture created during growth;* (3) therefore, if a previously normal adult joint becomes overloaded, its maintenance activities may determine whether or not arthrosis develops;*** and (4) many arthroses in people who become obese in adult life instead of during growth may stem from the latter phenomenon. That could apply to the facets and spinal stenosis in lordotic lumbar spines, and to hips and malaligned knees in obese patients [17].

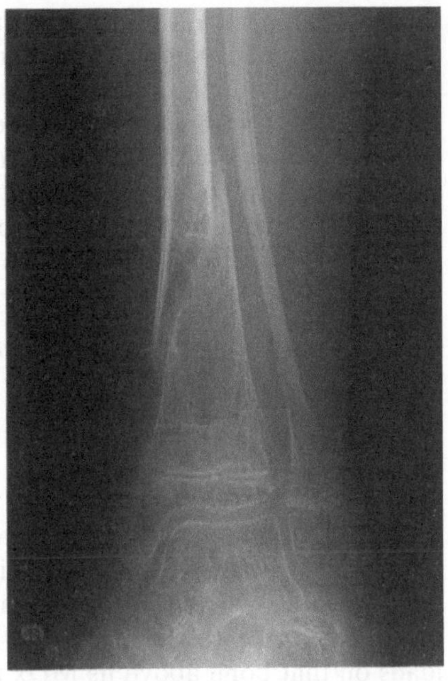

Fig. 15. Osteogenesis imperfecta. Congenitally increased modeling and remodeling setpoints in this disease cause the metaphyseal osteopenia (due to excessive loss of spongiosa) and decreased outside diaphyseal diameters (due to retarded modeling drifts) shown here. Normal usage of this osteopenic bone caused strains above the MDx threshold, which eventually caused this fracture. It then healed well

The setpoints for mechanically controlled articular cartilage and perichondral ring modeling are different because one can be abnormal but the other normal (Fig. 16).

MDx Repair. An elevated setpoint for the stimuli that turn MDx repair ON could let enough MDx accumulate to cause fatigue failures in affected bone, articular cartilage, or ligament [16,17,31]** in the presence of normal as well as abnormal amounts and types of structural tissues. It may require a stretch of the imagination to view chondrocalcinosis as a cause of impaired MDx repair in articular cartilage, and a degenerated intervertebral disc (as in Fig. 17) or osteoarthritic facet as likely results of that impairment. Dynamic histomorphometric studies of metabolic bone diseases, however, show that this kind of failure can happen in bone.* Clinical observations while repairing spontaneous tendon ruptures show it can happen in tendon as well.* Other clinicopathologic observations suggest that the same also applies to the annulus, the disc, and the articular cartilage in the facets.*** To repeat, many degenerated discs may result from elevated setpoints for the vital mechanism(s) that normally repair their MDx [17]. Another likely cause is an abnormality in composition or ultrastructure that makes the disc more susceptible to MDx. The biochemical and ultrastructural abnormalities in such discs are likely the result of these impairments, not the cause.

Microdamage and Grafts. MDx repair presumes that tissues have living cells which are able to detect and initiate repair [15].* Initially, large, devascularized autografts and all allografts lack the living cells needed to initiate MDx repair (so does dead cartilage). If they carry significant loads while still infarcted, they will develop MDx and can accumulate enough to cause fractures, which may heal poorly. Examples of this already appear in the bone allografts used in some total joint revisions, in oncologic surgery, and in ligament allografts. This could also explain why some spinal fusions tail, an idea supported by the better success associated with the use of effective internal fixation systems which markedly reduce the strains of healing grafts.

Load Focusing and Internal Fixation

Normal skeletal architecture has a strong tendency to transfer loads from one structure to another, and from one part of a given structure to another, in ways that prevent undue concentrations ("focusing") or increases of local unit loads [2,3,15,31].**

In that regard, most internal fixation devices used in spinal surgery do three things that can cause problems. First, they tend to concentrate or focus their mechanical loads on rather small areas of the bone around them, especially in osteopenic bone (as in most elderly adults).* Second, that can raise the unit loads on that bone above its MDx threshold, leading to enough MDx to loosen the devices and degrade any immobilization they provide.* Third, the devices usually load the bone surrounding them in the across-grain mode.* That could invoke the smaller across-grain MDx thresholds and accelerate loosening [93].

Minimizing such problems involves at least two considerations. First, devices should be designed so that their loads are to applied to larger bone surfaces to reduce the peak unit loads, and thus its MDx. Second, minimize loading on fixation devices postoperatively until the bone and fusion masses heal enough to begin carrying those loads themselves without overstraining (see below). At best, that can take months, and longer when healing is biologically impaired [4].

Mechanical Usage Windows

The responses of the spine's principal biologic mechanisms seem to vary according to increasing vigor of MU or increasing size of a tissue's typical peak strains [18].*** In a *disuse window*, strains stay small and the strength and

Fig. 17. The degenerated intervertebral disc. Note the narrowing and so-called vacuum sign, which is really a bubble of nitrogen in the disc space. Some time after skeletal maturity this disc disappeared due to local liquification and resorption instead of to mechanical herniation. That stemmed from impaired maintenance of the original disc. As a result, ultramicroscopic MDx in its collagen and proteoglycans began and accumulated. Those fragmented molecules became gradually resorbed in the surrounding annulus

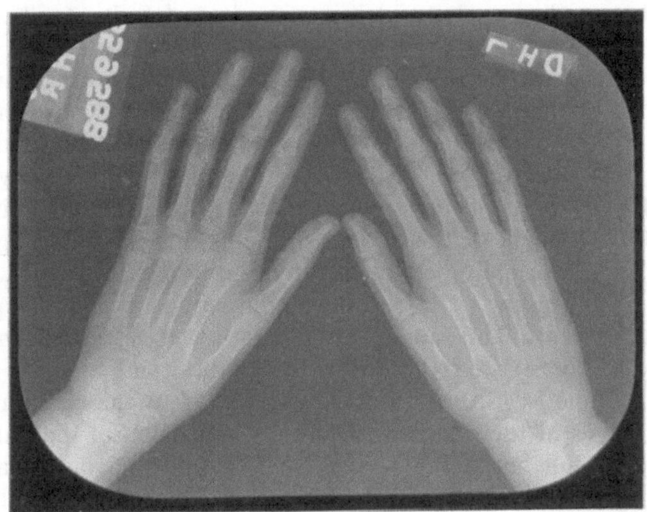

Fig. 16. Arachnodactyly. In this disease, bone and articular cartilage modeling respond normally to MU but the growth plate responses increase above normal. As a result, bones grow longer than normal for the patient's MU and muscle strength, but bone and joint diameters fit the MU normally. The result: bones that seem longer and more slender than normal. Here the setpoint for the MU effects on growth plates is subnormal because of a genetic defect (from [31] with permission)

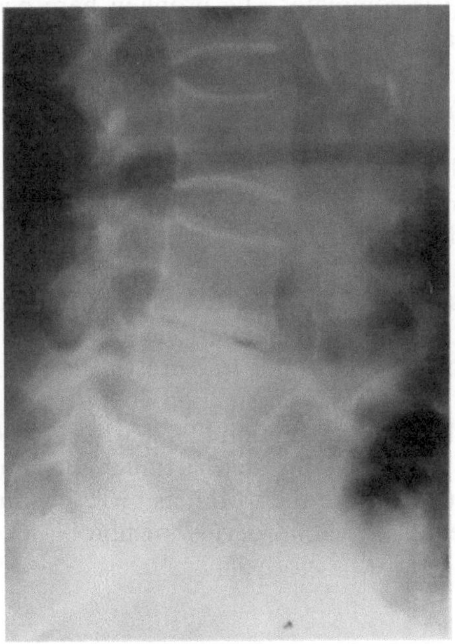

stiffness of bones, ligaments, and joints tend to deteriorate; bone becomes osteopenic and ligaments thinner. In an *adapted window*, a tissue's typical peak strains would stay within the boundaries between the disuse and the next window. Such a skeleton would already be adapted to its typical MU and need no major changes in architecture. This applies to normally active, healthy adults. In a *mild overload window*, strains would enter or mildly exceed the modeling MES setpoints of the structural tissues, so normal adaptive modeling would turn ON to begin stiffening and strengthening bone and ligament. The skeletons of most normally active, healthy children, and of growing animals too, stay in this window. The resulting adaptations eventually produce the normal adult skeleton and spine. In a *pathologic overload window*, tissue strains approach or exceed the MDx thresholds, and a RAP and clinical damage occurs. The MES thresholds should determine the boundaries of these windows. Changes in their setpoints may explain much of the pathology that can develop in adult and aging spines. Such setpoint changes may cause the longitudinal ligament problems well-known to Japanese orthopedic surgeons.

Mechanical Usage Windows for Healing Tissues. It is important to be aware that far smaller *loads* can strain a *healing* bone, ligament, or joint cartilage into its mild and pathologic overload windows than for normal, mature tissues. While straining a healing tissue into its pathologic window usually does impair or prevent good healing, *strains* that stay within the adapted or mild overload window of the tissue involved (equal to or less than its modeling MES) probably *help* the healing [4,17]. This could explain the empirical wisdom of starting *gentle* function early after an injury or operation, but deferring heavy loading until healing is complete. The problem here becomes knowing when healing ends and heavy loading can begin.***

Cytokines (and Other Agents)

The number of studies on cytokines has increased phenomenally, yet most of their functions *in intact patients* remain enigmatic. Nevertheless, many cytokines must help to control each activity described in this text. A future task of such research would be to determine the mechanism by which this occurs. Once this is accomplished, it should be possible to control vital biomechanical activities to fulfill numerous medical and surgical needs. In other words, instead of having merely to watch wounds and fractures heal, and bones, ligaments and joints adapt to their MU, clinicians may be able to take a more active role in the processes of healing and adaptation [23,28,41,92,94–96]. Table 3 lists some well-known agents that probably act as much or more by affecting how skeletons perceive and adapt to their MU, as by acting directly on effector cells like osteoclasts, osteoblasts, chondrocytes, or fibroblasts.

Table 3. Some agents that may exert their bone dffects either by changing modeling, remodeling, and other setpoints, or by combining that with direct actions on osteoclasts, osteoblasts, and other cells.

Adrenocortical steroids	Estrogens
Progestins	Parathormone
Growth hormone	Somatomedins
Testosterone	Calcitonin
Low serum calcium	Elevated serum calcium
Dietary calcium	Dietary phosphate
Thyroxine	Fluoride
Starvation	Vitamin D (+metabolites)
Bisphosphonates	Prostaglandins
Some cytokines	*The genome*
Metabolic acidosis	Metabolic alkalosis
Nonsteroidal antiinflammatory agents (NSAIDS)	

Predictive Models

Recent models can be used to predict some structural adaptations to mechanical usage (SATMU) challenges of skeletal tissues. They also suggest how to quantitate them and some mathematics to improve finite element analyses of skeletal problems that concern not just spine surgeons, but all orthopedic surgeons plus general, maxillofacial, ophthalmic, plastic and pediatric surgeons, neurosurgeons, pediatricians, rheumatologists, physiatrists, and sports medicine experts [7–10]. Learning how to apply them to clinical problems may be a challenge to our ingenuity.

Conclusion

This article offers clinicians who deal with spinal problems some concepts in the new skeletal paradigm that bear on their work, but which were previously buried in the area of basic science. There is much to learn, and I would like to offer four observations in point: (1) *The above material neither negates nor replaces what clinicians already know about such matters; it only adds to it*; (2) parts of it may seem new, yet it has probably remained unchanged since our species evolved; (3) the author's present contribution lay in organizing the work of many people to point out possible clinical applications. To other reviews of skeletal physiology, this one adds some belatedly perceived but vital biomechanics; and (4) many nonmechanical factors (hormones, cytokines, nutrition, drugs, genetics, etc.) can act by changing how skeletons perceive, adapt to, and endure their MU. That should not surprise us, since skeletons probably evolved to serve mechanical functions first, and were modified afterwards to help in other functions too (homeostasis, hematopoiesis).

Many authorities believe it is time for clinicians to begin learning and applying this material [97]. *Doing that requires knowing about the material first.* Hence this article.

Acknowledgments. The author is indebted to Mr. David Gavin for the drawings in this article, and to colleagues at the Southern Colorado Clinic and Pueblo's two general hospitals who allowed the time to write it. Others provided advice, experience and encouragement. They include Drs. L.V. Avioli, D.B. Burr, C. Hanson, H. Duncan, Z.F.G. Jaworski, D.H. Kimmel, W.S.S. Jee, R.B. Martin, A.M. Parfitt, E.S. Radin, R.R. Recker, L. Sokoloff, S. Stanisaljevic, H. Takahashi, and M.R. Urist. Prof. W.S.S. Jee deserves special thanks for permitting publication of some discussions at the famous Hard Tissue Workshops he has organized annually since 1965. Most material in this article had its first hearing and critique at those workshops, beginning in 1979.

The author is also indebted to the exceptional orthopedic surgeons trained at Henry Ford Hospital between 1957–1973 inclusive. Their aid in a time of great troubles made this work both possible and one of their contributions to orthopedic surgery and skeletal science.

References

1. Burr DB, Martin RB (1989) Errors in bone remodeling: Toward a unified theory of metabolic bone disease. Am J Anat 186:1–31
2. Frost HM (1987) The mechanostat: A proposed pathogenetic mechanism of osteoporoses and the bone mass effects of mechanical and nonmechanical agents. Bone Miner 2:73–85
3. Frost HM (1988) Vital biomechanics. Proposed general concepts for skeletal adaptations to mechanical usage. Calcif Tissue Int 42:145–155
4. Frost HM (1989) The biology of fracture healing. Clin Orthop Rel Res. Part I: 248: 283–293; Part II: 248:294–309
5. Frost HM (1989) Some ABCs of skeletal pathophysiology I: Introduction to the series. Calc Tiss Int 45:1–3
6. Frost HM (1989) Some ABCs of skeletal pathophysiology II: General mediator mechanism properties. Calc Tiss Int 45:68–70
7. Frost HM (1990) Structural adaptations to mechanical usage (SATMU): 1. Redefining Wolff's Law: The bone modeling problem. Anat Rec 226:403–413
8. Frost HM (1990) Structural adaptations to mechanical usage (SATMU): 2. Redefining Wolff's Law: The bone remodeling problem. Anat Rec 226:414–422
9. Frost HM (1990) Structural adaptations to mechanical usage (SATMU): 3. The hyaline cartilage modeling problem. Anat Rec 226:423–432
10. Frost HM (1990) Structural adaptations to mechanical usage (SATMU): 4. Mechanical influences on fibrous tissues. Anat Rec 226:433–439
11. Frost HM (1991) Some ABC's of skeletal pathophysiology. 5. Microdamage physiology. Calc Tiss Int 49:229–231

12. Frost HM (1991) Some ABC's of skeletal pathophysiology. 6. The growth/modeling/remodeling distinction. Calc Tiss Int 49:301–302
13. Frost HM (1991) Some ABC's of skeletal pathophysiology. 7. Tissue mechanisms controlling bone mass. Calc Tiss Int 49:303–304
14. Frost HM (1992) Perspectives: The role of changes in mechanical usage setpoints in the pathogenesis of osteoporosis. J Bone Miner Res 7:253–261
15. Frost HM (1992) Perspectives: On artificial joint design. J Long Term Eff Med Implants 2:9–35
16. Frost HM (1994) Introduction to Skeletal Physiology. I. Bone and Bones. Schuster's, Pueblo
17. Frost HM (1994) Introduction to Skeletal Physiology. II. Fibrous Tissue, Cartilage and Synovial Joints. Schuster's, Pueblo
18. Frost HM (1992) Nature's mechanical usage windows for bone. Schuster's, Pueblo
19. Jee WSS (1989) The skeletal tissues. In: Weiss L (ed) Cell and tissue biology. A textbook of histology. Urban and Schwartzenberg, Baltimore, pp 211–259
20. Jee WSS (1990) Local and systemic factors influencing bone formation. In: Takahashi H (ed) Bone morphometry Nishimura, Niigata, pp 284–289
21. Jee WSS, Li XJ (1990) Adaptation of cancellous bone to overloading in the adult rat: A single photon absorptiometry and histomorphometry study. Anat Rec 227: 418–426
22. Jee WSS, XJ Li, MB Schaffler (1991) Adaptation of diaphyseal structure with aging and increased mechanical usage in the adult rat. A histomorphometrical and biomechanical study. Anat Rec 230:332–338
23. Jee WSS, Mori X, Li X, Chan S (1990) Prostaglandin E2 enhances cortical bone mass and activates intracortical bone remodeling in intact and overiectomized female rats. Bone 11:253–266
24. Li XJ, Jee WSS (1990) Adaptation of diaphyseal structure to aging and decreased mechanical loading in the adult rat. A densitometric and histomorphometric study. Anat Rec 229:291–297
25. Li XJ, Jee WSS, Chow S-Y, Woodbury DM (1990) Adaptation of cancellous bone to aging and immobilization in the rat. A single photon absorptiometry and histomorphometry study. Anat Rec 227:12–24
26. Martin RB, Burr DB (1989) Structure, Function and Adaptation of Compact Bone. Raven, New York.
27. Martin RB, Burr DB, Radin EL (1983) Threshold values of the production of fatigue damage in bone in vivo. Orth Res Soc Abstr 29:69
28. Nordin RW, Jee WS, High WB (1990) The role of prostaglandins in bone in vivo. Prostaglandins Leukot Essent Fatty Acids 41:139–149
29. Recker RR (1983) Bone histomorphometry. Techniques and interpretation. CRC, Boca Raton
30. Schaffler MB (1985) Stiffness and fatigue of compact bone at physiological strain and strain rates. Thesis, West Virginia University, Morgantown
31. Frost HM (1986) Intermediary Organization of the Skeleton, vols I, II. CRC, Boca Raton
32. Nordin M, Frankel VH (1989) Basic biomechanics of the musculoskeletal system, 2nd edn. Lea and Febiger, Philadelphia
33. Burr DB, Stafford T (1990) Validity of the bulk staining technique to separate artifactual from in vivo microdamage. Clin Orthop Rel Res 260:305–308
34. Caler WE, Carter DR (1989) Bone creep-fatigue damage accumulation. J Biomech 22:625–635

35. Chamay A (1970) Mechanical and morphological aspects of experimental overload and fatigue in bone. J Biomech 3:262–270
36. Freeman MAR, Todd RC, Pirie CJ (1974) The role of fatigue in the pathogenesis of senile femoral neck fracture. J Bone and Jt Surg 56B:898–905
37. Frost HM (1960) Presence of microscopic cracks in vivo in bone. Henry Ford Hosp Med Bull 8:27–35
38. Frost HM (1963) An Introduction to Biomechanics. Charles C Thomas, Springfield.
39. Koszyca B, Fazzalari NL, Vernon-Roberts B (1989) Trabecular microfractures. Clin Orthop Rel Res 244:208–216
40. Shapiro F, Glimcher MJ (1980) Induction of osteoarthritis in the rabbit knee joint: Histologic changes following meniscectomy and meniscal lesions. Clin Orthop Rel Res 147:287–295
41. Takahashi H (1990) Bone morphometry (ed). Nishimura, Niigata.
42. Albright JA, Brand RA (1987) The scientific basis of orthopaedics 2nd edn. Appleton and Lange, Norwalk
43. Anderson WAD, Kissane JM (1977) Pathology, 7th edn. Mosby, St Louis
44. Courpron P (1981) Bone tissue mechanisms underlying osteoporoses. Orthop Clin N Am 12:513–546
45. Woodard JC (1991) Morphology of fracture nonunion and osteomyelitis. Vet Clin N Am 21:813–844
46. Biewener AA (1990) Biomechanics of mammalian terrestrial locomotion. Science 23:1097–1103
47. Carter DR (1987) Mechanical loading history and skeletal biology. J Biomech 20:1095–1109
48. Carter DR, Wong M (1988) The role of mechanical loading histories in the development of diarthrodial joints. J Orthop Res 6:804–816
49. Frost HM (1972) The Physiology of Bone, Cartilage and Fibrous Tissue. Charles C Thomas, Springfield
50. Frost HM (1973) Orthopaedic Biomechanics. Charles C Thomas, Springfield
51. Fondrk M, Bahniuk E, Davy D (1990) Transient creep behavior of cortical bone. ORS Abstracts 15:49
52. Frost HM (1986) Biomechanical determinants of the arthroses. Text distributed at the annual Hard Tissue Workshop organized by Prof WSS Jee
53. Duncan H, Frame B, Arnstein AR, Frost HM (1973) Migratory osteolysis of the lower extremities. Ann Int Med 66:1165–1173
54. Langloh ND, Hunder GG, Riggs BL, Kelley PJ (1973) Transient painful osteoporoses of the lower extremities. J Bone and Jt Surg 55A:1188–1196
55. Martin RB (1987) Osteonal remodeling in response to screw implantation in the canine femur. J Orthop Res 5:445–454
56. Duncan CP, Shim S (1977) The autonomic nerve supply of bone. J Bone Joint Surg 59B:323–324
57. Fuller M, Grigg P, Hoffman A (1990) Joint capsule mechanoreceptors: Sensors or strain or load? ORS Abstracts 15:3
58. Johansson H, Soika P (1991) A sensory role for the cruciate ligaments. Clin Orthop Rel Res 268:161–178
59. Miller MR, Kasahara M (1963) Observations on the innervation of human long bones. Anat Rec 145:13–17

60. Burstein AH, Reilly DT (1976) Aging of bone tissue: Mechanical properties. J Bone Joint Surg 58A:82–86
61. Akeson WH, Amiel D, Ing D, Abel MF, Garfin SR, Woo SL-Y (1987) Effects of immoblization on joints. Clin Orthop Rel Res 219:28–37
62. Jubb KVF, Kennedy PC, Palmer N (1985) Pathology of domestic animals. Academic, New York
63. Frost HM (1987) Osteogenesis imperfecta. The setpoint proposal. Clin Orthop Rel Res 216:280–297
64. O'Connor JA, Lanyon LE, MacFie H (1982) The influence of strain rate on adaptive bone remodeling. J Biomech 15:767–781
65. Pollack (1990) Electrical effects on bone: Relationship to bone remodeling. In: Bone morphometry. H Takahashi (ed). Nishimura, Niigata, pp 170–176
66. Rubin CT, Lanyon LE (1984) Regulation of bone formation by applied dynamic loads. J Bone and Jt Surg 66A:308–314
67. Johnson LC (1964) Morphologic analysis in pathology: The kinetics of disease and general biology of bone. In: Frost HM (ed) Bone Biodynamics. Little-Brown, Boston, pp 543–654
68. Takahashi H, Frost HM (1965) Correlation between body habitus and cross sectional area of ribs. Can J Physiol Pharmacol 43:773–782
69. Takahashi H, Frost HM (1966) Age and sex related changes in the amount of cortex in human ribs. Acta Orthop Scand 37:122–130
70. Anderson C, Cape RDT, Crilly RG, Hodsman AB, Wolfe BMJ (1984) Preliminary observations of a form of coherence therapy for osteoposis. Calcif Tissue Int 36:341–343
71. Compston J, Mellish RWE, Garrahan NJ, Croucher PI (1990) Structural mechanisms of trabecular bone loss in normal subjects. In: Takahashi H (ed) Bone histomorphometry. Nishimura, Niigata pp 371–374
72. Eriksen EF (1986) Normal and pathological remodeling of humant trabecular bone: Three-dimensional reconstruction of the remodeling sequence in normals and in metabolic bone disease. Endocr Rev 7:379–408
73. Frost HM (1964) Mathematical Elements of Lamellar bone Remodelling. Charles C Thomas, Springfield
74. Kimmel DB, Recker RR, Gallagher JC, Vaswani AS, Aloia JF (1990) A comparison of iliac bone histomorphometric data in postmenopausal osteoporotic and normal subjects. Bone and Min 11:217–246
75. Takahashi H, Epker BN, Frost HM (1964) Resorption precedes formative activity. Surg Forum 15:437–438
76. Mellish RW, Garrahan NJ, Compston JE (1989) Age-related changes in trabecular width and spacing in human iliac crest biopsies. Bone and Min 6:331–338
77. Smith EL, Gilligan C (1989) Mechanical forces and bone. Bone Miner Res 6:139–173
78. Uhthoff H, Jaworski ZFG (1978) Bone loss in response to long-term immobilization. J Bone and Jt Surg 60B:420–429
79. Hori M, Uzawa T, Morita L, Noda T, Takahashi H, Inoue J (1988) Effect of human parathyroid hormone (PTH(1–34)) on experimental osteopenia of rats induced by ovariectomy. Bone and Min 3:193–199
80. Arnold JS (1981) Trabecular patterns and shapes in aging and osteoporosis. In: Jee WSS, Paifitt Am (eds) Bone histomorphometry. Armour Montagu, Paris, pp 297–310

81. Cowin SC (1989) Bone Mechanics (ed). CRC, Boca Raton
82. Currey JD (1984) The mechanical adaptations of bones. Princeton University Press, Princeton
83. Duncan H, Jundt J, Riddle JM, Pitchford W, Christopher T (1987) The tibial subchondral plate. A scanning electron microscopic study. J Bone Joint Surg 69A:1212–1220
84. Amiel D, Akeson WH, Harwood FL, Frank CB (1983) Stress deprivation effect on metabolic turnover of the medial collateral ligament collagen. A comparison between nine- and twelve-week immobilization. Clin Orthop Rel Res 172:265–270
85. Dahners LE, Muller P (1988) The effects of the application of tension on ligament growth. OES Abstracts 13:56
86. Frank C, Bodie M, Anderson M (1987) Growth of a ligament. ORS Abstracts 12:42
87. Sumpio BE, Bres AJ, Link WG, Johnson G Jr (1988) Enhanced collagen production by smooth muscle cells during repetitive mechanical stretching. Arch Surg 123:1233–1236
88. Sutker B, Lester G, Banes A, Dahners L (1990) Cyclic strain stimulates DNA and collagen synthesis in fibroblasts cultured from rat medial collateral ligaments. ORS Abstracts 15:130
89. Wessels WE, Dahners LE (1988) Growth of the deltoid ligament in the rabbit. ORS Abstracts 13:199
90. Wilson CJ (1988) An examination of the mechanism of ligament contracture. Clin Orthop Rel Res 227:286–291
91. Woo SL-Y, Gomez MA, Sites TJ, Newton PO, Orlando CA, Akeson WH (1987) The biomechanical and morphological changes in the medial collateral ligament of the rabbit after immobilization and remobilization. J Bone and Jt Surg 69A:1200–1211
92. Adams ME, Billingham MEJ (1982) Animal models of degenerative joint disease. In: Berry CL (ed) Bone and Joint Disease. Springer, Berlin Heidelberg New York, pp 265–298
92a. Frost HM (1994) Perspectives: a vital biomechanical model of synovial joint design. Anat Rec 240:1–18
92b. Frost HM (1994) Perspectives: a vital biomechanical model of the pathogenesis of arthroses. Anat Rec 240:19–31
93. Burr DB, Schaffler MB, Yang KH, Wu DD, Lukoschek M, Kandzari D, Sivaneri N, Blaha JD, Radin EL (1989) The effects of altered strain environments on bone tissue kinetics. Bone 10:215–221
94. Evans RA (1987) Is there a need for whole body physiology? Bone Miner 2:243–244
95. Fulkerson JP, Edwards CC, Chrisman OD (1987) Articular cartilage. In: Albright JA, Brand RA (eds) The Scientific Basis of Orthopaedics, 2nd edn. Appleton and Lange, Norwalk, pp 347–372
96. Tada K, Yamamuro T, Okumura R, Kasai R, Takahashi H (1990) Therapeutic effects of h-PTH(1–34) on skeletons of osteoporotic rats with parathyroidectomy. In: Takahashi H (ed) Bone morphometry. Nishimura, Niigata, pp 448–451
97. These colleagues include Profs. C Anderson, LV Avioli, DB Burr, H Duncan, ZFG Jaworski, WSS Jee, DH Kimmel, RB Martin, F Melsen, RW Norrdin, EL Radin, L Raisz, RR Recker, G Rodan, MB Schaffler, L Sokoloff, H Takahashi, MR Urist, D van Sickle, JC Woodard, TJ Wronski

Morphological Changes and Stress Redistribution in Osteoporotic Spine

D.B. Burr[1], King H. Yang[2], Maureen Haley[3], and Hui-Chang Wang[2]

Abstract. Osteoporosis is characterized by a reduction in trabecular bone mass that results in vertebral fracture when increased stresses secondary to bone loss exceed the breaking strength of the vertebra. Non-uniform trabecular loss and adaptive changes in the cortical shell or bony endplate may compensate for, or accentuate, the mechanical effects of trabecular loss. Finite element techniques can be used to improve the diagnostic assessment of vertebral fracture risk in osteoporosis by examining relationships among the trabecular bone, cortical shell, and bony endplate. This paper reviews evidence for the contributions of the vertebral cortical shell, endplate, and posterior elements to the strength and fracture resistance of the vertebral body. It also presents a 3D finite element model of a lumbar motion segment that is used to calculate stress distributions in normal and osteoporotic vertebrae with variations in trabecular density, cortical shell thickness, and endplate thickness. The finite element modeling shows that the cortical shell takes 39% of the total axial load in normal vertebrae, while the posterior elements share 27%, and the trabeculae share 34%. With a 50% loss of trabecular mass, trabeculae share only 9% of the load, while cortical shell and posterior element contributions increase to 59% and 32%, respectively. A loss of bone in the vertebral body shifts loads to the posterior elements. These load shifts in osteoporotic vertebrae increase stresses on the cortical shell by 266% when two-thirds of the trabecular bone has been lost. If both trabecular and cortical bone are lost, cortical shell stresses quadruple. The maximum cortical stress occurred in the superior and anterolateral regions of the vertebral body, consistent with observations of

[1] Departments of Anatomy and Orthopedic Surgery, Biomechanics and Biomaterials Research Center, Indiana University School of Medicine, 635 Barnhill Drive, Indianapolis, IN 46202, USA

[2] Department of Mechanical Engineering, Wayne State University Detroit, MI 48202, USA

[3] Charleston Area Medical Center, Charleston, WV 25304, USA

wedge fractures in osteoporotic women. Loss of trabecular density or reduced cortical shell thickness can increase endplate stress more than seven times, significantly increasing the risk of endplate failure. Cortical thinning alone, without loss of trabecular mass or reduced endplate thickness will not reduce axial rigidity of the whole vertebra significantly, but will increase cortical bone stresses significantly.

Key Words. Osteoporosis, spine, stress, biomechanics, vertebrae, fracture, finite element modeling, bone mass, bone remodeling, endplate

Introduction

Osteoporosis is characterized by a reduction in trabecular bone mass that results in vertebral fracture when increased stresses secondary to bone loss exceed the breaking strength of the vertebra. Non-uniform trabecular loss [1–6] and adaptive changes in the cortical shell or bony endplate may compensate for, or accentuate, the mechanical effects of trabecular loss. Regional changes in the cortical shell or bony endplate can potentially compensate for significant loss in the trabecular compartment. In adults, adaptations to loss of trabecular number or contiguity can be made by adjusting the thickness and porosity of cortical bone. Mechanically, small changes in the cortical shell could have potentially large effects on strength even though bone mass is reduced significantly.

Compression (crush) fractures involve the bony endplate, but the relationship of the endplate and cortical shell to overall vertebral strength is controversial. Some believe that the cortical bone contributes little to compressive strength of the vertebra [7,8], but this does not take into account the role that the geometry of the whole vertebra, apart from mass density or absolute bone volume, plays in the strength and rigidity of the bone. The well known fact that neither trabecular bone mineral content (BMC), bone mineral density (BMD), or bone volume contributes more than 20%–50% to the variation in strength or fracture prevalence [9–12], but may contribute as much as 50%–80% when cortical bone is included [7,13–17] indicates that other considerations, including geometrical ones, may be relatively important to fracture risk assessments. Mosekilde et al. [15] showed that the loss of bone strength with age is greater than the loss of bone mass, indicating that other factors such as loss of trabecular continuity or regional factors are also important to fracture risk assessments. Consequently, redistribution of bone among horizontal and vertical trabeculae, or between trabecular and cortical compartments, can have a significant effect on mechanical behavior of the vertebral body even when bone volume remains unchanged [18].

Non-invasive methods such as single- and dual-photon absorptiometry (SPA and DPA), dual-energy X-ray absorptiometry, quantitative computed tomography (QCT), and neutron activation analysis are often used to determine changes in bone mass and geometry. However, changes detected by these methods currently provide only an incomplete picture of the change in overall vertebral strength because they do not reflect geometric parameters. Ott et al. [19] showed that bone mass measured using SPA, DPA, QCT, and neutron activation analysis correlated reasonably well with each other, but poorly with the severity of fracture. In some cases, geometric information is contained in the measurement, but needs to be extracted [20,21]. Although the relative risk of vertebral fracture doubles for every standard deviation decrease in bone mineral density [22], the power of density measurements to predict vertebral fracture is less in the axial skeleton than in the appendicular skeleton [23,24]. This may be due to limitations on accuracy with DPA [25], but may just as well be due to the failure to consider the more complex geometry of vertebral bone.

Non-invasive measurements can be made to reveal, in part, the morphological changes in the vertebrae, and can reflect to some extent the changes in the properties of its constituent materials. However, patterns of stress and strain in the vertebra that may reflect fracture risk cannot be reproduced using these methods alone. Finite element modeling (FEM) is the most suitable method to study the stress distribution of an object that has irregular geometry, has multiple material compositions, and is subjected to complex loading stiuations. Many FEMs have been used to link mechanical factors with the degeneration of the intervertebral disc and the etiology of low back pain [26–34], but fewer have addressed the mechanical response of an osteoporotic spine. Finite element techniques and mechanical property measurements of vertebral segments can be used to improve the diagnostic assessment of vertebral fracture risk in osteoporosis by examining relationships among the trabecular bone and the cortical shell and bony endplate of thoracic and lumbar vertebrae.

This paper reviews evidence for the significant contribution of the vertebral cortical shell, bony endplate, and posterior elements to the strength and fracture resistance of the vertebral body. Second, an FEM of a lumbar vertebra is developed and tested to evaluate the effects of changes in the cortical shell and bony endplate on stress redistribution to other parts of the vertebra, and on overall vertebral strength. The FEM provides some evidence for the significant role of the compact bone compartment in fracture prevention. Understanding the relationships among the various components of the vertebral complex will improve fracture risk prediction and may improve the assessment of therapeutic approaches for osteoporotic patients.

The Contribution of Cortical Bone to Vertebral Strength

Role of Structure in Bone Strength

One of the most important determinants of strength and stiffness of a bone is the nature of the distribution of the material within its cross-section [35,36].

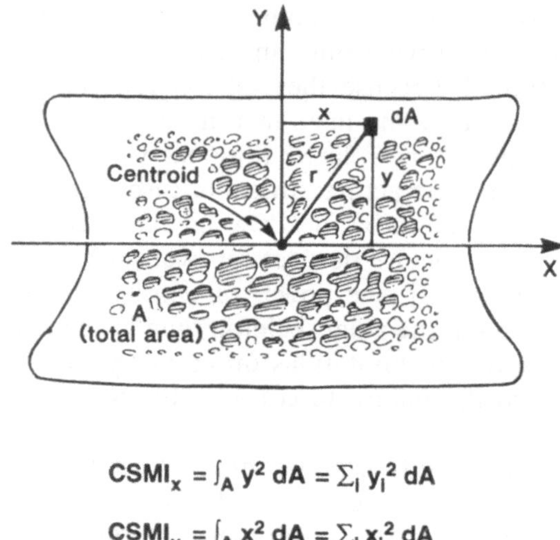

$$CSMI_x = \int_A y^2\, dA = \Sigma_i\, y_i^2\, dA$$

$$CSMI_y = \int_A x^2\, dA = \Sigma_i\, x_i^2\, dA$$

$$J = \int_A r^2\, dA = \Sigma_i\, r_i^2\, dA$$

Fig. 1. A sagitally sectioned lumbar vertebra shows how the cortical shell contributes significantly to overall vertebral strength. The *x-axis* points posteriorly, and the *y-axis* points superiorly. The rigidity of a structure is a function of both its mass and the distribution of the mass. The cross-sectional moment of inertia (CSMI) is proportional to the rigidity of bone in bending, and is calculated by summing each individual unit of area and its squared distance from the axis about which bending occurs (the neutral axis). The polar moment of inertia (*J*) is proportional to the rigidity of bone in torsion, and is calculated by summing each individual unit of area and its squared distance from the centroid of the section. Additions of small amounts of bone to the cortical shell can increase the bending and torsional rigidity of the vertebra even in the face of larger losses on trabecular surfaces, because cortical bone lies at a greater distance from the axis of bending and the centroid

Vertebral strength is not completely dependent on density or trabecular contiguity, but also depends on the geometrical distribution of bone within it. This distribution is quantified by the second moments of the area, also known as cross-sectional moments of inertia (CSMI), which are proportional to the rigidity of the bone in bending. Likewise, the distribution of material within the cross-section affects its torsional rigidity, which is proportional to the amount and distribution of material with respect to the centroid of the cross-section (Fig. 1).

It is well-known that additions of bone to the periosteal envelope result in much greater increases of bending and torsional strength than additions along trabecular or endocortical surfaces [37]. Assuming bone is homogeneous, isotropic, and linearly elastic (which of course it is not), this is because the structural strength of bone is broadly proportional to both its area (or volume) and the *squared* distance of that area from the axis about which bending occurs (the neutral axis) or from the centroid of the cross-section about which torsion occurs. Thus, the bending and torsional strength of the vertebra increase exponentially through additions of bone to the periosteal surface of the cortical shell, even when absolute bone volume and bone mineral density have decreased significantly. Significant increases in vertebral body diameter have, in fact, been shown to occur with age [38–40], reducing by 10%–15% the rate at which maximum vertical stress on the vertebral body increases with age following trabecular loss (from 57% to 46%). Diametric increases are particularly large in American blacks [38], perhaps partly explaining their lower vertebral fracture incidence. Geometric changes in the body partially, but not completely, compensate for trabecular loss.

Similar relationships do not hold for the behavior of bone under pure axial compression. Compressive strength is proportional to bone volume (or area of a cross-section) without regard to its distribution. Therefore, bone loss with aging could compromise the strength of the vertebra in axial compression, even though its strength in bending and torsion are maintained.

The implications of this for the importance of the cortical shell in the vertebrae are obvious. Large amounts of trabecular loss theoretically can be sustained without reducing the structural strength of the vertebra sufficiently to increase fracture risk. On the other hand, if cortical loss is a component of the osteoporotic condition, this could partly account for the observation that the loss of bone strength with age occurs much more quickly than the loss of bone mass [15,41]. Britton and Davie [41] showed that yield stress fell twice as fast as apparent density and yield energy declined 2.6 times faster than apparent density in a group that included both men and women. That is, the ability of the vertebrae to absorb energy declines more and faster with age than does bone loss. Nevertheless, the description and effect of *regional* losses and gains in the different compartments has not been examined critically, and so effects of such changes on regional distribution of stresses within the vertebrae are currently open to some speculation.

Experimental Studies of the Role of the Cortical Shell in Vertebral Strength

There has been lively debate about the contribution that the cortical shell makes in vertebrae to its overall strength and resistance to fracture. Evans [42] proposed that the cortical shell is of primary importance, while Bell et al. [13] and Bartley et al. [43] claimed that it is largely irrelevant. This debate continues today.

Rockoff et al. [44] tested lumbar vertebrae in compression with and without the cortex present. The cortex was removed from these specimens by grinding, so it is not clear whether only the cortex or also some of the trabecular bone was lost. In other cases, a transverse cut was made through the center of the vertebral body, keeping the cortex completely intact. These tests showed that the cortical shell contributes 45%–75% of the peak vertical compressive strength of the lumbar vertebrae, regardless of the degree of mineralization or physical density [44]. They showed that the importance of the cortical shell increases with age as trabecular bone is disproportionately lost. More of the load along the vertebral column was transmitted via the cortical shell in subjects older than 40 years (n = 18) than in those younger (n = 14). Unfortunately, only two of the nine subjects older than 60 years were women. Women lose more than twice as much compact bone from the vertebral body than men [45], and may be more dependent on this cortical bone to maintain vertebral strength in the face of the greater fractional trabecular loss [46]. This gender distribution could have led to an overestimation of the importance of the cortical shell in older individuals.

Compression testing of L1 and L3 by McBroom et al. [7], however, suggests that the cortical shell contributes only about 10%–15% of the strength of the vertebral body. These investigators tested a sample of lumbar vertebrae from 26 subjects between 63 and 99 years of age at the time of death. Most compressive failures occurred by fracture of the endplate, suggesting to them that the cortical shell contributed relatively little to overall vertebral strength.

Data from McBroom et al. [7] are inconsistent with what is known about BMC in the cortical and trabecular compartments, particularly when considered in light of the mechanically more important distribution of the cortical bone. In 99 women (mean age = 53.8 ± 13.0 years, range 26–79 years), Pacifici et al. [47] found that cortical BMC accounted for about 35% of the total bone in the anterior three-quarters of the L_1 or L_2 vertebral body. Others have estimated the cortical component to contribute <20% [48], 20%–30% [49–51], 30%–45% [44,52,53], or 60%–80% [54–57]. The estimates by Nottestad and Jones may be too high because they used an older sample in which substantial amounts of trabecular bone may already have been lost. This was not true of Sandor et al. [57], however, who performed CT scans of 139 lumbar vertebrae from 50 women between the ages of 20 and 83 years (mean = 53.8 years). In any event, because the cortical bone is at the outer margin of the vertebral body, it will contribute more to bending and torsional strength than it contributes to the fractional volume of the vertebral body it composes. Yoganandan et al. [48] found that the cortical shell contributed less than 20% of the total cross-sectional area in both men and women, but bore 35%–45% of the total load. In the osteoporotic spine, the cortical shell accounted for 74% of the total vertebral strength. Therefore, even if the cortical shell only accounts for a fraction of the total bone in the lumbar vertebra, it will contribute much more than this to the bending or torsional strength of the vertebra.

If preferential loss of trabecular bone accounts for overestimates of the contribution of cortical bone in the vertebrae, it suggests that trabecular bone is lost at a much faster rate than cortical bone [55,58], an assertion not borne out by all studies [57]. In actuality, the rate of cortical bone loss with age more likely has been underestimated both by extrapolation from appendicular

Table 1. Cortical and trabecular bone loss in lumbar vertebrae of normal aging men and women.

Absolute loss (mg/ml/yr)		Percent loss (/yr)					
Cortical	Trabecular	Cortical	Trabecular	Gender	Age	N	Reference
−3.15	−2.21	−1.01	−1.84	Female	20–83 (53.8)[a]	50	Sandor et al. 1992
−2.20	−1.82	−0.32	−1.51	Female	<20–>80 (40–49)[b]	139	Kalender et al. 1989[c]
—	−2.05	−0.58	−1.16	Female	26–79 (53.8)[a]	99	Pacifici et al. 1987
−3.24	−2.50	−1.44	−2.08	Female	50–70 (58.7)[a]	12	Jones et al. 1987
−2.86 (0.47)	−2.15 (0.25)	−0.84 (0.43)	−1.65 (0.35)	Mean (S.D.)			
−0.94	−1.70	−0.75	−1.39	Male	<20–>80 (40–49)[b]	135	Kalender et al. 1989[c]

[a] Mean age
[b] Median age range
[c] Anterior half of vertebra measured only

cortical bone sites [47,59] and by presenting the loss in terms of fractional loss rather than absolute loss. The fractional loss of trabecular bone in the vertebrae in women (1%–2% per year) is nearly double the fractional loss in cortical bone (0.5%–1% per year) [45,57], but the absolute rate of loss of cortical bone (about 3 mg/cm^3/yr) is greater than the absolute loss of trabecular bone (about 2 mg/cm^3/yr) (Table 1) [12,45,57,60].

There is no difference in the absolute amount of trabecular loss by gender [4,45], but women have a higher fractional rate of loss than men [45] because of their lower initial bone mass. There are, however, large differences between men and women in cortical bone loss with age. Although cortical thickness decreases in both men and women [46], women lose about 2.5 times more cortical bone in the lumbar spine than men [45]. Women with increased cortical loss appear at greater risk of fracture [61] even though their bone mass may only be reduced by 10%–15% overall. This suggests that older women are more dependent on maintenance of the cortical shell than men to prevent fracture following a substantial loss of trabecular volume. Differences in cortical bone loss between men and women may account for some of the variance in fracture risk.

The cortical shell becomes more important to vertebral strength in patients in whom significant bone loss has occurred [40,46], and contributes *more* to the strength of the vertebra in osteoporotic patients than in normal subjects. Both men and women who sustained a vertebral osteoporotic fracture have significantly ($P < 0.03$) thinner cortices than a group of nearly the same age who did not have any fractures [62]. Details of the measurement in relation to the timing of the fracture were not given, so it is possible that some bone loss occurred subsequent to the fracture, rather than causing the fracture. Vesterby et al. [46] found that, following age and gender, cortical thickness and trabecular star volume were significant predictors of vertebral compressive strength. Faulkner et al. [63] found a 12% contribution of the cortex to yield stress in lumbar vertebrae from non-osteoporotic patients, but a 56% contribution in subjects with previous vertebral fractures. Moreover, in patients who already have a fracture, the cortex supports as much as 67% of the entire load.

The importance of cortical bone also may be indicated by data on vertebral density and fracture following sodium fluoride therapy. Increased vertebral density resulting from sodium fluoride therapy failed to protect against fractures [64,65]. One reason may be that sodium fluoride increases bone density in the trabecular compartment, not the cortical compartment, and this is less effective at improving the mechanical characteristics of the bone. Riggs et al. [64] found that sodium fluoride increased trabecular BMD in the lumbar spine by 35%, but failed to prevent losses of cortical bone up to 4% at appendicular sites. Mosekilde et al. [15] found a 17% increase in cancellous bone density without a change in compressive strength, stiffness, or energy absorption. Cortical bone changes were not measured. These data suggest that bone mass changes are not, and should not be, the only indicator of vertebral competence or fracture risk.

Regional Variation Within a Vertebra

Non-uniform loss of trabecular or cortical bone in the vertebrae can create stress concentrations that could increase fracture risk and accelerate failure [1]. The anterior margin of the vertebral body is subjected to especially high compressive loads under conditions in which loads are reduced on the facets [29,66–69], as in forward flexion. Preferential bone loss in the anterior half of the vertebra would reduce the mechanical loadbearing properties of the vertebra much more greatly than predicted by a simple bone mass measurement averaged over the entire vertebra.

Both autopsy studies and studies using QCT in vivo show that trabecular loss occurs at different rates across the vertebral body [39,70]. Jones et al. [55] found significant reductions of trabecular BMD in the anterior half of the vertebra in both osteoporotic men and women compared to normal subjects, and a significant reduction of the BMD of the anterior cortical shell in osteoporotic men. Compact bone BMD in osteoporotic women was not significantly less than in age-matched normal women. Likewise, Kalender et al. [45] found significant decreases in both trabecular and cortical BMD in the anterior lumbar vertebral body in women without signs of osteoporosis. Edwards et al. [71] showed that trabecular bone apparent density of the anterior centrum of lumbar vertebrae was less than two-thirds the density of the posterior centrum.

These data are consistent with measurements of significantly lower compressive rigidity in the anterior vertebral body in older subjects of both genders [71]. Edwards et al. [71] reported that the anterior lumbar vertebral body is less than half as strong in compression as the posterior centrum. Moreover, they found that a significant portion of the variance in strength ($r^2 = 0.63$, $P < 0.0001$) could be explained by apparent density alone. This suggests that trabecular bone loss in the anterior part of the vertebral body is both significant mechanically and important to assessing fracture risk.

Anterior wedge fractures are common among older women. The risk of such a fracture occurs both from excessively high anterior compressive stresses, shown to occur from FEMs of the spine [68,69,72], and from the reduced regional compressive strength consequent to accelerated bone loss and reduced BMD in the anterior region of the vertebra. BMD measurements that include the entire vertebra or vertebral body may mask losses that are more mechanically significant in the anterior vertebral body. Regional analyses of BMD in aging men and women are indicated.

Contributions of the Bony Endplate to Vertebral Strength

A number of investigators have shown that the endplate and adjacent cancellous bone are the weakest part of the intervertebral joint [14,73,74]. Granhed et al. [74] and others [75,76] showed that the endplate was the first part of the vertebra to fail when subjected to combined compression-flexion loads within "physiologic limits". This may be particularly true in osteoporotic individuals [77].

The contribution of the bony endplate to vertebral strength and fracture risk is difficult to assess because it depends on a number of factors. In particular, stress distribution varies according to the inclination of the endplates under compressive loads, and to the severity of intervertebral disk degeneration. These factors are difficult to assess using standard radiologic techniques.

Biconcave vertebral fractures [17] have been attributed to high stresses on the endplate beneath the intervertebral disk [78]. However, Horst and Brinckmann [79] used mechanical testing to show that, if the intervertebral disk is not degenerated, stress on the vertebral endplate is constant. Stress concentrations are only created if the region below the anulus is stressed more than the central region due to eccentric loading caused by disk degeneration. The experimental work of Rolander and Blair [77] generally supports this. Hansson and Roos [80], on the other hand, have shown that disk degeneration has no effect on mechanical strength of the vertebral body.

Whether the disk is degenerated or not, eccentric loading of the spine will cause local stress concentrations on the endplate. Most in vivo loading of the spine does not occur in axial compression, (although most experimental loading does because it is easier to perform). Forward flexion and twisting motions would create eccentric loading on the vertebral endplates that could potentially create stresses significant enough to cause fracture.

All in all, these data are contradictory and confusing, and shed little light on the role that the endplate plays in the fracture process. Epistatic relations between various components of the vertebra have not been addressed either mechanically or analytically, but could be potentially important to the mechanical strength of the osteoporotic vertebra. It is likely that when these interactions are addressed, the role of the endplate will become better defined.

Contribution of the Posterior Elements to Vertebral Strength

Using an intradiscal pressure transducer, Nachemson [81] estimated that the facets carry approximately 20% of the total vertical load borne by the spine. Although he retracted this statement 3 years later [82], many other investigators have found that the posterior elements bear significant loads. Adams and Hutton [83] corroborated Nachemson's original data, finding that the facet joints transmit about 16% of the load in the standing position. Hakim and King [68] also demonstrated significant facet loads when a spinal segment was loaded either statically or dynamically.

Facet load transmission is dependent on geometry. This creates significant discrepancy among measurements, which depend upon the orientation of the facets and the position of the body. For example, Adams and Hutton [83] found that in the erect sitting posture, the facet joints carry no load. Yang and King [28] measured the facet loads in the lumbar vertebrae and reported that the facets carried an average of 22% of the total load when the vertebra was loaded 10mm anterior to its center, 25% when loaded at the center, and 30% when loaded 10mm posterior to its center. While there is some variation among these values, a reasonable estimate is that the facet joints transmit 15%–30% of the total vertical load on the lumbar vertebrae.

Finite Element Analysis of Vertebral Bone

Why Use Finite Element Modeling for Analysis of Vertebral Stress?

The vertebral column, and even a single vertebra, is such a complex structure that it can be helpful to use computational techniques to evaluate the change in stress distribution following simulations of bone loss or under various conditions of loading. These data are difficult to collect experimentally, and FEMs that predict where failure may occur can be useful in formulating hypotheses about fracture risk. While non-invasive measurements can reveal, in part, the morphological changes of the vertebra and changes of constituent properties, stress and strain cannot be determined from these measurements. The finite element method is the most suitable method to study the stress distribution of an object that has irregular geometry, multiple material compositions, and is subjected to complex loading situations. Finite element techniques and mechanical property measurements of vertebral segments can be used to improve the diagnostic assessment of vertebral fracture risk in osteoporosis by examining relationships among the trabecular bone and the cortical shell and bony endplate of thoracic and lumbar vertebrae.

Hakim and King [68] developed a three-dimensional (3D) model of a normal vertebra, including the posterior elements and intervertebral disk. They validated the model by controlled ex vivo static and dynamic loading experiments in which strain was monitored at various locations on the cortex of the vertebra. For normal vertebrae, they predicted the highest strain on the anterior cortex of the vertebral body at mid-centrum, with strains superior and inferior to this being 20%–80% of this maximum strain. They also found regions of high stress at the junction of the pedicles with the vertebral body, and at the junction of the lamina with the inferior facet.

While interesting, these data tell us nothing about stress changes in the osteoporotic spine or about possible fracture modes. Faulkner et al. [63] developed a 3D FEM to assess the effect of bone distribution on vertebral strength. This analysis stressed the importance of the cortical shell to overall vertebral strength, but neglected to examine the interrelationship between the cortical shell, regional patterns of trabecular loss, and the bony endplate. Yet adaptive changes in any of these structures may compensate for, or accentuate, the mechanical effects of trabecular loss.

Finite Element Modeling of Stress Redistribution in the Osteoporotic Spine

Model Formation. A 3D FEM of a spinal motion segment was developed to calculate the stress distribution of a normal and of an osteoporotic vertebra. The model consisted of two lumbar vertebral bodies, the intervertebral disk between them, facet joints, and all posterior elements. The model geometry was digitized from a cadaver L_2–L_3 motion segment [28]. The model consisted of 506 nodes and 358 elements (Table 2). Three-dimensional 4-node shell elements were used to simulate vertebral endplates, transverse and spinous processes, and vertebral cortical bone. The trabeculae were modeled by isotropic solid elements (Table 2). Three dimensional orthotropic solid elements were used to simulate the anulus fibrosus. The nucleus pulposus was simulated by 3D fluid elements. The posterior and anterior longitudinal ligaments were not simulated because the segment was loaded in pure compression and no moment was created.

Six representative cases were compared (Table 3). Four cases (I, III, V, and VII) considered normal trabecular density, while the other four (II, IV, VI, and VIII) incorporated reduced trabecular density simulating osteopenia. Cases III, IV, VII, and VIII incorporated reduced cortical thickness into the model (with or without reduced trabecular density), and cases V–VIII

Table 2. Material properties and element types used in the finite element model.

Structure	Element Type	No. of Elements	Elastic Modulus (MPa)	Poisson ratio	Thickness (mm)
Cortical bone	Quadrilateral shell	68	11 032	0.30	0.635
Trabecular bone (healthy)	Isoparametric solid	120	87.44	0.30	—
Trabecular bone (osteoporotic)	Isoparametric solid	120	7.67	0.30	—
Endplate	Quadrilateral shell	80	12 480	0.28	0.512 (central) 0.812 (periph.)
Posterior elements	Quadrilateral shell	10	12 480	0.28	—
Pedicles, laminae facets	Isoparametric solid	36	11 032	0.25	—
Facet joint	Interface contact	4	—	—	—
Anulus fibrosus	Isoparametric solid	24	40.0	0.45	—
Nucleus pulposus	Fluid	16	2 255 (bulk mod.)	—	—

periph., Peripheral

Table 3. Cases simulated by the finite element model.

Case	Trabecular bone density	Cortical bone thickness	Endplate thickness
I	Normal	Normal	Normal
II	Osteoporotic	Normal	Normal
III	Normal	50% Normal	Normal
IV	Osteoporotic	50% Normal	Normal
V	Normal	Normal	50% Normal
VI	Osteoporotic	Normal	50% Normal
VII	Normal	50% Normal	50% Normal
VIII	Osteoporotic	50% Normal	50% Normal

simulated a reduced endplate thickness (with and without reduced trabecular density and cortical thickness).

Material property values used for the disk were taken from the literature. The bulk modulus of water was used as the bulk modulus for the nucleus pulposus. The anulus was assumed to have a modulus of 40 MPa [30].

Values for trabecular density were taken from averages for young women determined by QCT (173 mg/ml) [84]. Using this density, we calculated the trabecular bone compressive strength using regression equations proposed by McBroom et al. [7] to simulate a healthy spine, and determined a value of 3.76 MPa for healthy trabecular bone, within the range reported by Yamada [85]. Buchanan et al. [84] reported that when the QCT density was reduced to

50 mg/ml the vertebra has a 70% chance of fracture. The corresponding trabecular bone strength calculated from the 50 mg/ml density was used to simulate trabecular loss (0.33 MPa). Because the average percentage of compressive contraction is 4.3%, the modulus of the trabecular bone in the vertebral body used for healthy trabecular bone was 87.44 MPa (cases I, III, V, and VII), while a value of 7.67 MPa was used for osteoporotic vertebrae (cases II, IV, VI, and VIII) (Table 2).

The modulus for cortical bone was based on an average of several studies [44,86–88]. A value of 11 032 MPa was used for the cortical shell of the vertebral body, as well as the spinous and transverse processes (Table 2). The latter were not available in the literature, but their moduli should be close to that of cortical bone.

A physiologic static loading simulating a person lifting a 40 N weight was applied to the model using the calculation of Schultz and Andersson [89], with 80% of the load applied to the vertebral body and 20% through the facet joints [28]. This is a relatively low level of loading compared to other physical activities. This new model, improved from a previous one [72], includes a more realistic representation of the facet joint contact. Previously, the facet was assumed to stick to the pars interarticularis of the inferior vertebra once contact occurred. The new model allows the tip of one vertebral facet to slide on the pars interarticularis of an adjacent vertebra. Post-processing was accomplished using the commercially available FEM package ANSYS.

Model Validation. The model was validated by comparing the axial stiffness and intradiscal pressure with experimental data. The stiffness of the normal spine calculated by the model was 3935 N/mm, within the same range of magnitude as experimentally determined from previous studies [90,91]. The facet load predicted by the model also was similar to that reported by Yang and King [28]. In addition, the maximum cortical bone stress determined from the model of the healthy spine was nearly the same as the average peak strength for subjects under 40 years old [44].

Results. Reduced trabecular mass caused >20% reduction in axial compressive stiffness in the motion segment regardless of the thickness of the cortical shell or endplate. On the other hand, cortical thinning alone, without loss of trabecular mass or reduced endplate thickness (case III) did not reduce axial stiffness significantly. Likewise, a thinner endplate had no effect on stiffness if trabecular mass was normal.

In the healthy spine, the model predicts that the posterior elements share 27% of the axial load while the cortical shell shares 39% and the trabeculae 34% (Fig. 2). This value for cortical load sharing agrees with those reported by others [44,48,92], but is considerably higher than predicted by some [7]. With trabecular loss, the load on the cortical shell increases, so that the cortical shell supports nearly 60%, the posterior elements about 32%, and the trabeculae only about 9% of the total load. Reduced cortical shell or endplate thickness had no effect on loads borne by the posterior elements; in all cases of cortical

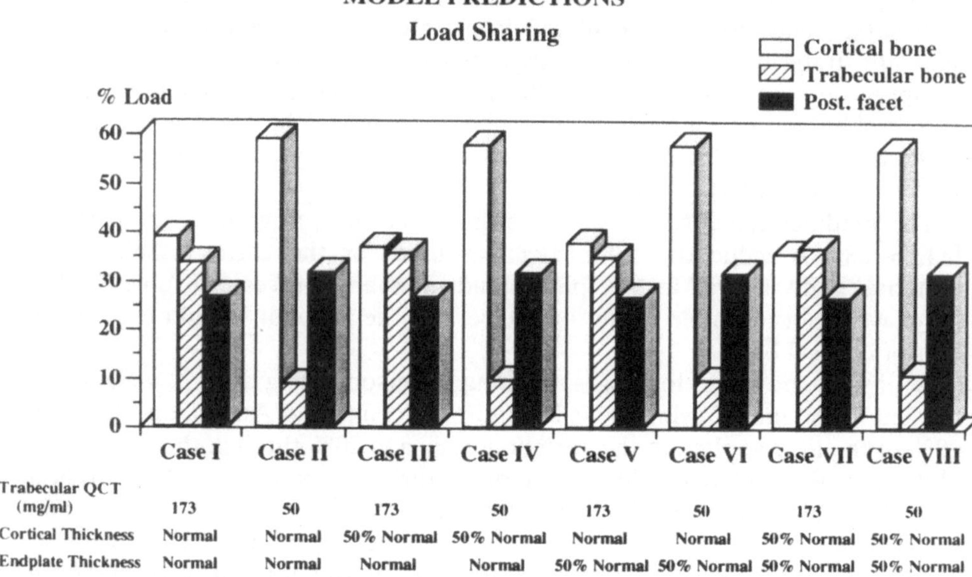

Fig. 2. Model predictions for load sharing by the cortical shell, trabecular bone, and posterior (*post*) elements of a lumbar vertebra for eight cases simulated by the finite element model. *QCT*, quantitative computed tomography

and endplate thinning, loads were redistributed between the cortical and the trabecular compartments.

The increased load on the posterior elements with trabecular loss caused a 100% increase in posterior element stresses (Fig. 3). When the model simulated both trabecular and cortical loss (case IV), posterior element stresses more than doubled compared to the healthy spine. In the osteoporotic spine, the posterior elements bear a greater load and develop significantly greater stress than in the healthy spine. This is consistent with the frequent fractures between the pedicles and vertebral body observed in osteopenic patients.

With normal cortical thickness but reduced trabecular mass, cortical bone stresses more than triple (Fig. 3). However, if both trabecular and cortical bone are lost, cortical shell stresses are more than four times greater than in the non-osteoporotic vertebra. The maximum cortical stress occurred in the superior and anterolateral regions of the vertebral body. This is consistent with clinical observations of wedge fractures in osteoporotic patients. Thus, while losses of trabecular bone alone can significantly increase vertebral fracture risk, concurrent losses in both the trabecular and cortical compartments may nearly assure that the bone will exceed its breaking strength.

Cortical thinning alone, without loss of trabecular mass or reduced endplate thickness will not reduce axial rigidity of the whole vertebra significantly, but will increase cortical bone stresses significantly.

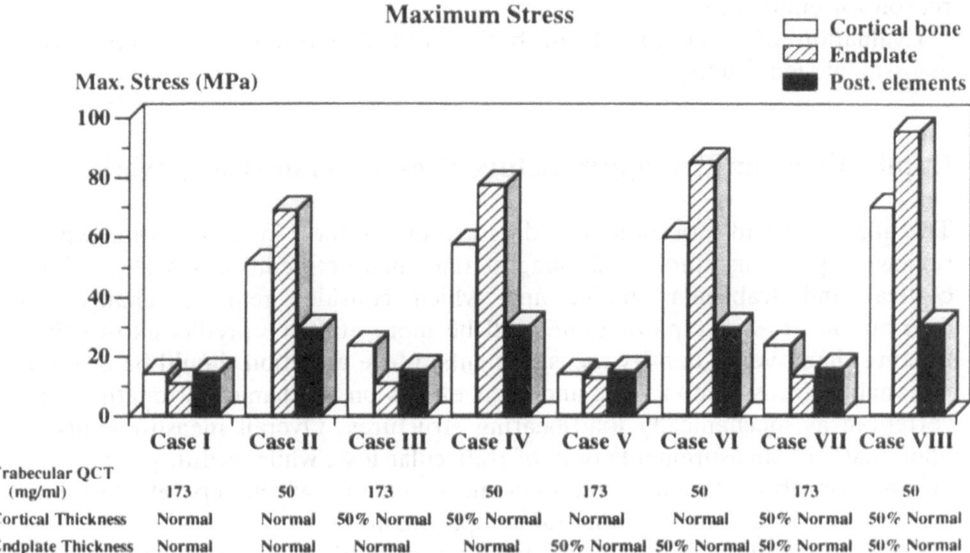

Fig. 3. Model predictions for maximum stress on the cortical shell, trabecular bone, and posterior elements of a lumbar vertebra for the eight cases simulated by the finite element model

The cortical bone stress was not affected by reduced endplate thickness (Fig. 3). However, the loss of trabecular bone causes endplate stresses to increase by sevenfold. This suggests that loss of trabecular density results in increased bony endplate stress, increasing the likelihood of endplate failure. This is independent of any loss in the cortical shell or reduced thickness in the endplate itself. This is consistent with observations from ex vivo biomechanical testing of vertebral motion segments, in which endplate fractures are relatively common [77].

If bone is lost from all compartments (case VIII, Fig. 3), the maximum stresses for both endplate and cortical shell increase even more than those described above.

Model Predictions. These data show that if trabecular loss is large enough (≥67%), the risk of vertebral wedge or compression fractures increases even without concurrent loss of bone from the cortical shell. However, concurrent loss of bone from the cortical and trabecular compartments may increase stresses on the cortical shell above the fracture threshold. This could be one reason for vertebral crush fractures (either compression fractures or biconcave fractures).

The model also predicts that loss of trabecular density will increase endplate stresses above its breaking strength and can cause subchondral fracture.

Combinations of reduced trabecular mass and endplate thinning could be one reason for endplate fractures.

Evaluation of bone loss from both areas should improve fracture risk assessment significantly.

Implications for Therapy/Fracture Prevention in Osteoporosis

The analytical and morphological data presented here, in combination with a review of previous studies, all suggest that measurements which assess both cortical and trabecular bone, and which consider regional changes in distribution of each type of bone, will be more effective predictors of spinal fracture than overall density measurements. More attention should be given to regional patterns of bone loss and their effects on mechanical strength of the vertebrae as mechanically load-bearing structures. Overall measurements of bone mass, or measurements only of trabecular loss, while useful, provide less information about fracture risk than measurements which separate loss into trabecular, cortical, or subchondral compartments.

Because simultaneous loss of bone from both trabecular and cortical envelopes can accelerate fracture, agents which act to restore bone or prevent loss on only one compartment, sometimes at the expense of the other, will be less effective clinically at preventing fracture than agents which prevent loss from both compartments. In this regard, it is unlikely that sodium fluoride, which acts primarily on the trabecular envelope, will ever be an effective agent to completely prevent vertebral fragility. Both estrogen and some bisphosphonates, on the other hand, may have a positive effect on trabecular bone mass and prevent loss from the compact bone compartment. Calcium, through its action to reduce porosity in compact bone, may be effective in some cases in which calcium deficiency is a concern.

Agents which cause addition of cortical bone to the outer shell of the vertebra may also be more effective in established osteoporosis. Once trabeculae are lost, they are difficult to re-establish. Lamellar bone formation requires a substrate upon which to deposit. Because of this, treatments which supplement the normal age-related expansion of the vertebral cortical shell, but also prevent loss on the endocortical surface, would hold great promise for preventing the degradation of mechanical properties in the spine of postmenopausal women.

References

1. Parfitt AM, Duncan H (1982) Metabolic bone disease affecting the spine. In: Rothman R, Simeone F (eds) The spine. W.B. Saunders, Philadelphia, pp 775–905
2. Aaron JE, Makins NB, Sagreiya K (1987) The microanatomy of trabecular bone loss in normal aging men and women. Clin Orthop 215:260–271

3. Mosekilde L (1988) Age-related changes in vertebral trabecular bone architecture—assessed by a new method. Bone 9:247–250
4. Mosekilde L (1989) Sex differences in age-related loss of vertebral trabecular bone mass and structure—biomechanical consequences. Bone 10:425–432
5. Mellish RWE, Garrahan NJ, Compston JE (1989) Age-related changes in trabecular width and spacing in human iliac crest biopsies. Bone Miner 6:331–338
6. Parfitt AM (1992) Implications of architecture of the pathogenesis and prevention of vertebral fracture. 13:S41–S47
7. McBroom RJ, Hayes WC, Edwards WT, Goldberg RP, White AA III (1985) Prediction of vertebral body compressive fracture using quantitative computed tomography. J Bone Joint Surg 67A:1206–1214
8. O'Keefe D (1991) Morphometry. Radiol Clin N Am 29:165–174
9. Brassow F, Crone-Munzebrock W, Weh L, Kranz R, Eggers-Stroeder G (1982) Correlations between breaking load and CT absorption values of vertebral bodies. Eur J Radiol 2:99–101
10. Brinckman P, Biggemann M, Hilweg D (1984) Prediction of the compressive strength of human lumbar vertebrae. Clin Biomech 4:S1–S27
11. Mosekilde L, Bentzen SM, Ortoft G, Jorgensen J (1989) The predictive value of quantitative computed tomography for vertebral body compressive strength and ash density. Bone 10:465–470
12. Block JE, Smith R, Blueer C-C, Steiger P, Ettinger B, Genant HK (1989) Model of spinal trabecular bone loss as determined by quantitative computed tomography. J Bone Miner Res 4:249–257
13. Bell GH, Dunbar O, Beck JS, Gibb A (1967) Variations in strength of vertebrae with age and their relation to osteoporosis. Calcif Tissue Res 1:75–86
14. Hansson T, Roos B, Nachemson A (1980) The bone mineral content and ultimate compressive strength of lumbar vertebrae. Spine 5:46–55
15. Mosekilde L, Kragstrup J, Richards A (1987) Compressive strength, ash weight, and volume of vertebral trabecular bone in experimental fluorosis in pigs. Calcif Tissue Int 40:318–322
16. Ericksson SAV, Isberg BO, Lindgren JU (1989) Prediction of vertebral strength by dual photon absorptiometry and quantitative computed tomography. Calcif Tissue Int 44:243–250
17. Kanis JA, McCloskey EV (1992) Epidemiology of vertebral osteoporosis. Bone 13:S1–S10
18. Recker RR, Smith RT, Kimmel DB (1992) Loss of trabecular connectivity in osteoporosis demonstrated with independent methods. Presented at the 6th International Congress on Bone Morphometry, Lexington KY, October
19. Ott SM, Kilcoyne RF, Chesnut CH III (1988) Comparisons among methods of measuring bone mass and relationship to severity of vertebral fractures in osteoporosis. J Clin Endocrinol Metab 66:501–507
20. Beck TJ, Ruff CS, Warden KE, Scott WW Jr, Rao GU (1990) Predicting femoral neck strength from bone mineral data. A structural approach. Invest Radiol 25:6–18
21. Yoshikawa T, Turner CH, Markwardt P, Burr DB (1992) Cross-sectional moment of inertia of the femoral neck measured using DEXA. J Bone Miner Res 7:S135
22. Mazess RB (1990) Fracture risk: A role for compact bone. Calcif Tissue Int 47:191–193

23. Ross PD, Wasnich RD, Heilbrun LK, Vogel JM (1987) Definition of a spine fracture threshold based upon prospective fracture risk. Bone 8:271–278
24. Odvina CV, Wergedal JE, Libanati CR, Schulz EE, Baylink DJ (1988) Relationship between trabecular vertebral body density and fractures: A quantitative definition of spinal osteoporosis. Metabolism 37:221–228
25. Kanis JA, McCloskey EV, Eyres KS, O'Doherty D, Aaron J (1990) Screening techniques in the evaluation of osteoporosis. In: Drift JO, Studd JWW (eds) HRT and osteoporosis. Springer, Berlin Heidelberg New York, pp 135–147
26. Kulak R, Belytschko T, Schultz A, Galante J (1976) Nonlinear behavior of the human intervertebral disc under axial load. J Biomech 9:377–386
27. Shirazi-Adl SA, Shrivastava SC, Ahmed AM (1984) Stress analysis of lumbar disk-body unit in compression. Spine 9:120–134
28. Yang KH, King AI (1984) Mechanism of facet load transmission as a hypothesis of low back pain. Spine 9:557–565
29. King AI, Yang KH (1985) Biomechanics of the lumbar spine. In: Schmid-Schonbein G, Woo S, Zweifach B (eds) Frontiers in applied mechanics and biomechanics. Springer, Berlin Heidelberg New York, pp 210–214
30. Spilker RL, Jacobs DM, Schultz AB (1986) Material constants for a finite element model of the intervertebral disk with a fiber composite annulus. J Biomech Eng 108:1–11
31. Ueno K, Liu YK (1987) A three-dimensional nonlinear finite element model of lumbar intervertebral joint in torsion. J Biomech Eng 109:200–209
32. Natali A, Meroi E (1990) Nonlinear analysis of intervertebral disk under dynamic load. J Biomech Eng 112:358–363
33. Sharma M, Rodriguez J, Largrana N (1991) Effect of the wedge angle on lumbar intervertebral discs under compressive load. In: Vanderby (ed), 1991 Advances in Bioengineering, American Society of Mechanical Engineers, New York, pp 133–136
34. Kasra M, Shirazi-Adl A, Drouin G (1992) Dynamics of human lumbar intervertebral joints—experimental and finite element investigations. Spine 17:93–102
35. Wainwright SA, Biggs WD, Currey JD, Gosline JM (1982) Mechanical design in organisms. University Press, Princeton, NJ
36. Allen WC, Piotrowski G, Burstein AH, Frankel VH (1968) Biomechanical principles of intramedullary fixation. Clin Orthop 60:13–20
37. Martin RB, Atkinson PJ (1977) Age and sex-related changes in the structure and strength of the human femoral shaft. J Biomech 10:223–231
38. Ericksen MF (1978) Aging in the lumbar spine. III. L5. Am J Phys Anthropol 48:247–250
39. Pesch HJ, Scharf HP, Lauer G, Seibold H (1980) Der altersabhängige Verbundabbau der Lendenwirbelkörper. Virch Arch Pathol Anat Histol 386:21–41
40. Mosekilde L, Mosekilde L (1986) Normal vertebral body size and compressive strength: Relations to age and to vertebral and iliac trabecular bone compressive strength. Bone 7:207–212
41. Britton JM, Davie MWJ (1990) Mechanical properties of bone from iliac crest and relationship to L5 vertebral bone. Bone 11:21–28
42. Evans FG (1957) Stress and strain in bones. CC Thomas, Springfield, IL
43. Bartley MH Jr, Arnold JS, Haslan RK, Jee WSS (1966) The relationship of bone strength and bone quantity in health, disease, and aging. J Geront 21:517–521

44. Rockoff SD, Sweet E, Bleustein J (1969) The relative contribution of trabecular and cortical bone to the strength of human lumbar vertebrae. Calcif Tissue Res 3:163–175
45. Kalender WA, Felsenberg D, Louis O, Lopez P, Klotz E, Osteaux M, Fraga J (1989) Reference values for trabecular and cortical vertebral bone density in single- and dual-energy quantitative computed tomography. Eur J Radiol 9:75–80
46. Vesterby A, Mosekilde L, Gunderson HJG, Melsen F, Mosekilde L, Holme K, Sorensen S (1991) Biologically meaningful determinants of the in vitro strength of lumbar vertebrae. Bone 12:219–224
47. Pacifici R, Rupich RC, Avioli LV (1990) Vertebral cortical bone mass measurement by a new quantitative computer tomography method: Correlations with vertebral trabecular bone measurements. Calcif Tissue Int 47:215–220
48. Yoganandan N, Myklebust JB, Cusick JF, Wilson CR, Sances A Jr (1988) Functional biomechanics of the thoracolumbar vertebral cortex. Clin Biomech 3:11–18
49. Johnson LC (1964) Morphologic analysis in pathology: The kinetics of disease and general biology in bone. In: Frost HM (ed) Bone biodynamics. Little and Brown, Boston, pp 543–654
50. Weissberger MA, Zamenhof RG, Aronow S, Neer RM (1978) Computed tomography scanning for the measurement of bone mineral in the human spine. J Comput Assist Tomogr 2:253–262
51. Eastell R, Mosekilde L, Hodgson SF, Riggs BL (1990) Proportion of human vertebral body bone that is cancellous. J Bone Miner Res 5:1237–1241
52. Mazess RB (1983) Noninvasive methods for quantitating trabecular bone. In: Avioli LV (ed) The osteoporotic syndrome: detection, prevention, and treatment. Grune and Stratton, New York, pp 85–114
53. Wahner HW, Dunn WL, Offord KP, Riggs BL (1983) Dual photon absorptiometry: Clinical considerations. In: Frame B, Potts JT (eds) Clinical disorders of bone and mineral metabolism. Excerpta Medica, Amsterdam, pp 34–38
54. Nottestad SV, Baumel JJ, Kimmel DB, Recker RR, Heaney RP (1987) The proportion of trabecular bone in human vertebrae. J Bone Miner Res 2:221–229
55. Jones CD, Laval-Jeantet A-M, Laval-Jeantet MH, Genant HK (1987) Importance of measurement of spongious vertebral bone mineral density in the assessment of osteoporosis. Bone 8:201–206
56. Van Berkum FNR, Birkenhager JC, Van Veen LCP, Seelenberg J, Birkenhager-Frankel DH, Trouerback WT, Stinen T, Pols HAP (1989) Noninvasive axial and peripheral assessment of bone mineral content: A comparison between osteoporotic women and normal subjects. J Bone Miner Res 4:679–685
57. Sandor T, Felsenberg D, Kalender WA, Clain A, Brown E (1992) Compact and trabecular components of the spine using quantitative computed tomography. Calcif Tissue Int 50:502–506
58. Cann CE, Genant HK, Kolb FO, Ettinger B (1985) Quantitative computed tomography for prediction of vertebral fracture risk. Bone 6:1–7
59. Mazess RB (1982) On aging bone loss. Clin Orthop 165:239–252
60. Pacifici R, Susman N, Carr PL, Birge SJ, Avioli LV (1987) Single and dual energy tomographic analysis of spinal trabecular bone: A comparative study in normal and osteoporotic women. J Clin Endocrinol Metab 64:209–214
61. Smith DM, Khairi MRA, Johnston CC (1975) The loss of bone mineral with aging and its relationship to risk of fracture. J Clin Invest 56:311–318

62. Vesterby A, Ullerup R, Kristensen BI, Melsen F (1991) Cortical bone: A major determinant for fracture risk in vertebral osteoporosis. J Bone Miner Res 12:S274
63. Faulkner KG, Cann CE, Hasegawa BH (1991) Effect of bone distribution on vertebral strength: Assessment with patient-specific nonlinear finite element analysis. Radiology 179:669–674
64. Riggs BL, Hodgson SF, O'Fallon WM, Chao EYS, Wahner HW, Muhs JM, Cedel SL, Melton LJ III (1990) Effect of fluoride treatment on the fracture rate in postmenopausal women with osteoporosis. New Engl J Med 322:802–809
65. Kleerekoper M, Peterson EL, Nelson DA, Phillips E, Schork MA, Tilley BC, Parfitt AM (1991) A randomized trial of sodium fluoride as a treatment for postmenopausal osteoporosis. Osteoporosis Int 1:155–161
66. Prasad P, King AI (1974) An experimentally validated dynamic model of the spine. J Appl Mech 41:546–550
67. Prasad P, King AI, Ewing CL (1974) The role of articular facets during $+G_z$ acceleration. J Appl Mech 41:321–326
68. Hakim NS, King, AI (1979) A three dimensional finite element dynamic response analysis of a vertebra with experimental verification. J Biomech 12:277–292
69. Ranu HS (1990) A vertebral finite element model and its response to loading. Med Prog Tech 16:189–199
70. Sandor T, Felsenberg D, Kalender WA, Brown E (1990) Global and regional variations in the spinal trabecular bone: Single and dual energy examinations. J Clin Endocrinol Metab 72:1157–1168
71. Edwards WT, McBroom RC, Hayes, WC, Goldberg R, White AA III (1986) Variation of density in the vertebral body measured by quantitative computed tomography. Trans ORS 11:205
72. Yang KH, Sofranko R, Burr DB (1988) Stress redistribution of osteoporotic spine. In: Spilker RL, Simon BR (eds) Computational methods in bioengineering. ASME, New York, pp 427–436
73. Hansson T, Keller TS, Spengler DM (1987) Mechanical behavior of the human lumbar spine. II. Fatigue strength during dynamic compressive loading. J Orthop Res 5:479–487
74. Granhed H, Jonson R, Hansson T (1989) Mineral content and strength of lumbar vertebrae: A cadaver study. Acta Orthop Scand 60:105–109
75. Lin HS, Liu YK, Ray G, Nikravesh PE (1978) Systems identification for material properties of a lumbar intervertebral joint. J Biomech 11:1–14
76. Yoganandan N (1986) Biomechanical identification of injury to an intervertebral joint. Clin Biomech 3:149
77. Rolander SD, Blair WE (1975) Deformation and fracture of the lumbar vertebral end plate. Orthop Clin N Am 6:75–81
78. Coventry MB, Ghormley RK, Kernohan JW (1945) The intervertebral disc: Its microscopic anatomy and pathology. Part III. Pathological changes in the intervertebral disc. J Bone Joint Surg 27A:460–474
79. Horst M, Brinckmann P (1981) Measurement of the distribution of axial stress on the end-plate of the vertebral body. Spine 6:217–232
80. Hansson T, Roos B (1981) The relation between bone mineral content, experimental compression fractures and disc degeneration in lumbar vertebrae. Spine 6:147–153
81. Nachemson A (1960) Lumbar intradiscal pressure. Acta Orthop Scand (Suppl) 43:1–104

82. Nachemson A (1963) The influence of spinal movements on the lumbar intradiscal pressure and on the tensile stress in annulus fibrosus. Acta Orthop Scand 33:183–207
83. Adams MA, Hutton WC (1980) The effect of posture on the role of the apophysial joints in resisting intervertebral compressive forces. J Bone Joint Surg 62B:358–362
84. Buchanan JR, Myers C, Greer RB, Lloyd T, Varano LA (1987) Assessment of the risk of vertebral fracture in menopausal women. J Bone Joint Surg 69A:212–218
85. Yamada J (1970) Strength of biological materials. Williams and Wilkins, Baltimore
86. McElhaney JH (1966) Dynamic response of bone and muscle tissue. J Appl Physiol 21:1231–1236
87. Wu HC, Rao RF (1976) Mechanical behavior of the human annulus fibrosus. J Biomech 9:1–7
88. Carter DR, Hayes WC (1977) The compressive behavior of bone as a two-phase porous structure. J Bone Joint Surg 59A:954–962
89. Schultz AB, Andersson GBJ (1981) Analysis of loads on the lumbar spine. Spine 6:76–82
90. Rolander SD (1966) Motion of the lumbar spine with special reference to the stabilizing effect of posterior fusion. Acta Orthop Scand (Suppl) 90:1–144
91. Markolf KL (1972) Deformation of the thoracolumbar intervertebral joints in response to external loads. J Bone Joint Surg 54A:511–533
92. Myklebust JB, Yoganandan N, Sances A Jr (1987) Failure biomechanics of thoracolumbar vertebrae. ASME Adv Bioeng, pp 99–100

Bone Density, Distribution, and Estimated Strength

CHRISTOPHER E. CANN, J. KEENAN BROWN, and ALAN IWASHITA[1]

Key Words. Bone mineral density, computed tomography, structural analysis, bone strength, finite element analysis, osteoporosis, mathematical models

Introduction

The definition of osteoporosis as a disease or process has remained imprecise. It is defined by the NIH Consensus Panel on Osteoporosis as "an age-related disorder characterized by decreased bone mass and by increased susceptibility to fractures in the absence of other recognizable causes of bone loss". There are many techniques available to assess "bone mass", but no exact definition exists for "decreased bone mass", because all of the methods used show a substantial overlap between values obtained in the non-fracture population and the clinically osteoporotic (fracture) population [1,2]. Many investigators define osteoporosis relative to an absolute threshold level for bone mass below which fractures are observed in some patients. Depending on the technique used, this level can classify between 30% and 80% of the normal age-matched elderly population as osteoporotic. Bone mass or bone density measurements are important, but they are not sufficient to predict which patients will sustain atraumatic fractures. Other factors must also contribute significantly to increased susceptibility to fractures due to osteoporosis.

Conventional bone measurements do not identify the individual at risk for fracture. Current efforts comparing the "sensitivity and specificity" of one measurement technique with another in population studies assume that population-based risk assessments will translate into better management of

[1] Department of Radiology and Bioengineering Graduate Group, University of California, San Francisco, CA 94143, USA

patients [3,4]. From a public health perspective this may be true—i.e., a 10% improvement in specificity for a population may save millions of dollars by determining which patients do not need treatment. As with most clinical tests, bone assessment (by mineral density or other properties) divides the population into three groups: (a) not at risk or minimal risk, (b) high risk, and (c) equivocal. The greatest gains in terms of public health can be achieved by narrowing the "equivocal" range, so that more patients must be classified as either non-risk (therefore no treatment) or high risk (definitely requiring treatment), thus eliminating the costs associated with unnecessary prophylactic treatment.

Bone density is like serum cholesterol; it is a risk factor which can be used to determine the need for further testing. If serum cholesterol is high, a patient is referred to a cardiologist for further assessment. The patient may be sent for a stress test to determine the capability of the heart to handle abnormal loads. Myocardial perfusion at rest may be normal, but under the stress of exercise, the blood flow may be reduced to such an extent that the risk of heart attack increases dramatically. The stress test identifies the individual patient at risk of heart attack under conditions likely to be experienced in normal life.

There are no "stress tests" to identify osteoporotic patients, however. An individual with osteoporosis is identified clinically as one who has reduced bone mass and has had a minimally traumatic fracture. In other words, the patient's bones have already suffered their first "heart attack". The utility of routine bone density measurements is similar to that of serum cholesterol measurements, or at best, of basal myocardial perfusion studies. At present, there are no noninvasive methods for determining a defect in bone strength due to osteoporosis. Our recent work has been directed toward the development of an osteoporosis stress test whereby the individual patient can be evaluated for her or his bone fracture risk under normal living conditions.

Bone Mass and Bone Strength

Estimation of the risk of fracture of a particular bone requires the ability to relate measurable properties of the bone to its strength as well as some knowledge of the expected loading conditions. In the laboratory, experiments have been done isolating a portion of a bone, measuring some mechanical properties of the bone tissue under a defined set of loading conditions, and then comparing the mechanical properties with some other parameter, typically mass or density. Numerous experiments of this type have been done [5–14], but even under the best conditions, the mineral density of an individual piece of bone cannot be used to predict with a high degree of accuracy what its individual mechanical properties will be. Compact bone shows a closer relationship between bone mineral density (BMD) and strength than does trabecular bone, where the material does not follow the normal engineering assumptions of homogeneity.

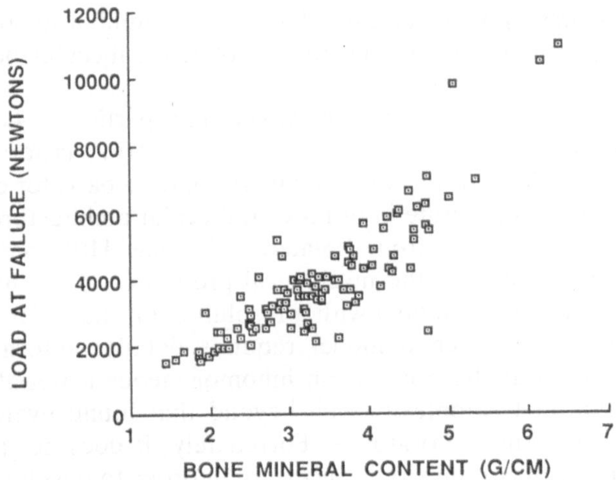

Fig. 1. Bone strength as a function of bone mineral content. The relationship was determined by mechanical testing of vertebral specimens obtained at autopsy from non-fracture individuals. Note that for the same bone mineral content, the load at failure can vary by factors of 2 to 3, but that there is a general nonlinear relationship which corresponds to that seen in isolated bone cubes or cylinders. (From [16], with permission)

A second class of experiments has been done in an attempt to relate measurable properties of whole bones (mass or density) to their strength [15–20] under conditions approximating the in vivo situation. The hypothesis in these experiments is that a measurement of bone mass done in vivo can be used to estimate the strength of the whole bone, and by inference, its resistance to fracture. Again, even under carefully controlled laboratory conditions, BMD and strength are not related closely enough to allow the strength of an individual bone to be predicted from its mass with a high degree of accuracy, with only 50%–60% of the variance (r = 0.7–0.8) explained by the hypothesized relationship in most experiments (Fig. 1). In addition, these laboratory results can be extrapolated to the clinical situation only to a very limited extent because little is known about the exact loading conditions on the bones in vivo.

Analysis of bone using engineering principles requires explicit knowledge of its material properties, including modes of elastic (reversible) and plastic (irreversible) deformation, as defined by modulus and geometrical distortion on loading, the stress at which deformation becomes mostly plastic (yield stress), and the relationship between these properties in all dimensions being analyzed. The literature on orthopedic biomechanics that has been published over the past 20 years provides a large body of information about these properties, most of which is contained in studies of trabecular or compact bone around prosthetic implants or as part of their design. The recent interest in bone structure in osteoporosis research has led to a number of studies of bone properties in isolated specimens, mostly in isolated trabecular bone or whole bones [16–21].

For the most part, the data on bone mechanical properties has been generated with specimens large enough to satisfy the engineering criterion of homogeneity. Therefore, these results are not an appropriate basis for constructing a model of a bone that is accurate in terms of trabecular architecture. To do this, we would have to use data from isolated trabeculae [10] combined with a known architecture, estimate the mechanical properties of the intertrabecular spaces, and construct a 3-D model with a resolution on the order of 10–20 μm. However, validation of such a model requires detailed information at the microscopic level about the bone as an inhomogeneous material as well as a level of computational complexity well beyond that found even in the most sophisticated engineering laboratories. Fortunately, it does not appear at the present time that such complexity is necessary in order to develop macroscopic models of whole bones.

Simple application of engineering principles to the measurement or analysis of bone properties dictates that the distribution of bone mineral will affect the strength of a whole bone. Normalization of mineral density by cross-sectional area in the vertebrae [15] and various methods for analysis of the proximal femur [22,23] have been shown in vitro to be helpful in better estimating bone strength. Recent work [24] has shown that including a large number of regional BMD measurements when comparing bone mineral and whole bone strength in the vertebrae adds significantly to the predictive capability of BMD, to the point that up to 80%–90% of the variance can be explained. Such in vitro work is of necessity limited to only a small number of specimens used to study the relationships, and even in the most complex analyses, only a small amount of the available information about bone distribution is used, further limiting the application of engineering principles to the case where the patient closely matches the laboratory experiment.

Mathematical Models for Bone Structural Analysis

Mathematical modeling can help extend in vitro results to the in vivo situation. If a problem or a structure can be described mathematically, a set of tools exists with which the results of the single experiment of set of experiments can be extrapolated to the class. Modeling is applied in one of two ways: (1) using the results of a series of experiments as input to develop an output related to the class, or (2) using a generic description to learn something about the elements which make up the class. The first application is the one used classically in orthopedics, for example, to design prostheses that are useful in a certain class of patients. The second application is illustrated by physiological modeling studies such as calcium tracer kinetics, where data from an individual is input into a specified model of calcium homeostasis to obtain results related to the individual.

The requirements for these applications of modeling are different: In the first case, the accuracy of the model is most important because any output of the model must conform to a set of specifications, whereas in the second case, the information sought can be relative within the class, and it is more important to analyze each element in the same way than to try to optimize analysis for each element by changing the model in search of a more "accurate" result.

Numerical or analytical modeling is an efficient means of including bone distribution in the analysis of BMD and its relationship to bone strength. Many bones may be modeled as simple structures, but in doing so, the important information about heterogeneous bone mineral distribution may be lost as discrete elements are averaged in order to minimize the complexity of the model. Alternatively, developing a model of an individual bone to high accuracy restricts the results to that particular bone, reducing its utility as a model for the whole class containing that bone. A clinically useful tool from which conclusions about individual patients can be drawn requires a physiological model in which the relative contributions of the structure's principal load-bearing components reflect the known situation in the specific population to be studied. At the same time, the model must be sufficiently general to allow for the biological variability within that population.

The physiological modeling approach to bone as a structure and the use of that result to evaluate patients has been very limited. Most modeling of bone has been undertaken from an engineering perspective, to try to produce an accurate result. Any attempt to develop an accurate engineering model of real bones in a large number of patients is bound to be compromised from the start. In vivo loading is not measured directly. Physical properties of the bone and associated tissues—i.e., hydration, tension in ligaments, microarchitecture, and resiliency of the bone tissue—cannot be determined noninvasively. The amount of work required to develop accurate mathematical or numerical models to describe each bone individually would be prohibitive. Thus, any attempt to use physiological modeling of bone in a clinical setting must first reduce the problem to a few important and measurable parameters which have clinical significance, i.e., which are useful in the evaluation of the individual patient. When these parameters have been defined, a model that can be generalized to a class of patients can be developed and validated using classical engineering tests.

Of what clinical use is a mathematical model of a single bone in a patient? If we can estimate the strength of a bone more accurately by including distribution as well as bone density, we should in theory be able to better separate patients with a high risk of fracture from the low-risk group. This diagnostic sensitivity is important, but it may be of limited clinical value because most patients in the high risk groups are identified by means other than bone density. Thus, the addition of a complex numerical modeling step to patient workup may not be cost-effective by itself. If, however, an osteoporosis stress test with data for an individual patient can be used to simulate changes in the amount and distribution of bone within the envelope for which the model has been developed, then the altered data set can be tested to see if the "strength" of the bone has been altered.

A method of this kind has two clinical uses. First, the key to treating osteoporosis is prevention, and therapies are available to prevent postmenopausal bone loss as well as, in some cases, other osteoporoses. Prophylactic therapy is expensive, however, and may also be contraindicated in some individuals. A method whereby the bone structure of an individual patient could be "aged" by applying average alterations in the distribution of bone, and then tested to see if the individual may be at risk for fracture at some time in the future, could minimize the need for therapy; it could also be used to determine optimal timing for serial bone mass measurements. The second clinical requirement for such a test comes from the partial efficacy of newer treatments for established osteoporosis. The goal of such therapies is to prevent further osteoporotic fractures. The pharmaceuticals and hormones currently under investigation have been shown to add bone or prevent bone loss differentially between compact and trabecular bone, and this may be one of the major reasons that clinical trials have shown mixed results. With the exception of prospective fracture incidence studies, there is no way at present to determine whether added mineral also adds significantly to the strength of the bone, and these studies are very time-consuming and expensive. In addition, there is no way of telling whether an individual patient may benefit more from one therapy than from another, thus requiring a "guesswork" approach to treatment. The use of a model of a bone to "add" bone mathematically and then determine whether it increased in strength could be used in the choice of therapy for an individual osteoporotic patient.

Methods and Analysis

We have used 3-dimensional quantitative computed tomography (3-D QCT) as the BMD determination method for our studies because it reveals the complete three-dimensional distribution of bone at a spatial resolution of about 1 mm and because, in our laboratory, it has a reproducibility for BMD of about 0.7%. The methods we have developed for structural analysis are applied to this 3-D data set but can be applied to 2-D bone mineral data sets from dual-energy X-ray absorptiometry (DEXA) as well. Our initial work used the finite element method of analysis (FEA) as a tool for structural analysis; more recently, we have developed simplified methods which can reduce the computation time significantly, allowing us to use complex model geometries to more accurately represent the bones. Results from a comparison of these methods are also given here.

Virtually all QCT work is done using a simplified method whereby a single scan is taken through each of several vertebrae [2]. This method ignores

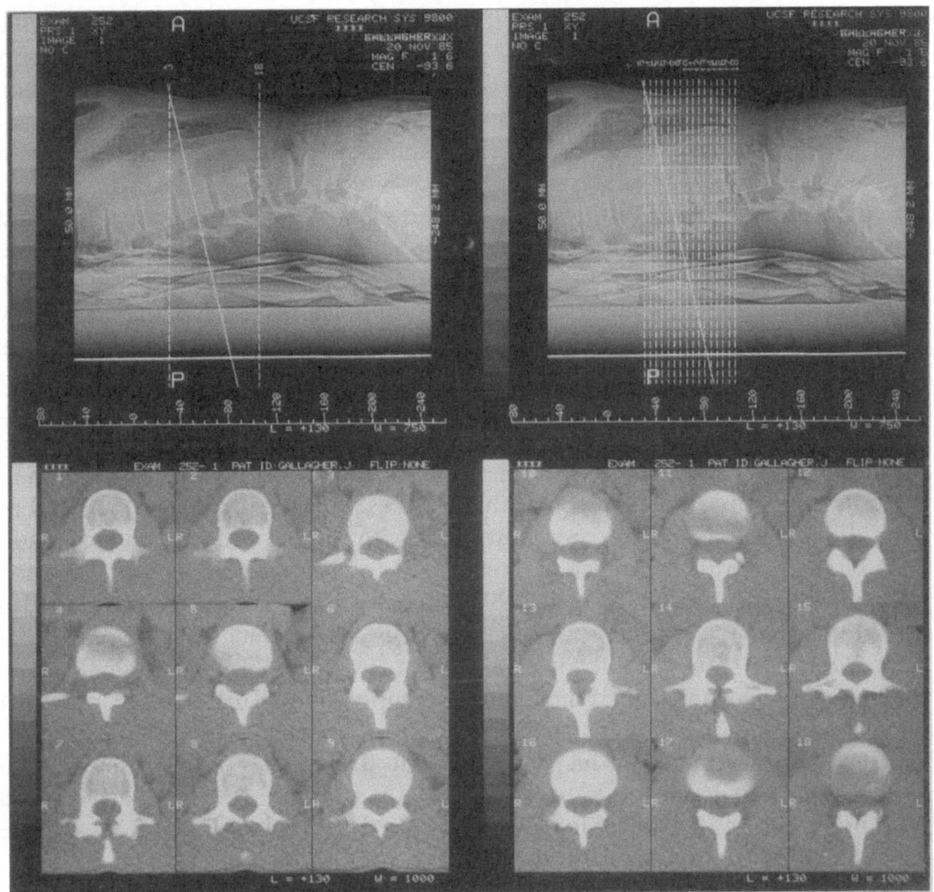

Fig. 2. 3-D quantitative computed tomography (QCT) technique uses a set of contiguous CT scans covering two complete vertebrae to acquire a 3-D data set with resolution of approximately 1 mm in each dimension. Resulting data can be rotated to any configuration and automatically registered to scans of the same vertebrae done at subsequent times, eliminating positioning errors for region-of-interest analysis

vertebral structure. The 3-D QCT method, which was first developed in the late 1970s [25–27], has been in continual use by our laboratory since that time; it is currently capable of measuring trabecular mineral density with a reproducibility of 0.7%–0.8% [28,29] (Fig. 2). Total vertebral mineral can be measured with a reproducibility of 1.0% [28]. Regional mineral density can also be measured, to a resolution on the order of 1–2 mm. CT data are acquired using the 3-D technique at low radiation dose and in a total scanning time of under 2 min. The data obtained are converted to BMD using a standard K_2HPO_4 calibration phantom, then interpolated and rotated in 3-D to provide a standard and reproducible geometry for regional mineral analysis and stress analysis. For multiple studies, the 3-D CT data sets are automatically superimposed to a resolution of about 0.5 mm, virtually eliminating repositioning errors in serial studies. This methodology has been a key facet in our development work, because these BMD measurements make a small contribution to the overall error in our analysis, simplifying interpretation of the data.

Finite element analysis is a well-developed method for structural analysis and computational fluid dynamics. Instead of attempting to model a complete object analytically, FEA relies on the assumption that any structure can be divided into a large number of substructures, or elements, each defined uniquely by its material properties, its position within the overall structure, and its connectivity to neighboring elements. Thus, it is ideally suited as a method to analyze quantitative data obtained from 2-D or 3-D imaging. While FEA is a very powerful tool, it also has significant drawbacks. The primary problem is the fact that, as the number of elements in the model gets larger, the computer time required to solve the problem scales with the square of the number of nodes. Thus, a 1000-element problem with simple 8-noded cubic geometry becomes intractable when converted to 2000 elements of 20-noded isoparametric geometry. In order to approach this problem, we developed a simple mathematical formalism which replaces a 32-element matrix representing each 1-mm axial slice through a vertebra with an equivalent single node when loading is maintained in uniaxial compression. This has the effect of reducing a complex 3-dimensional problem to a linear array of simple springs, and the solution time is reduced from about 10 h to only a few minutes. We have tested the simple model relative to FEA and found that under standard conditions, the results for "yield" of a vertebra are virtually identical, and the reproducibility of analysis is on the order of 1%–1.5% (Fig. 3).

Finite element analysis or other structural analysis requires data on material properties; 3-D QCT measures BMD. Following thorough study, we chose to use the data of Carter and Hayes [11] as the best estimate for the relationship between BMD, elastic modulus, and yield stress of bone. As a test of the adequacy of this choice, we (mathematically) isolated cubes of trabecular bone from the center of osteoporotic and normal vertebrae and subjected them to incremental loading to failure in the FEA. The results showed excellent agreement with theoretical predictions [30,31]. We also compared the FEA-determined yield stress of these trabecular cubes with other investigators' published yield stress data determined in cylindrical autopsy specimens of vertebral trabecular bone by in vitro mechanical testing [21]. For the same range of trabecular mineral density (30–200 mg/cm^3), our computer-determined yield of 0.02–2.4 MPa compared favorably with the published data for yield stress in the vertical direction of 0.1–2.7 MPa. Further tests using very simple finite element models for the vertebrae (3 × 3 × 5 mm brick elements, about 600 per vertebral body) showed similar results. Computer-determined yield stress ranged from 0.8 to 2.8 MPa in normal subjects and 0.2 to 1.0 MPa in osteoporotics, with little overlap in the data compared to the large overlap in

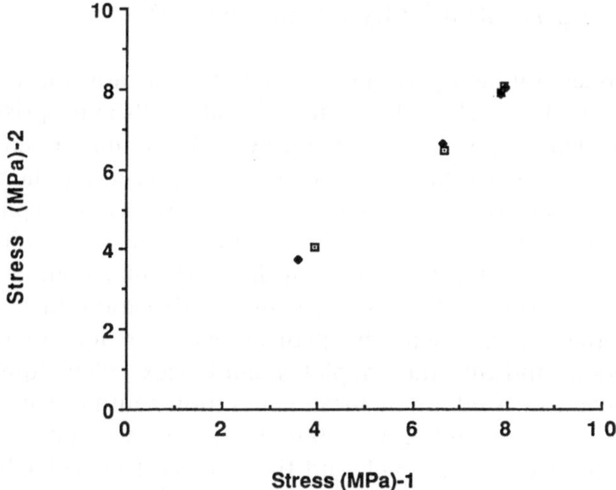

Fig. 3. Reproducibility of yield stress determined from duplicate CT scans done on the same day in patients. Average precision is about 1.5%, both for finite element analysis (FEA) and a simplified dynamic model which simulates the FEA measurement. Note the excellent correspondence between the simple and FEA analyses, allowing the simplified model to be used in most routine cases. *Open squares with dots*, stress FEA; *solid squares*, simplified model

total bone mineral content [28,29]. These results can be compared to published data from in vitro mechanical testing of whole vertebral bodies by Hansson et al. [16]; failure stresses for his work for the 39 L1 and L2 vertebrae from non-osteoporotic women aged 34–74 years old were 1.0 to 4.9 MPa, again showing good agreement of our data with in vitro testing.

We also tested the capabilities of FEA to conduct regional analysis in the bone, again using very simple models [32]. Previous studies by Rockoff et al. [33] have shown that the vertebral cortex contributes 45%–75% of the peak vertebral strength, while McBroom et al. [15] concluded the contribution was only 10%. We tested whole vertebral bodies "intact", then again following mathematical removal of the vertebral cortex; the difference in total load at "yield" was defined as the cortical contribution to vertebral strength. In the 9 normal vertebrae tested (mean trabecular mineral density [TMD] 160 mg/cm^3), average contribution due to the cortex was 12.4% of yield stress, while in the 9 vertebrae from osteoporotic individuals (mean TMD 39 mg/cm^3) the cortex contributed an average of 56%. Perhaps a more significant finding was that in patients with osteoporosis, the total load estimated to be borne by the cortex relative to the trabecular core was constant for all values of trabecular mineral density, at a ratio of about two-thirds load on the cortex and one-third in the trabecular bone, whereas in normals there was no such relationship.

Results Using an Anatomically Accurate Model

We have extended our early results using a significantly more complex but anatomically correct model of the vertebral body with appropriate separation of those regions which may respond variably to a stimulus. Each individual 1-mm-thick section is divided into 32 elements, 16 representing the cortex and 16 representing internal trabecular bone. This allows us to separate out the endplates, the anterior and posterior cortex at different vertical levels, and the anterior as well as the left and right posterior trabecular bone at those levels. This division was prompted in part by our observation that a number of patients lose bone rapidly near the pedicles while maintaining the anterior trabecular portion, and that the endplates and cortex behave quite differently as well. We have now used a new mesh generation routine, with the "cortex" represented by a shell including the 400–600-μm-thick compact bone and the transition region between this shell and the internal trabecular body, and the trabecular core, represented by larger elements (Fig. 4). The mesh is designed to fit the three-dimensional geometry of any patient's vertebra, deforming as necessary. This new geometry is a much better representation of the real

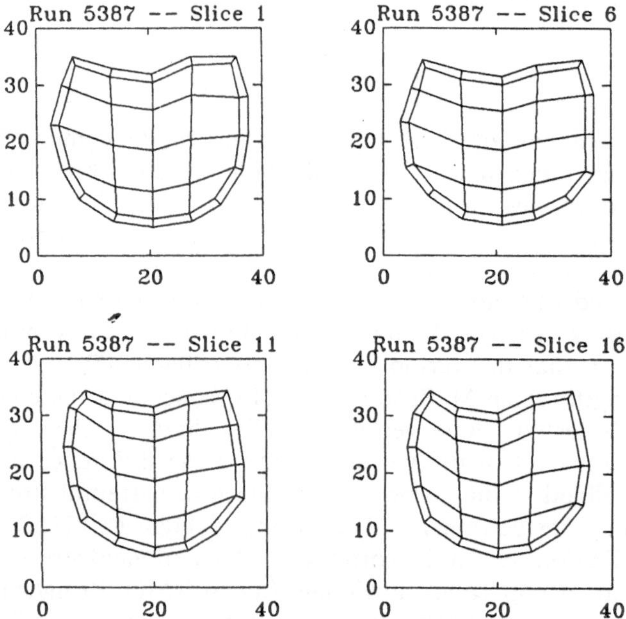

Fig. 4. Diagram of FEA mesh generated automatically at four of the typical 30 levels in the vertebral body. "Cortex" is comprised of 16 elements and central "trabecular" area is the other 16 elements. Conversion of bone density to material properties for each element is done using the relationship of Carter and Hayes [11]

vertebra, but it introduces significant complexity in the mesh generation, the connectivity matrix, and the extraction of results from the output data file. However, even with these complicating factors, it is a more accurate model for analysis, because vertebrae from all patients have the same number of elements with the same relationship among elements, and isolation of the cortical shell, transition zone, and trabecular core is much more accurate.

We have tested this new model geometry using loading conditions similar to those seen in vivo, where the vertebral body is loaded on both endplates, not just the superior one, and the stresses propagate through both endplates into the center of the vertebral body. By fixing the vertebral model at the pedicles, cumulative stresses in the central portion of the vertebra can be measured, as well as the point at which this plane undergoes plastic (irreversible) deformation. We have analyzed the relationship between stress and the volume of the whole vertebral body which has undergone plastic deformation in a number of data sets. We found that a vertebral stress-strain curve can be divided into three regions: as a vertebral model is loaded, it undergoes elastic deformation up to a point where the first element yields (volume of plastic deformation equals zero); as loading continues to increase, there can then be a gradual increase in the volume of bone which has made the transition from elastic to plastic deformation; and finally, the energy stored within the bone reaches a point where only a slight increase in load is required to cause rapid yield of a significant volume of the bone. Physically, the last region can be thought of as the point where the bone fractures, with the few percent of volume undergoing plastic deformation corresponding to a 10% or greater decrease in anterior vertebral height, similar to the definition of fracture used clinically. For the sake of definition, we have adopted a criterion we call "model failure", where 50% of the volume of a 5-mm contiguous segment of the vertebral body has made the transition from elastic to plastic deformation. This physical correspondence between model deformation and clinical fracture modes appears to provide a more realistic definition of "yield" than does a yield stress definition based on laboratory testing, but it is in no way intended to represent an actual value of the failure stress or load of that bone if it was subjected to in vitro testing under controlled conditions. Another important point in favor of this analysis is the fact that it is model-independent, that is, the whole bone is always considered, rather than merely a specific plane or specified elements in the model, and it can thus be used to analyze any bone under any loading conditions.

With incorporation of these modifications into the computer analysis of 3-D QCT data sets, we have solved many of the problems we had in our initial studies. Figure 3 shows that the reproducibility of the computer-predicted "model failure" is on the order of 1%–2% instead of the 13% we had obtained at the outset. We have analyzed a series of data sets similar to the one used in our earlier studies. The results are shown in Figs. 5 and 6. When we analyzed pre- and postmenopausal normal and osteoporotic women, we saw the expected decrease of TMD with age and existence of fracture. We also saw that our "model failure" criterion separated the non-fracture from fracture cases better than TMD. Of particular interest is the fact that while postmenopausal women without fractures lost the expected 20%–25% in TMD from age 50 to 60, representing a total vertebral mass decrease of 10%–12%, the "yield strength" decreased over 50% [34] (Fig. 7). While it can be argued that the modeling may not provide an accurate estimate of the true bone strength, these data clearly support the use of a "physiological model" of the vertebral body.

Discussion

Conventional measurements of bone mineral density can be used to help in the management of patients suspected to be at risk for osteoporosis, primarily by classifying them as "at some risk" or "at no risk" at the time of the exam. They are not sufficient, however, to identify with accuracy the absolute risk of an individual patient for the future development of fractures, nor can they be used to try to predict such future risk. Bone density measurements can be used to measure the change in total bone mass with therapy, but extrapolation of bone mass change to a corresponding change in bone strength requires major assumptions about the relationship between bone mass and bone strength in vivo.

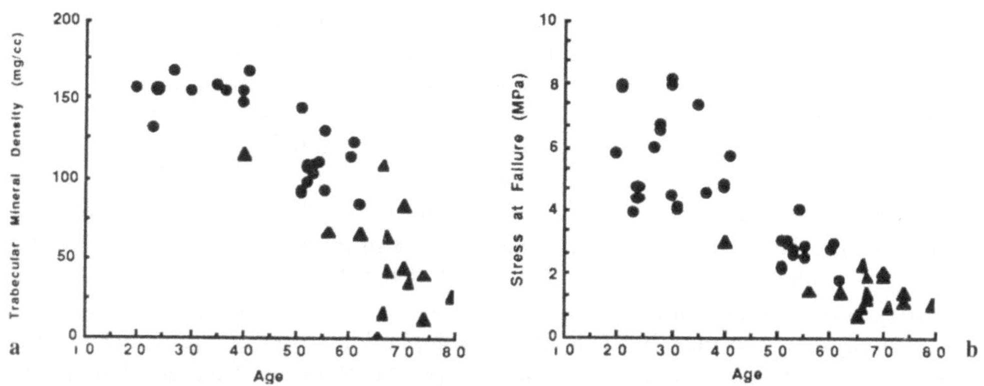

Fig. 5.a Relationship of trabecular density (normal QCT) to age in women. *Circles*, non-fracture; *triangles*, fracture. The normal 10%–20% decrease due to menopause is noted at about age 50, as is the normal threshold level of 110–120 mg/cc, below which vertebral fractures begin to occur. **b** Estimated vertebral strength in the same women as a function of age. Note that there is a wide variation in strength in premenopausal women even when the trabecular mineral density (TMD) is similar (ages 20–40). Also note that there is a large decrease in whole bone strength at the menopause even though the loss in TMD is only 10%–20%. This indicates that the loss of interior trabecular bone may be the primary factor in reduced bone strength in postmenopausal osteoporosis. *Circles*, non-fracture; *triangles*, fracture

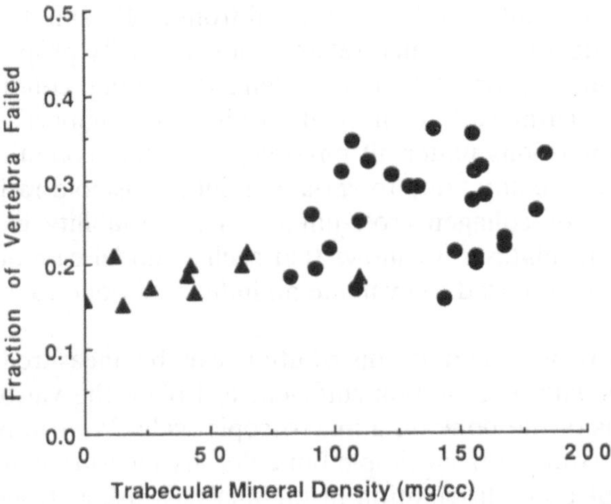

Fig. 6. Fraction of whole vertebra "failed" at the point that 50% of a contiguous 5-mm-thick region has collapsed, similar to the clinical appearance of a fracture. In osteoporotics, the failure is very uniform, with failure almost always resulting in a collapse of 15%–20% of the whole bone. In contrast, vertebrae from normal patients fail at higher loads and with no apparent relationship to density. *Circles*, non-fracture; *triangles*, fracture

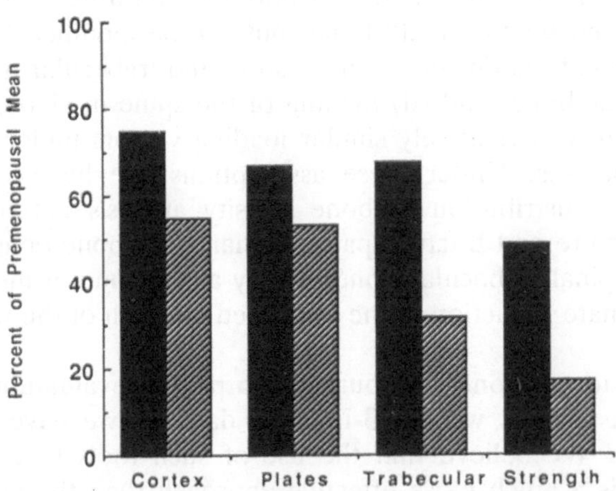

Fig. 7. Change in mineral density and strength in the vertebral cortex, regions near endplates, and central trabecular region relative to premenopausal women shows regional bone loss with menopause and osteoporosis. Estimated strength of whole bone shows a greater decrease than mineral density of any of the individual compartments. Measured bone density in any compartment can be mathematically "changed" for an individual patient, then the strength reestimated to see the effect of adding or subtracting bone regionally. *Solid bars*, postmenopausal women; *hatched bars*, osteoporotic women

Absolute bone strength could be estimated from BMD and its distribution by using a mathematical model which relates known density properties to known engineering material properties under defined loading conditions. Such a model requires accurately known relationships for compact and trabecular bone in three dimensions under all physiologic loading conditions and for all variations in bone "quality" due to variable mineral: osteoid ratio, crystal size, microarchitecture, or collagen cross-linking. The variability in the published density to strength relationship shows that such a model cannot be developed at the present time and used to evaluate an individual bone to a high degree of accuracy.

Bone mineral density and its distribution can be measured accurately in three dimensions with a resolution sufficient to isolate the various structurally important regions of the bone on a macroscopic scale. We can improve on the estimate of bone strength from simple bone density measurements by including information about bone distribution in the analysis, using structural engineering analysis tools. However, it must be recognized that any such model will be restricted in its accuracy by the same problem noted above, i.e., that the variability in the relationship between density and strength, even under laboratory conditions, is large. We have developed and tested such a model under the following assumptions: (a) bone density and bone material properties are related globally as given in the literature from materials testing experiments, (b) compact and trabecular bone are treated as a continuum of variable porosity, as is done in the orthopedic literature, (c) the published properties are given for "normal" bone, but can be modified for "abnormal" bone using published relationships, such as isolated trabecular bone strength in normal *vs* fluorotic bone, and (d) loading of the spine in vivo occurs within a specific range and with relatively similar loading vectors under normal conditions in most humans. Under these assumptions, we have shown that the inclusion of bone distribution in bone density analysis better discriminates between non-fracture and fracture patients than does bone density alone, and that the loss of spinal trabecular bone density at the time of menopause leads to a disproportionate reduction in the estimated strength of the whole vertebral body.

The incorporation of bone distribution into patient evaluations can be done with 2-D DEXA data as well as 3-D QCT data, as we have done, using a similar approach. We believe that the use of such tools to evaluate the individual patient is a much more effective approach than the use of statistical analysis to determine population-based optimal evaluation or treatment. While epidemiological studies can give useful information about those factors which contribute a small but significant risk to the development of osteoporosis, the heterogeneity of osteoporosis makes it even more necessary to be sure that those factors which can contribute a highly significant risk for the individual patient are included in the evaluation. Clinical medicine is still involved in the treatment of the individual patient, and with better recognition of the individual at risk we will be able to treat the population as a whole more efficiently.

Summary. The relationship between bone mineral density (BMD) and the actual strength of a bone depends not only on the amount of bone but also on the distribution of bone substance within the structure. Bone geometry and bone distribution are optimized by the normal loads placed on the bone during growth and development; osteoporosis results when the amount and distribution of bone are not sufficient to support these normal loads. Conventional bone density measurements do not use available information about bone distribution in the evaluation of patient data. By combining these measures with structural analysis methods, however, an estimate of relative bone strength can be obtained.

Traditional engineering analysis of bone has sought to obtain highly accurate models which can be used to predict the loads which will develop when prostheses are placed in the bone. These models require accurate material properties and use well-defined loading conditions to predict the forces within the bone and its process of remodeling to reduce internal stresses to normal. A different approach is used for the relative analysis of bone function, where instead of predicting the actual forces in the bone, it suffices to define a criterion which accurately predicts the clinical endpoint, i.e., fracture. This is similar to a myocardial stress test, where cardiac perfusion is only estimated but the patient is classified relative to a population of at-risk patients.

We have developed a similar osteoporosis stress test by coupling 3-D bone measurements with structural analysis. The analysis better separates fracture from non-fracture patients than does BMD alone and can be used to predict a future relative risk of fracture from mathematical analysis of a current BMD study. It will also be useful in determining the optimal drug therapy for individual patients instead of relying on population-based studies.

References

1. Riggs BL, Wahner HW, Seeman E, Melton LJ III, Mazess RB (1982) Changes in bone mineral density of the proximal femur and spine with aging. Differences between the postmenopausal and senile osteoporosis syndromes. J Clin Invest 70:716–723
2. Cann CE, Genant HK, Kolb FO, Ettinger B (1985) Quantitative computed tomography for prediction of vertebral fracture risk. Bone 6:1–7
3. Wasnich RD, Ross PD, Heilbrun LK, Vogel JM (1987) Selection of the optimal site for fracture risk prediction. Clin Orthop 216:262–268
4. Reinbold WD, Genant HK, Reiser UJ, Harris ST, Ettinger B (1986) Bone mineral content in early postmenopausal and postmenopausal osteoporotic women: Comparison of measurement methods. Radiology 160:469–478
5. Williams JL, Lewis JL (1982) Properties of an anisotropic model of cancellous bone from the proximal tibial epiphysis. J Biomech Eng 104:50–56
6. Weaver JK, Chalmers J (1966) Cancellous bone: Its strength and changes with aging and an evaluation of some methods for measuring its mineral content. J Bone Joint Surg 48A:289–298

7. Galante J, Rostoker W, Ray RD (1970) Physical properties of trabecular bone. Calcif Tiss Res 5:236–246
8. Behrens JC, Walker PS, Shojo H (1974) Variations in strength and structure of cancellous bone at the knee. Biomechanics 7:201–207
9. Chatterji S, Wall JC, Jeffery JW (1981) Age-related changes in the orientation and particle size of the mineral phase in human femoral cortical bone. Calcif Tissue Int 33:567–574
10. Mente PL, Lewis JL (1989) Experimental method for the measurement of the elastic modulus of trabecular bone tissue. J Orthop Res 7:456–461
11. Carter DR, Hayes WC (1977) The behavior of bone as a two-phase porous structure. J Bone Joint Surg 59A:954–962
12. Mosekilde Li (1989) Sex differences in age-related loss of vertebral trabecular bone mass and structure-biomechanical consequences. Bone 10:425–432
13. Mosekilde Li, Viidik A, Mosekilde Le (1985) Correlation between the compressive strength of iliac and vertebral trabecular bone in normal individuals. Bone 6:291–295
14. Kuhn JL, Goldstein SA, Choi K, London M, Feldkamp LA, Matthews LS (1989) Comparison of the trabecular and cortical tissue moduli from human iliac crests. J Orthop Res 7:876–884
15. McBroom RJ, Hayes WC, Edwards WT, Goldberg RP, While AA (1985) Prediction of vertebral body compressive fracture using quantitative computed tomography. J Bone Joint Surg 67A:1206
16. Hansson T, Roos B, Nachemson A (1980) The bone mineral content and ultimate compressive strength of lumbar vertebrae. Spine 5:45–55
17. Mosekilde Li, Bentzen SM, Ortoft G, Jorgensen J (1989) The predictive value of quantitative computed tomography for vertebral body compressive strength and ash density. Bone 10:465–470
18. Dannucci GA, Martin RB, Cann CE (1987) Relationship between CT derived bone mineral content and the compressive mechanical properties of the canine lumbar spine. J Biomech 20:898
19. Martin RB, Burr DB (1984) Non-invasive measurement of long bone cross-sectional moment of inertia by photon absorptiometry. J Biomech 17:195–201
20. Young DR, Howard WH, Cann CE, Steele CR (1979) Non-invasive measures of bone bending rigidity in the monkey (m. Nemestrina). Calcif Tiss Int 27:109–115
21. Mosekilde Li, Mosekilde Le, Danielsen CC (1987) Biomechanical competence of vertebral trabecular bone in relation to ash density and age in normal individuals. Bone 8:79–85
22. Beck TJ, Ruff CB, Warden KE, Scott WW, Rao GU (1990) Predicting femoral neck strength from bone mineral data. Invest Radiol 25:6–18
23. Leichter I, Margulies JY, Weinreb A (1982) The relationship between bone density, mineral content, and mechanical strength in the femoral neck. Clin Orthop 163:272–281
24. Cody DD, Goldstein SA, Flynn MJ, Brown EB (1991) Correlations between vertebral regional bone mineral density (rBMD) and whole bone fracture load. Spine 16:146–154
25. Cann CE, Genant HK, Boyd DP (1978) Spinal bone mineral determination in patients using dual-energy computed tomography. Presented at Radiological Society of North America 64th Scientific Assembly, Chicago

26. Cann CE, Genant HK, Young DR (1980) Comparison of vertebral and peripheral mineral loss in disuse osteoporosis in monkeys. Radiology 134:525–529
27. Cann CE, Genant HK (1980) Precise measurement of vertebral mineral content using computed tomography. J Comput Assist Tomogr 4:493–500
28. Cann CE, Henzl M, Burry K (1987) Reversible bone loss is produced by the GnRH agonist nafarelin. In: Cohn DV, Martin TJ, Meunier PJ (eds) Calcium regulation and bone metabolism: Basic and clinical aspects, vol. 9, Elsevier, pp 123–127
29. Cavanaugh DJ, Cann CE (1988) Brisk walking does not stop bone loss in post-menopausal women. Bone 9:201–204
30. Faulkner, KG, Cann CE (1989) Quantitative computed tomography and finite element modeling to predict vertebral fractures. J Bone Min Res 4:S234
31. Faulkner KG, Cann CE (1989) Patient-specific finite element models for analysis of vertebral strength. Radiology 173(P):415
32. Faulkner KG, Cann CE, Hasegawa BH (1991) The effect of bone distribution on vertebral strength using patient-specific nonlinear finite element analysis. Radiology 179:669–674
33. Rockoff SD, Sweet E, Blenstein J (1969) The relative contribution of trabecular and cortical bone to the strength of human lumbar vertebrae. Calcif Tiss Res 3:163–175
34. Cann CE, Brown JK (1991) In vivo vertebral strength is highly dependent on average trabecular bone density, but not total bone mineral content. J Bone Min Res 6:S-175

Stress Analysis of the Lumbar Spine Using the Finite Element Model

YOSHISHIGE ARAI[1], HIDEAKI E. TAKAHASHI[1], and HIROYUKI SUZUKI[2]

Key Words. Lumbar spine, biomechanics, stress analysis, finite element method, three-dimensional model

Introduction

At present, it is almost impossible to accurately measure the stress distribution of bones directly. The stress distribution of a normal spine should be investigated to identify the weak points of the spinal column, and analysis of the influence of trauma, degenerative changes, and surgical procedures including instrumentation are also important. The finite element method (FEM) is a simulation technique that could provide a significant advantage to achieve these purposes [1–3]. Two- and three-dimensional FEM models were employed to simulate and evaluate the behavior of a normal lumbar spine before and after surgery.

Subjects

The two-dimensional (2-D) model contains all the motion segments including five intervening discs. Therefore, changes in stress were observed in some static postures. However, the three-dimensional (3-D) model has only one motion segment, including two vertebrae and an intervening disc; it could not simulate changes in postures, so an intact normal model, a laminectomy model, and a hemifacetectomy model were simulated within the limits of the 3-D model.

[1] Department of Orthopedic Surgery, Niigata University School of Medicine, Asahimachi-dori 1-757, Niigata, 951 Japan
[2] Department of Orthodontics, Nagasaki University, Nagasaki, Japan

Materials and Methods

Two-Dimensional Model

The X-ray films of a healthy 31-year-old man in three postures, standing, sitting, and sitting cross-legged, were traced on paper. The cross-legged sitting posture was selected because it is common in Japanese life. A mesh composed of 355 elements and 843 nodal points was hand-drawn over the figures. The six-node isoparametric triangular elements were used as bony structure, annulus fibers, nucleus, cartilaginous end-plate, and joint cartilage of facets, and the two-node cable element was used as back muscle and ligamentous tissue. Geometrical data were accurately obtained using a digitizer (Fig. 1a).

Boundary conditions were: lower half of sacral element was fixed, uniform axial compressive loads applied on each node of the upper surface of L1 vertebra. The calculations were done using the mainframe computer (Fujitsu M-760 model 30, Fujitsu, Tokyo, Japan) at Nagasaki University by Suzuki.

Three-Dimensional Model

Subsequently, a 3-D model was made from computed tomography (CT) of the fresh autopsy lumbar spine of a 57-year-old man, who died from bronchial asthma and had been free of any discal or bony abnormalities. The slices of L3 were scanned using a graphic scanner (Epson Image Scanner GT-100, Epson-Seiko, Tokyo, Japan) and divided into mesh using an original program. The same geometrical data were transformed by adjustment to the alignment in the scout CT films. It contains 813 elements composed of an isoparametric 20-node

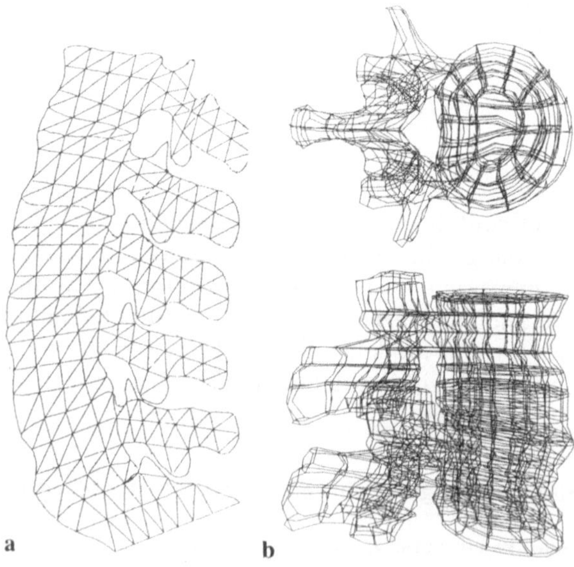

Fig. 1a,b. Mesh of models. **a** Two-dimensional model. **b** Three-dimensional model

Table 1. Material properties of three-dimensional model.

Material	Young's modulus (MPa)	Poisson's ratio	Shear modulus (MPa)	Reference
Cortical bone	12000	0.3	4615	[4]
Cancellous bone	100	0.2	417	[5]
Bony post. element	3500	0.25	1400	[3]
Cartilaginous end-plate	24	0.4	8.57	[5]
Annulus fibrosus (ground substance)	4.2	0.45	1.45	[6]
Nucleus pulposus	1667	0.48	563	[7]
Ligamentous Structure (torus)	24	10[a]		
Connection of the facet	300	10[a]		

post., Posterior
[a] Cross-sectional area

cubic element, 15-node prism element, and a 2-node cable element used as a ligamentous tissue and contains 4158 nodes (Fig. 1b). Nonhomogeneous disc structure was considered to be divided by the annulus fibers and the inner nucleus.

This model was compared to material properties of other models reported in the literature and used in other finite element models (Table 1). The posterior complex could not be divided into shell and core, so that an intermediate value was selected, as in the report by Shirazi-Adl [3]. Axial compressive loads were applied on the upper surface of the vertebral body and on the superior facets of the upper vertebra rectangularly, and the lowest nodes of the lower vertebra were fixed.

Results

Two-Dimensional Model

The maximum principal stress in each posture was distributed, as shown in Fig. 2. The length of the line represents the magnitude of stress in each element, the triangular terminator shows compressive stress, and lines without terminators show tensile stress. The minimum principal stress is represented by the line crossing the maximum principal stress line at right angle.

Compressive principal stress was intense at the anterior cortex of the body at L1 or L2. Compressive stress was intense at the superior facet of the lower vertebra. A comparison of the stress in each posture showed that compressive stress at the anterior cortex of the vertebral body increased in proportion to the degree of flexion and at the lower superior facets and interarticular portion in proportion to the degree of extension.

Statistically, the correlation of the stress distribution between L1 and L2 was weaker than that between L3 and L4. This was thought to be because

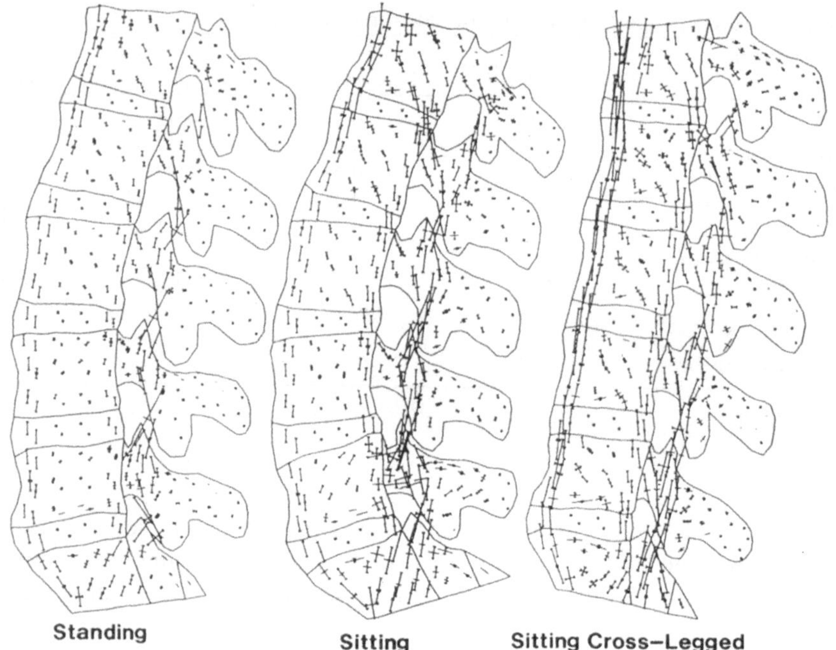

Fig. 2. Principal stress in each posture

loaded vertebrae respond differently to mechanical stress in comparison with nonloaded vertebrae.

Three-Dimensional Model

The results of the 2-D model were taken into account, so only the calculated data of the lower vertebra was evaluated and stored for statistical evaluation, especially the data from the posterior column. Principal stress was well-dispersed in the lower vertebra, as in the two-dimensional model. It seems that the shell structure of the bone and the microstructure of spongy bone may play an important role, but it is geometrically too complicated to apply the 3-D finite element method. The calculated stresses were divided into three columns for comparison. Slight tensile stress was observed in the cartilaginous end-plate above the disc. There were no significant changes between the normal and operated models.

In the anterior column, the principal and shear stress was conentrated at the posterior inferior cortex. A similar result was observed in the middle column (Fig. 3). In the posterior column, loaded facets and interarticular portions showed considerable stress, especially in the joint cartilage (Fig. 4). In the surgical treatment models, the superior facet seemed to have larger stress.

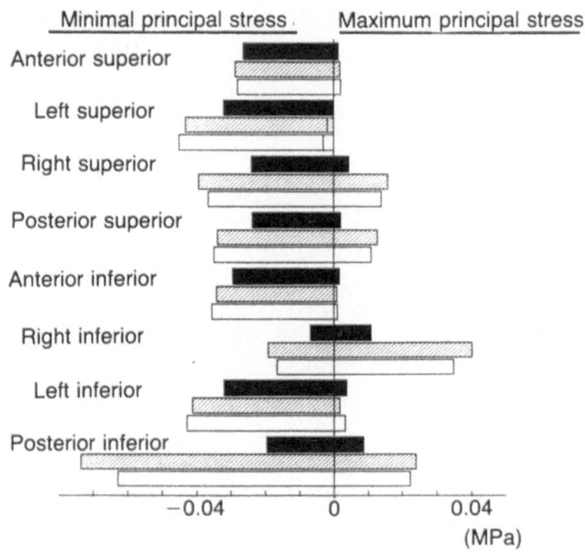

Fig. 3. Principal stress of anterior cortex. *Solid bars*, normal; *hatched bars*, laminectomy; *open bars*, facetectomy

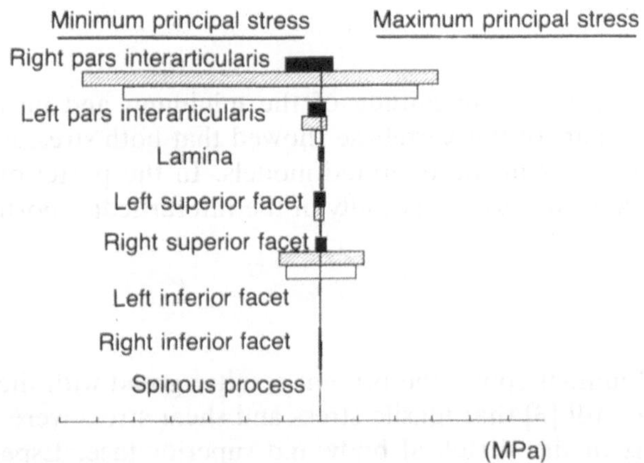

Fig. 4. Principal stress of posterior cortex. *Solid bars*, normal; *hatched bars*, laminectomy; *open bars*, facetectomy

In the axial view, maximum principal stress in the anterior superior cortex appeared to be increased (Fig. 5). In the middle slice of the lower vertebra, at the interarticular portion of hemifacetectomy, compressive principal stress and shear stress were increased. In the lower slice of the vertebral body, there were no significant changes, even in the operated models.

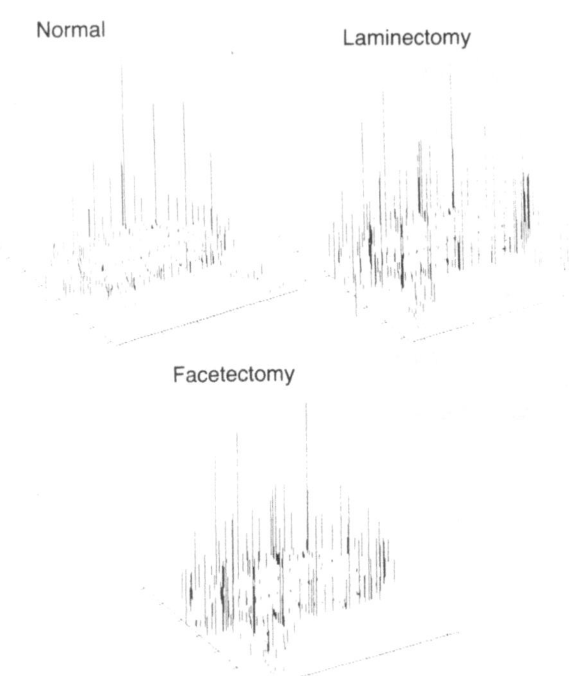

Fig. 5. Axial view of principal stress

A comparison of the magnitude of the minimum and maximum principal stresses in each part of the vertebrae showed that both stresses were increased in the inferior cortex in the operated models. In the posterior complex, both stresses were concentrated, especially in the interarticular portion.

Discussion

In the normal lumbar spine, the present results agreed with the result of Ueno [2] and Shirazi-Adl [3] that tensile stress and shear stress were concentrated in the upper part of the vertebral body and superior face. Especially the latter result is interesting in terms of the common disc degeneration at the lower lumbar spine.

The advantages of the FEM model are accurate geometrical simulation, and the ability to build a complex of various mechanical properties, even if both of the material properties and the geometry are complex. However, the validation of the model is not easy because of the difficulty of measuring the stress of wet bone precisely and of determining the material properties of soft tissue and of an intervertebral disc. However, current research is advancing our knowledge of intradiscal pressure, the amount of disc bulge, axial compression force, displacement after loading and so on.

Another problem is the long processing time required to perform the calculation and to produce a realistic simulation using isoparametric elements nonlinearly, and to consider the soft tissue. The models described so far are not accurate in this regard, but such models may elucidate the features of the normal spine and may give us a better understanding of the mechanics of the spine.

Conclusions

Two-Dimensional Model

1. Two adjacent vertebrae showed similar stress distributions except when one was loaded.
2. Compressive stress was intense at the anterior cortex of the upper level and superior facets of the lower level.

Three-Dimensional Model

Laminectomy and/or hemifacetectomy caused:

1. Increased compressive stress at the cortex near the intervertebral disc and facet joints
2. Tensile strain at the posterior cortex and annulus fibrosus
3. Shear stress at the remainder facet joint

References

1. Spilker RL, Suh J, et al. (1990) Effect of friction on the unconfined compressive response of articular cartilage: a finite element analysis. J Biomech Eng 112:138–146
2. Ueno K, Liu VK (1987) A three dimensional nonlinear finite element model of lumbar intervertebral joint in torsion. J Biomech Eng 109:200–206
3. Shirazi-Adl A, Ahmed AM, et al. (1986) Mechanical response of a lumbar motion segment in axial torque alone and combined with compression. Spine Eng 11: 914–927
4. Carter DR, Caler WE, et al. (1981) Resultant loads and elastic modulus calibration of long bone cross sections. J Biomech Eng 14–11, 739–745
5. Yamada H (1970) Strength of Biological Materials: Edited by Evans FG, Williams and Wilkins 73–78
6. Wu HC, Yao RF (1976) Mechanical behavior of the human annulus fibrosus. J Biomech Eng 9:1–7
7. Lim TH, Goel VK, Kim YE (1990) Possible role of stresses in inducing spinal stenosis-A long-term complication following disk excision. J Biomech Eng 112: 478–481

A New Biomechanical Analysis of the Degenerative Spine

SHUNJI MATSUNAGA[1], TAKASHI SAKOU[1], TOKUTAROU NAGAYAMA[1], and KENJI NAKANISHI[2]

Abstract. New computer programs for spinal alignment and strain distribution of the intervertebral discs were used to study biomechanical changes in degenerative spines.

Biomechanical data from lateral view X-ray films were fed into a computer by a digitizer. The difference between individual spinal alignments and ideal smooth alignments were calulated mathematically. Furthermore, the characteristic value "A" representing the degree of spinal curvature change, were also calculated. The value "A" can be available to characterize the spinal alignment. True strain distributions among the intervertebral discs were calculated by using the computer program. Thirty patients with lumbar disc herniation were analyzed and compared to 40 similarly aged normal subjects.

The spinal alignments of normal subjects showed little difference from the ideal with "A" values at $(11.7 \pm 3.4) \times 10^{-5}$. Strain was distributed almost evenly throughout the entire intervertebral disc in 38 normal subjects (95%). The "A" values of 20 patients with herniated discs (67%) were beyond the normal range, and strain was concentrated on the herniated discs.

Although there are no established biomechanical programs for clinical use, the present analysis represented the biomechanical characters of the subjects accurately and is convienient for clinical use. The method may be used to clarify the biomechanical influence of spinal surgery, spinal instability, and other studies of the spine.

Key Words. Spinal alignment, stress distribution, lumbar disc herniation

---

[1]Department of Orthopaedic Surgery, Faculty of Medicine, [2]Department of Engineering, Faculty of Manufacturing and Engineering, Kagoshima University, 8-35-1 Sakuragaoka, Kagoshima, 890 Japan

Introduction

The recent progress in computer technology has contributed greatly to the advancement of the basic orthopedics. Evaluation of changes in various parts of the body associated with tissue degeneration requires analysis from biomechanical approaches. Although the natural history of vertebral discs is a matter of considerable uncertainly, epidemiological and biomechanical studies indicate that mechanical factors may play a prominent role [1,2]. However, measurements alone may not be sufficient to clarify the nature of correlation between mechanical factors and disc disorders. We developed a new method for biomechanical analysis of the spinal alignment and the strain distribution of intervertebral discs, and studied the significance of its clinical application.

The results of the study are expected to contribute to the understanding of some aspects of mechanics and pathology of the degenerative spine.

Materials and Methods

Dynamic lateral X-ray films of the lumbar spine were fed into a microcomputer with a digitizer for image analysis. The analysis was made automatically by running a program for the spinal alignment and the strain of the disc on the microcomputer (Fig. 1). About 2 min were needed from the data input to the end of the analysis.

For the analysis of the spinal alignment, an ideal alignment, in which the stress is evenly distributed without concentrating at particular points, was calculated mathematically in each subject with a polynomial expression by the least square method (Fig. 2). This alignment curve was differentiated twice, and the degree of bending at the site where the curvature reversed was determined and expressed numerically as the "A" value (Fig. 3). As the "A" value increases, the alignment at the site of disease or injury is considered to be more sharply altered, and the dynamic stress to be more concentrated.

The strain of the intervertebral disc was analyzed by the use of a technological true strain formula on the assumption that the disc is an aggregate of line

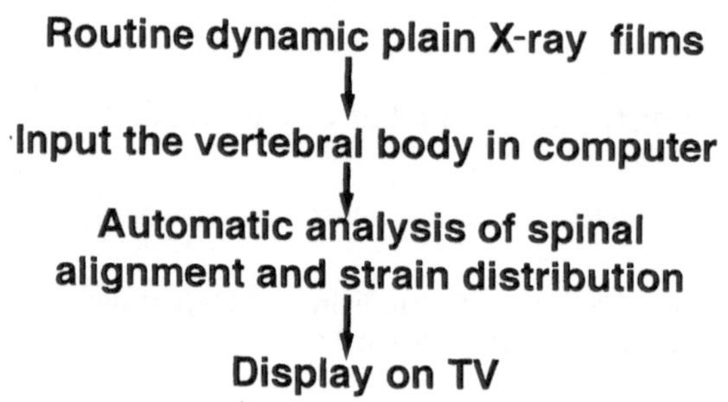

Routine dynamic plain X-ray films

↓

Input the vertebral body in computer

↓

Automatic analysis of spinal alignment and strain distribution

↓

Display on TV

Fig. 1. Analytical methods

Fig. 2. Analysis of spinal alignment

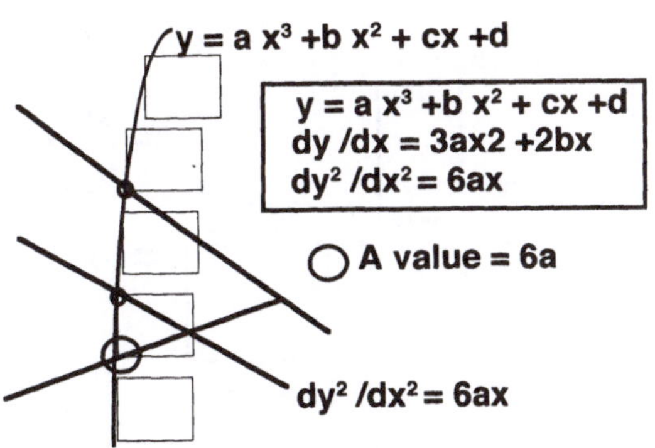

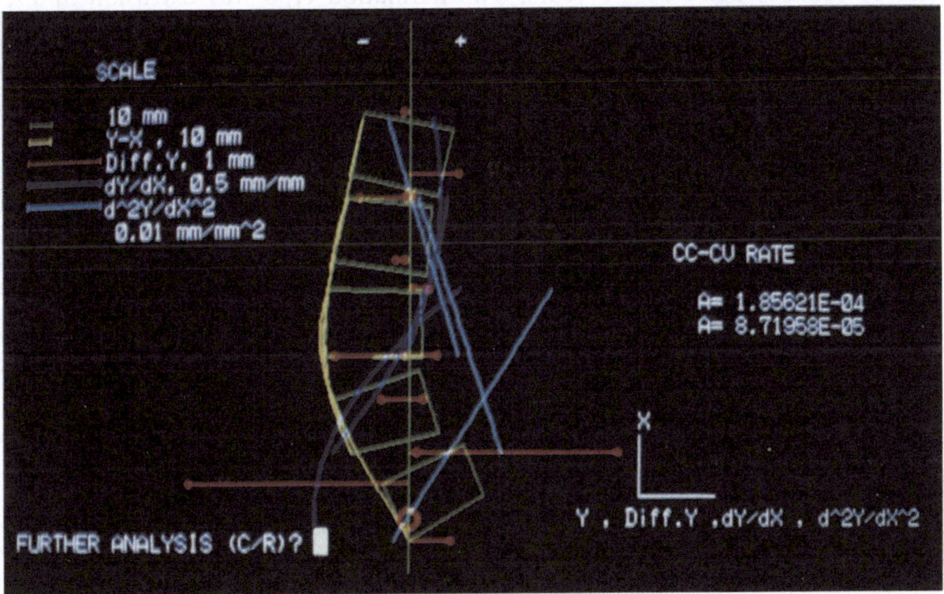

Fig. 3. The real display of "A" value

components [3]. The lower surface of the vertebral body was divided into 200 equal segments, and the strain gradient was calculated with a computer to quantitatively assess the strain. The degree of the strain was indicated visually with separate colors for tension and compression (Fig. 4).

The analysis was performed first in 40 normal subjects 20 males and 20 females, aged 15–60 years without a history of low back pain or lower limb pain who showed no abnormalities on radiograms. This analysis was also done

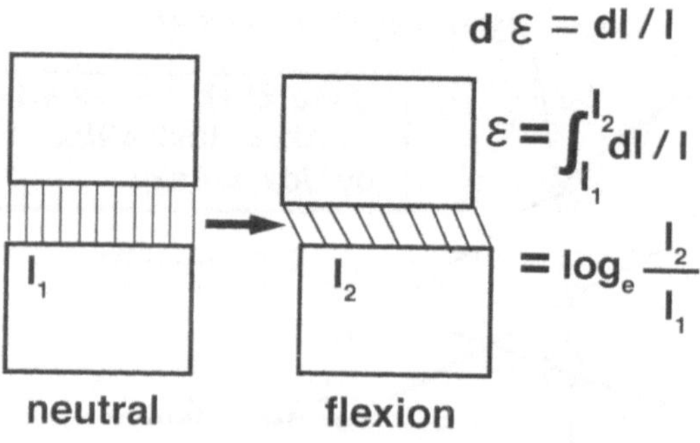

Fig. 4. Strain analysis of intervertebral discs

in 30 patients with disc herniation at the L4/5 level. They consisted of 19 males and 11 females aged 16–51 years. The herniation type was extrusion in 19, protrusion in 7, and sequestration in 4.

Results

Analysis of Normal Subjects

A value of "A" that indicates changes in the alignment at L4/5 level was mean 11.7×10^{-5} at all ages and showed no marked changes with anteroposterior bending (Fig. 5). The strain was also distributed evenly from tension to compression at all disc levels. Such even strain distribution was observed in 95% of the 40 subjects (Fig. 6).

Analysis for Patients with Lumbar Disc Herniation

Concerning the vertebral alignment at the L4/5 level, "A" value that indicates the degree of stress concentration was significantly greater in the hernia pa-

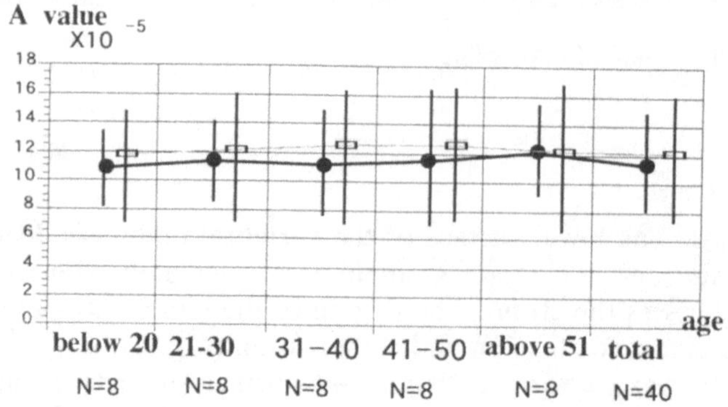

Fig. 5. "A" value of normal subjects. *Closed circles*, male; *open boxes*, females

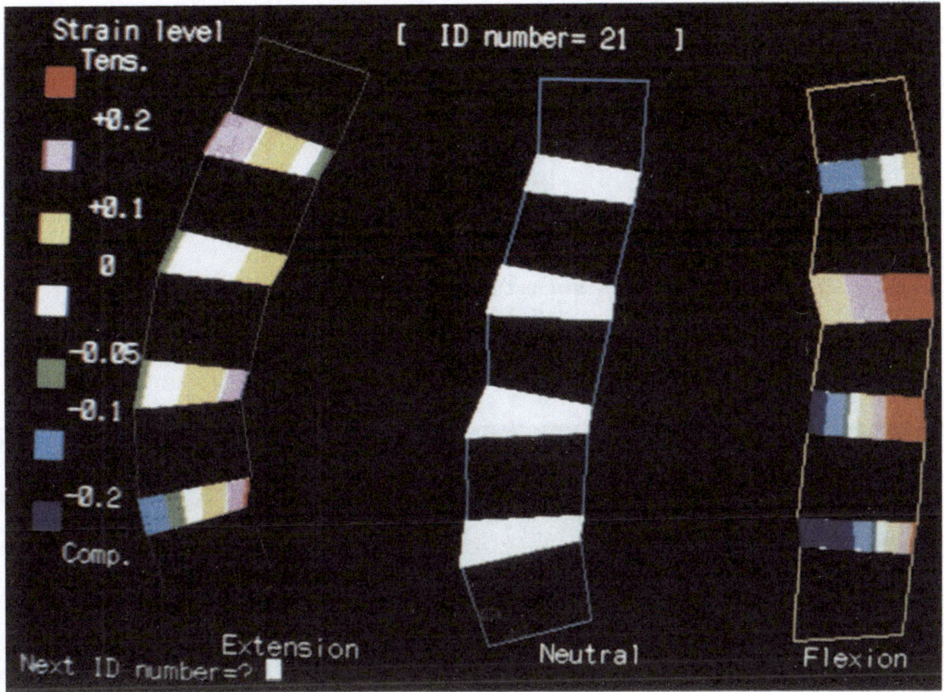

Fig. 6. Strain distribution of normal subjects

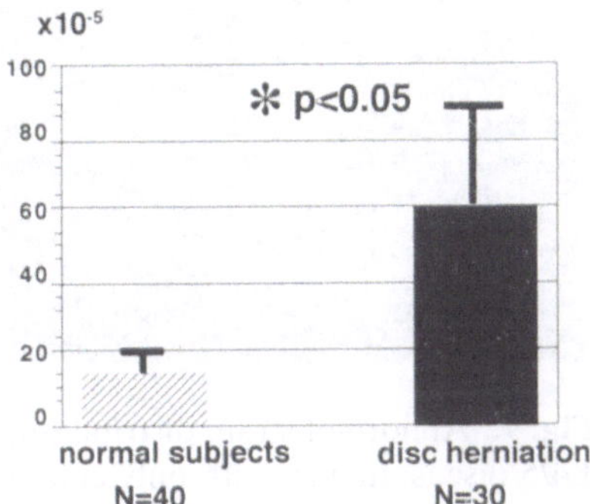

Fig. 7. "A" value of lumbar disc herniation

tients than in the normal subjects, and 67% of the patients showed values exceeding the range in the normal subjects (Fig. 7). Patients with sequentration type disc herniation had large "A" values compared with other types of herniation (Fig. 8). The distribution of the strain in the disc was uneven in the hernia patients, unlike the normal subjects (Fig. 9), with only tension or compression being observed in 75% of the 30 subjects.

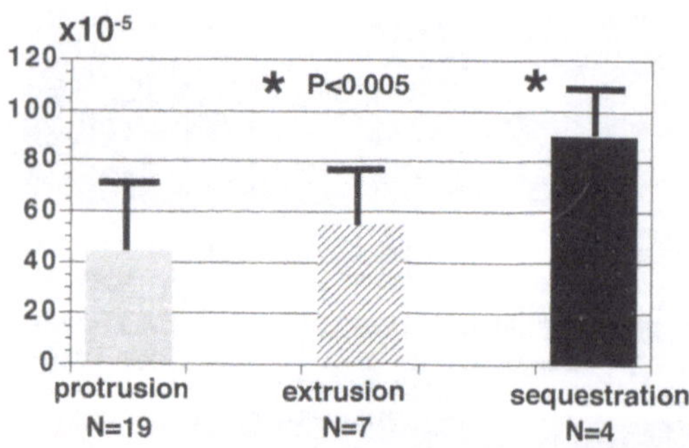

Fig. 8. "A" value and the type of herniation

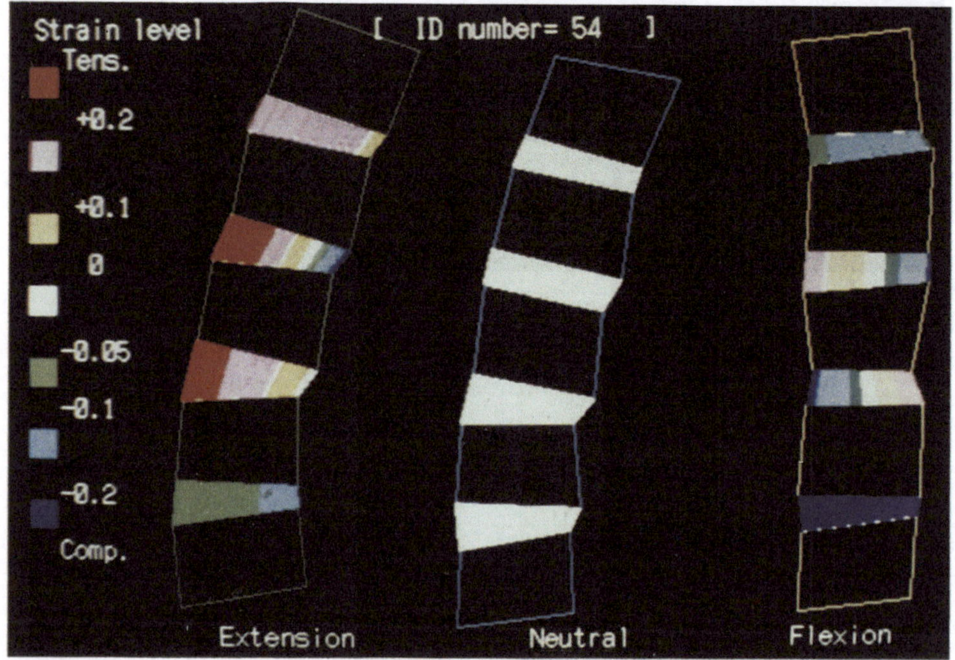

Fig. 9. Abnormal strain distribution of a herniated disc. The distribution of the strain in L4/5 disc is uneven with only compression

Discussion

Biomechanical analysis of the spine has generally been made by the finite element method [4–7]. However, the results of such analysis have not been consistent among reports because this method uses artifical models and because differences in the conditions of model input affect all results of the analysis

[8]. In addition, this technique requires a very complicated procedure, which makes its clinical application impractical. A new method that is more clinically applicable is needed for biodynamic analysis of changes associated with spinal degeneration. We developed a new method for biomechanical analysis of the spinal alignment and the strain distribution of intervertebral discs. Since the radiographic information is directly input for this analysis, the analysis reflects the characteristics of individual cases. Although the program itself is complicated, the simplicity of the actual analytical procedure makes it practical for clinical use. This biomechanical analysis showed that both spinal alignment and strain distribution were abnormal in patients with lumbar disc herniation. Patients with degenerative discs had large "A" values compared with patients without disc degeneration. This suggests that the present biomechanical analysis is applicable to study degenerative changes of the spine.

This analytical method is considered to be applicable to a wide range of clinical use including the evaluation of preoperative and postoperative changes in degenerative diseases of the spine, differences in their outcome according to the surgical procedure, and condition of the neighboring vertebrae that have been surgically fixed to the affected vertebra.

Conclusion

A new method was devised for biomechanical analysis of changes in the lumbar spine associated with spinal degeneration, and its clincial significance was evaluated. This method is simpler and more clinically practical than the finite element method, and is considered to be applicable to a wide variety of studies of spinal diseases.

References

1. Kelsy JL (1978) Epidemiology of radiculopathies. Adv Neurol 19:385–398
2. White AA III, Panjabi MM (1978) Clinical biomechanics of the spine. J.B. Lippincott, Philadelphia, pp 1–86
3. Outa T (1983) Material engineering. Sankaidou, Tokyo, pp 4–22
4. Arai Y, Takahashi E, Arai H, Suzuki H (1990) Stress analysis of the lumbar spine in the different posture. Proceedings of 1990 Annual Meeting of Japanese Society for Orthopaedic Biomechanics 12:145–148
5. Belytschko TB, Kulak RF, Schultz AB, Galante JO (1974) Finite element stress analysis of an intervertebral disc. J Biomech 7:27–285
6. Yamamoto I, Kaneda S, Tanno S, Ishikawa H (1989) Stress and deformation analysis of the whole lumbar spine by qusai three-dimensional finite element method. Proceedings of 1989 Annual Meeting of Japanese Society for Orthopaedic Biomechanics 11:17–20

7. Yamamoto I, Kaneda S, Tanno S, Ishikawa H (1990) Influence of the lumbar spinal fusion to the adjacent vertebral joint. Proceedings of 1989 Annual Meeting of Japanese Society for Orthopaedic Biomechanics 12:149–152
8. Shirazi-Adl SA, Shrivastava SC, Ahmed AM (1984) Stress analysis of the lumbar disc body unit in compression: A three-dimensional nonlinear finite element study. Spine 9:120–133

Fracture Mechanism and Acoustic Emission of the Osteoporotic Vertebral Body

SHIGEO TANAKA[1], TOSHIAKI HARA[2], KAZUHIRO HASEGAWA[3], and HIDEAKI E. TAKAHASHI[3]

Key Words. Biomechanics, acoustic emission, osteoporosis, vertebral body, trabecula

Introduction

Acoustic emission (AE) may be defined as the elastic stress waves generated by microcracks, dislocation movements, etc. during loading in a material. The AE from bone under loading was first reported by Hanagud et al. in 1973 [1], and other reports on the AE properties of bone have been published [2,3]. The aim of this study is to identify the influence of osteoporosis on the fracture mechanism of vertebral bodies using the AE method. We performed quasi-static compression tests on eight osteoporotic lumbar vertebrae and determined stiffness and maximum load from load-deformation curves. Simultaneously, AE from the vertebral body during the compression test was measured by an AE sensor, and the AE, event count rate and AE energy distribution were analyzed. We herein discuss the relationship between the fracture mechanism of vertebrae and AE involving various grades of osteoporosis, which was determined by the value of bone mass density (BMD) and by X-ray findings.

[1] Japan Advanced Institute of Science and Technology, Hokuriku, Asahidai 15, Tatsunokuchi, Ishikawa, 932-12 Japan
[2] Department of Mechanical and Productive Engineering, Faculty of Engineering, Niigata University, Ikarashi 2-nocho, Niigata, 950-21 Japan
[3] Department of Orthopedic Surgery, Niigata University School of Medicine, Asahi-machi-dori 1-757, Niigata, 951 Japan

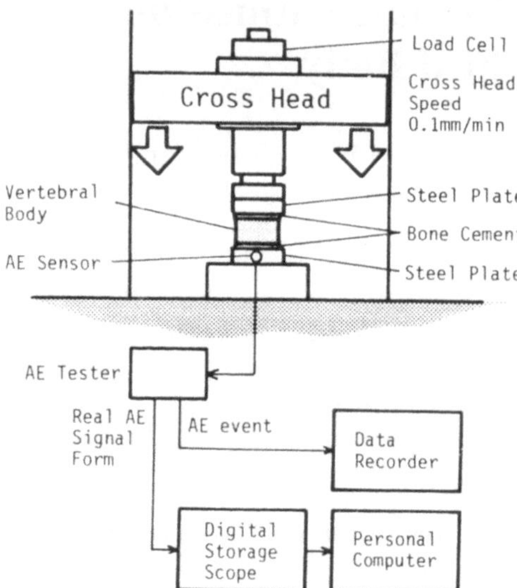

Fig. 1. Experimental apparatus

Materials and Methods

The osteoporotic third lumbar vertebrae taken from eight embalmed cadavers (from 60 to 89 years of age at the time of death) were used. Before the mechanical testing, BMD was measured by dual-energy X-ray absorptiometyr (DEXA) (Hologic, Inc., Waltham, Mass., QDR-1000) from the lateromedial view to evaluate the grade of osteoporosis quantitatively. Quasi-static compression testing was performed on an Instron type testing machine (Shimadzu Corp., Kyoto, Japan, AUTOGRAPH AG-25TD) at a cross-head speed of 0.1 mm/min. We determined stiffness and maximum load from the load-deformation curves. AE was monitored by a flat response piezoelectric transducer (NF Electronic Instr., Yokohama, Japan, AE-900S-WB) attached to a lower steel plate. We recorded the AE event signals to determine the cumulative AE event count and the real AE wave form signals to calculate the AE energy distribution. A schematic diagram of test setup is shown in Fig. 1. AE energy is defined by the following equation:

$$E = \int_0^T f(t)^2 dt \tag{1}$$

where T is the duration of 1 event and f(t) is the instantaneous magnitude of the real AE wave form signal. The AE energy distribution of the AE events was determined using log-log plots as shown in Figs. 2b, 3b, and 4b, in which E is the AE energy and N(E) represents the number of events whose AE energy exceeds E. If it is assumed that the relation between N(E) and E is linear on a

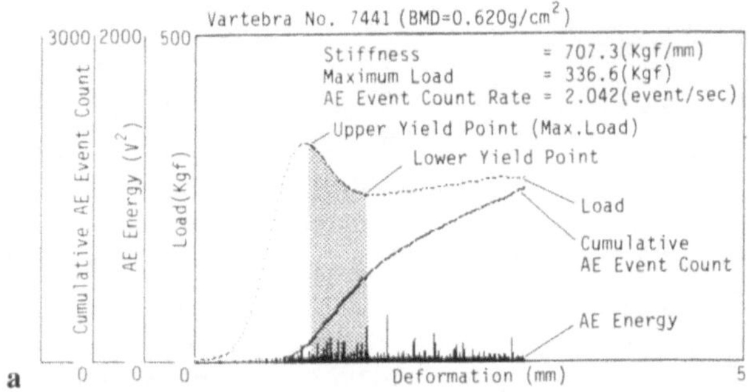

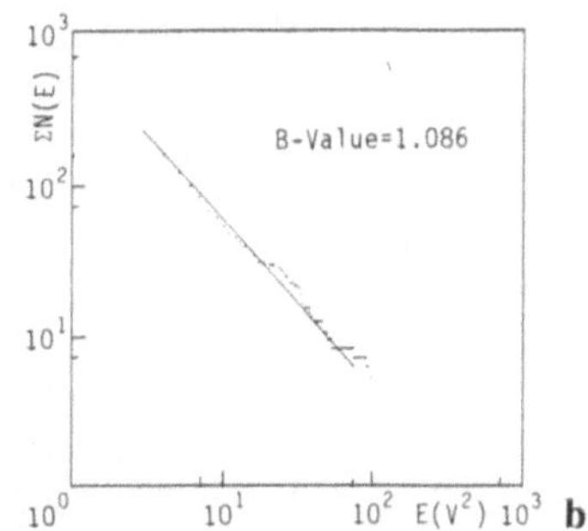

Fig. 2a,b. Mechanical behavior and AE of low grade osteoporotic vertebrae. **a** Load, AE energy, and cumulative AE event count versus deformation. **b** Cumulative AE energy distribution

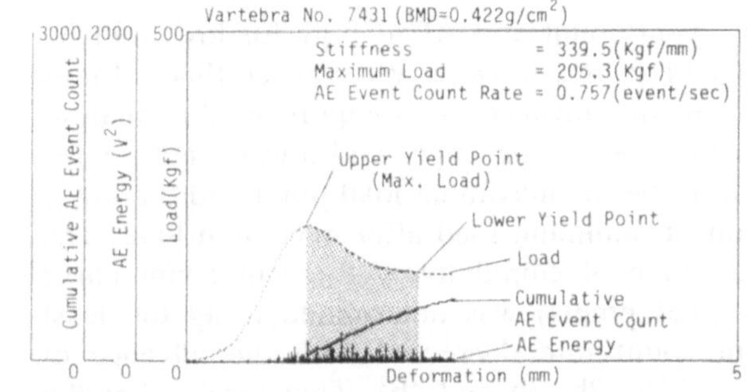

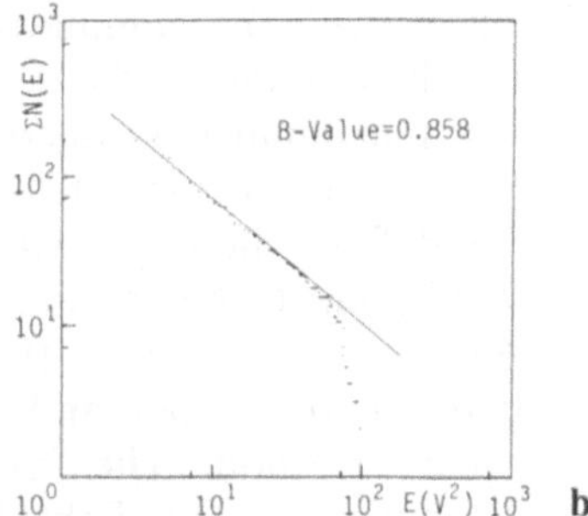

Fig. 3a,b. Mechanical behavior and AE of middle grade osteoporotic vertebra. **a** Load, AE energy, and cumulative AE event count versus deformation. **b** Cumulative AE energy distribution

log-log scale, it can easily be shown that the cumulative AE energy distribution gives

$$\Sigma N(E) = K \cdot E^{-m} \tag{2}$$

where $-m$ is the slope of the regression straight line and k is a constant. We defined the b-value obtained from the absolute grade value of the slope of the regression straight line to evaluate the AE energy distribution quantitatively. The higher the b-value, the greater the percentage of a low AE energy event.

Results

Figures 2–4 show the results for typical low, middle, and high grade osteoporotic vertebrae, respectively. Figures 2a, 3a, and 4a show the load-deformation

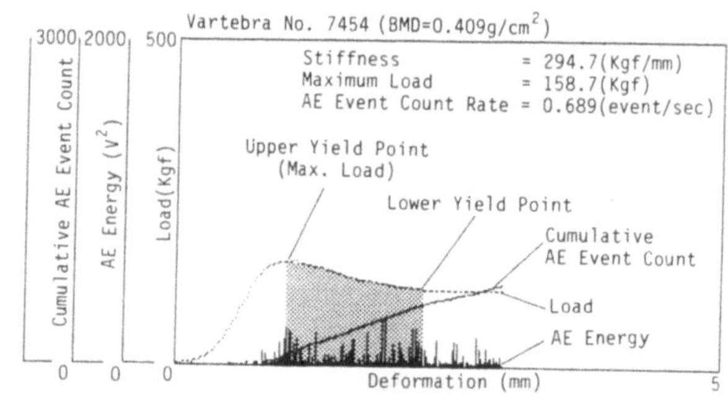

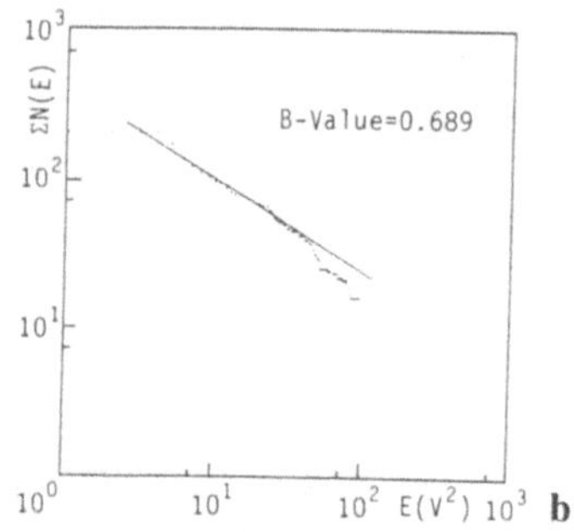

Fig. 4a,b. Mechanical behavior and AE of high grade osteoporotic vertebrae. **a** Load, AE Energy, and cumulative AE event count versus deformation. **b** Cumulative AE energy distribution

curves with the cumulative AE event count and AE energy for low, middle, and high grade osteoporotic vertebrae, respectively. We can see that stiffness and maximum load decreased with the advance of osteoporosis. AE analysis was applied to the AE event data between the upper and lower yield points. We defined the upper yield point to be the maximum load point and the lower yield point to be the initial point of minimum load after maximum load. The AE event count rate (i.e., the slope of cumulative AE event count curve between the upper and lower yield points) was determined using the least square method. The AE event count rate decreased with the advance of osteoporosis, as did the b-value (Figs. 2b, 3b and 4b). That means that the percentage of high energy AE events increases with the advance of osteoporosis. Stiffness ($r = 0.975$, $P < 0.01$), maximum load ($r = 0.895$, $P < 0.01$), AE event count rate ($r = 0.773$, $P < 0.05$), and b-value ($r = 0.695$, $P < 0.1$) have significant positive correlations with BMD.

Discussion

The trabeculae disappear with the advance of osteoporosis. In particular, transverse trabeculae disappear to a greater extent than do longitudinal trabeculae, as shown schematically in Fig. 5. The decrease in stiffness and maximum load with the advance of osteoporosis may be caused by the decreased buckling load of the longitudinal trabeculae due to the disappearance of the transverse trabeculae [4]. The AE energy distribution had a tendency to increase the percentage of high energy AE events with the advance of osteoporosis. In high grade osteoporotic vertebrae, the complete fracture of longitudinal trabeculae may be caused by buckling. This type of trabecular fracture produces high energy AE events. On the other hand, it is unlikely that the longitudinal trabeculae of low grade osteoporotic vertebrae will fracture completely as a

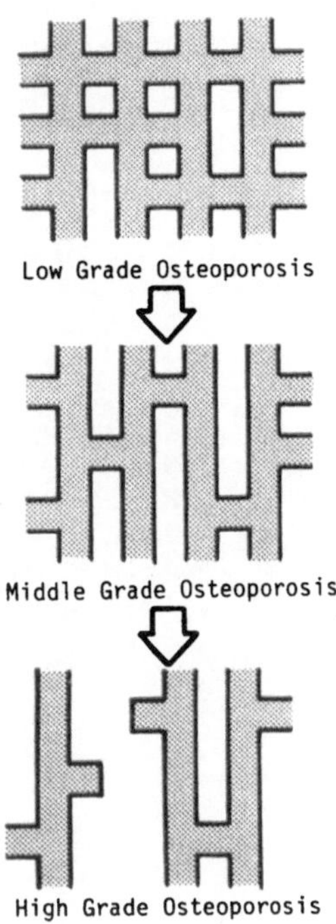

Fig. 5. Schematic model of cancellous bone in osteoporosis

result of buckling because many transverse trabeculae remain. In this case, relatively low energy AE events are more common.

References

1. Hanagud S, Clinton R, Lopez JP (1973) Acoustic emission in bone substance. Proceedings of biomechanics symposium of american society of mechanical engineering, p 79
2. Wright TM, Vosburgh F, Burstein AH (1981) Permanent deformation of compact bone monitored by acoustic emission. J Biomech 14:405–409
3. Fischer RA, Arms SW, Pope MH, Seligson D (1986) Analysis of the effect of using two different strain rates on the acoustic emission in bone. J Biomech 19:119–127
4. Townsend PR, Rose RM (1975) Buckling studies of single human trabeculae. J Biomech 8:199–201

Part III.

Bone Mineral Measurement

Bone Densitometry in Research and Practice

Robert R. Recker[1]

Abstract. This symposium honors the 75th anniversary of the Department of Orthopedics at Niigata. It is a distinct pleasure to honor 75 years of achievement. The most important bone disease in the world is osteoporosis, a condition of excessive skeletal fragility. Over one half million fractures occur each year in the United States due to osteoporosis at a cost of over $10 billion. Bone density is the most important determinant of skeletal fragility, and measurement of bone density has become a basic tool in clinical practice and research in this area. Dual-energy X-ray absorptiometry is the most commonly used method of measuring bone density and is the subject of this discussion.

Key Words. Bone mass, bone density, dual-energy X-ray absorptiometry, precision, osteoporosis, fractures, DEXA, diagnosis of osteoporosis, bone loss, osteoporosis treatment

Importance of Bone Densitometry

The most important bone disease in the world is osteoporosis. This is a condition of excessive skeletal fragility which is responsible for 1.2 million fractures per year in the United States. This includes 538 000 fractures of the vertebrae, 229 000 of the hip, 172 000 of the forearm, and 283 000 others [1]. The economic impact of hip fracture is huge. In 1986, there was an estimated 238 000 hip fractures in the US treated at a cost of $7.2 billion [2]. We will have an estimated 512 000 in the year 2040 treated at a cost of $16 billion without inflation and $240 billion at 5% inflation in health care costs. We have not seen

---

[1] Creighton University, Center for Hard Tissue Research, 601 North 30th Street, Suite 5740, Omaha, NE 68131, USA

an inflation rate in health care in the US as low as 5% for more than two decades.

Bone mass, or bone density, is an important determinant of the risk of fracture as shown by Hui et al. [3]. In the age range above 50, there is a progressive and striking increase in the risk of fracture with reductions in bone mineral density.

Bone Density, Measurement Technology

Over the past three decades, we have arrived at a point where dual-energy X-ray technology (DEXA) has replaced most of the earlier methods [4]. Quantitative computed tomography [5] also enjoys considerable use, but not as extensive as DEXA because of the expense and the high radiation exposure. This discussion will be limited to DEXA which permits measurement of bone density of any area of the body as well as the total body. DEXA technology employs an X-ray tube for a source of photons. The X-rays are highly collimated and filtered so that two photo peaks emerge from the tube and are detected by two detectors. The energies of the photo peaks are approximately 100 KeV and 44 KeV.

By analyzing the attenuation of these two energy peaks and by using a mathematical solution of simultaneous equations, the mineral and soft tissue densities can be calculated. The patient lies on a table while a scanning yoke containing the X-ray tube beneath the table and the detectors above the table pass over the body in a Raster fashion. While the machine can be used to measure density at any location, the most commonly measured sites are the spine, hip, forearm, and total body. The density data are displayed on a computer screen and can be printed or stored electronically.

A bone mineral density expression is given as the grams of mineral in the region selected (g/cm^2), and as the bone mineral content divided by the area of the region of interest present on the screen. This is not a true density measurement but an estimate of density. It is a two-dimensional rather than a three-dimensional expression. Software is also available for measurement of total bone mineral in animals such as the laboratory rat.

Precision

Table 1 shows a summary of the precision analysis performed on our Norland DEXA machine (Fort Atkinson, WI) when it was first installed. The data were obtained between 1988 and 1990. This analysis of precision included only healthy women whose ages ranged between 25 and 65. The method of determining precision was to obtain a mean and standard deviation for the scans of each site in each individual. Then for each site, the standard deviations of each of the 12 patients were expressed as percents of the mean and

Table 1. Summary of precision analysis (Norland DEXA Machine). $n = 12$, months = 1–27, scans/subj = 5–21.

	Precision (%)	
Site	*BMD*	*BMC*
Spine	1.89	2.36
Ward's triangle	5.81	5.81
Trochanter	2.83	9.32
Femoral neck	2.86	3.50
Total body		2.62

averaged. The average percent is expressed here as the precision. The bone mineral content (BMC) measurements had less precision in every case than the bone mass density (BMD) ones, and the femoral neck precision was less than the spine or total body in every case. These precision data were developed prior to certain improvements that have been installed in both the hardware and software in our machine, and we anticipate they will be much better when repeated. The degree of precision shown here is less than the usually optimistic estimates published by the manufacturers, whose precision standards are rarely achieved in the clinical or research setting. One must always perform precision analysis in one's own laboratory.

Impact of Precision

The precision of these instruments impacts greatly on their usefulness. It is a statistical fact that if precision is equal to 2%, then the smallest difference between two measurements in the same individual that is significant (reject the null hypothesis at $P < 0.05$) is 5.6%. The inference, then, is that this technology is not very useful in detecting differences over time in an individual patient or detecting treatment effects within an individual patient.

On the other hand, detecting changes within groups is a different matter. The machine can be quite powerful in detecting group change with time, but attention must be paid to the method of analyzing these changes. Two general methods have been used.

Fractional Change by Visit

In this method, each measurement of bone density of each member of a study group done on each visit is expressed as a fraction of the original value. Then, for each visit, the fractional changes for the group are averaged and plotted. Various statistical tools can be applied to the series of mean fractional changes in order to determine significant changes with time. Alternatively, each measurement can be expressed as a fraction of each member's mean of all measurements.

This method is ideal for displaying the results of a study on a graph. However, the power to detect significant change is less than other methods.

Mean Slopes of Change

In this method, each measurement from an individual is expressed as a fraction of that individual's mean. A regression of the fractions is plotted on time of observation for each individual, and the group changes are expressed as the average of the slopes of the group. The mean slopes can then be compared.

This method is quite sensitive in detecting changes between groups. However, the length of observation must be at least 1 year for each subject in order to minimize the variation in the measurement and achieve optimal statistical power.

Machine Drift

The use of DEXA technology or any other bone density measurement over time requires that the instrument remain stable as time passes. Indeed, these instruments are reasonably stable, however, caution must be taken in an individual laboratory to assure that lack of machine stability does not confound measurements. Figure 1 demonstrates the results of daily spine phantom scans over nearly 2 years of machine use.

Some of the more important uses of DEXA are outlined in Table 2. First, it can be used in determining risk for an individual. This is important in deciding on whether to use long-term estrogen replacement in a healthy person who presents at or near the time of menopause. If bone mass is below the 50th percentile or perhaps below the 25th percentile, then it is likely that the benefits of estrogen replacement therapy outweigh the risks. On the other hand, with bone mass well above the 50th percentile, the risk of long-term estrogen replacement may not be worth taking.

Use of DEXA can also determine whether or not bone-active drugs are appropriate. When corticosteroid use is contemplated, a bone mass measurement may help make the decision as to whether the risk of corticosteroid use is worthwhile and how long the corticosteroid use may take place before serious risk accrues to the skeleton.

The most common use of the machinery in the United States is detecting changes in groups during interventions. Most often, this occurs in treatment trials in which one treatment is compared with another or with an untreated control population over a period of time.

It can also be used to follow population groups or in population studies in which there is no intervention but in which secular trends in bone mass are examined.

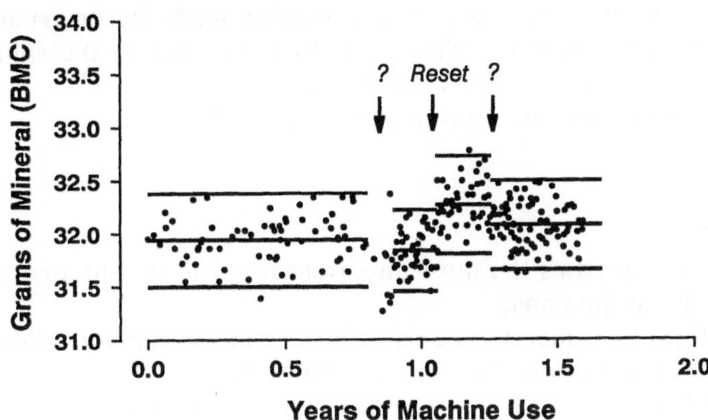

Fig. 1. The solid lines subtend plus or minus 2 standard deviations. One standard deviation is approximately 0.5% of the mean. For nearly 1 year, the measurements were fairly consistent, but at about 10 months they began falling below the −2 standard deviation level. At that point, we recalibrated the X-ray tube. We found a small but statistically significant change in the values during the ensuing period of time compared to the earlier period. At the word "reset" and an arrow, there was installation of new software and a change in hardware to include a dynamic filtering device to accommodate variation in soft tissue thickness among patients. After that, a long self-calibration of the instrument was performed, done by activating the manufacturer's software instructions. Again there was a change in the machine's baseline. Still another change occurred in the phantom measurements at the second question mark. It is interesting that nearly all of the phantom measurements, no matter which era, were within the manufacturer's acceptable limits for quality assurance, which is 0.5%. The changes in the phantom measurements will be accommodated when the results of ongoing studies are analyzed by correcting scans made during various eras to a single era

Table 2. Uses of DEXA.

1. Determining risk for an individual
   Decision on long-term estrogen replacement
   Decision on treatment with bone-active drugs
2. Detecting changes in groups during intervention
   Treatment trials
   Population studies
3. Aid in diagnosis
   Recent solitary compression fracture
   History of malignancy
4. Animal research

It can be used as an aid in diagnosis. A recent solitary compression fracture may be a puzzling diagnostic problem. If the vertebral bone mass is high, then the suspicion of an alternate cause of compression might be entertained. For example, a malignancy might declare itself by metastasis to the spine which shows up as a recent solitary compression fracture.

Finally, the machine can be used in animal research.

Summary

1. DEXA has emerged as the most important tool for measurement of bone density in vivo in humans;
2. DEXA will provide measurements of bone mineral content (BMC, g) for the entire skeleton or any local area of interest;
3. DEXA will provide two-dimensional measurements of "bone mineral density" (BMD, g/cm^2) for the entire skeleton or any local area of interest;
4. The precision and safety of DEXA are acceptable;
5. DEXA is useful for predicting risk of fracture for an individual patient and as an aid in diagnosis for an individual patient;
6. DEXA is useful for monitoring change in groups of patients as in treatment trials of pharmaceutical agents;
7. DEXA is not useful in the definitive diagnosis of osteoporosis in an individual patient (examination of the patient and the patient's radiographs are better for this);
8. DEXA is not useful in detecting change in bone mass over time in an individual patient;
9. During long-term use of DEXA, an external phantom should be monitored in order to correct for machine drift in the baseline; and
10. Further refinements are anticipated which will improve the speed, accuracy, and precision of the instruments.

References

1. Riggs BL, Melton LJ III (1986) Involutional osteoporosis. N Engl J Med 314:1676–1686
2. Cummings SR, Rubin SM, Black D (1990) The future of hip fractures in the United States—numbers, costs, and potential effects of postmenopausal estrogen. Clin Orthop 252:163–166
3. Hui SL, Slemenda CW, Johnston CC Jr (1988) Age and bone mass as predictors of fracture in a prospective study. J Clin Invest 81:1804–1809
4. Mazess RB, Barden HS (1988) Measurement of bone by dual-photon absorptiometry (DPA) and dual-energy X-ray absorptiometry (DEXA). Ann Chir Gynaecol 77:197–203
5. Block JE, Smith R, Glueer CC, Steiger P, Ettinger B, Genant HK (1989) Models of spinal trabecular bone loss as determined by quantitative computed tomography. J Bone Miner Res 4:249–257

Influence of Bone Mineral Density on the Mechanical Stability of Transpedicle Screwing

Koichiro Okuyama[1], Kozo Sato[1], Eiji Abe[1], Hajime Murai[1], Yoichi Shimada[1], Hitoshi Inaba[1], Shinichi Kamata[2], and Hidehiko Nagata[2]

Key Words. Bone mineral density, osteoporosis, insertion torque, transpedicle screwing, mechanical stability

Introduction

Recently, transpedicle screwing has been widely used in surgery for many spinal disorders, including the segmental instability caused by spondylolisthesis, trauma, tumors, and others.

Numerous positive results have been clinically reported. Some complications, however, have also been presented. When this fixation is carried out for degenerative lumbar diseases, such as degenerative spondylolisthesis, screw loosening, or loss of correction which is caused by insufficient mechanical stability in the bone-screw interface, it is sometimes found in an osteoporotic subject that has low bone mineral density (BMD) of the vertebra [1–3].

However, no specific guidlines have been objectively proposed regarding the risk of screw loosening or loss of correction in osteoporotic cases, and the current methods of fixing the bone-screw interface are not satisfactory.

The purposes of this study are to reveal: (1) how BMD of the lumbar vertebrae affected the stability in transpedicle screwing, and (2) whether the maximum insertion torque of the screw can predict the mechanical stability of transpedicle screwing.

[1] Department of Orthopaedic Surgery, School of Medicine, Akita University, 1-1-1 Hondo, Akita, 010 Japan
[2] Department of Engineering Materials and Applied Chemistry, Mining College, Akita University, 1-1 Tegata Gakuen-machi, Akita, 010 Japan

Materials and Methods

The third, fourth, and fifth lumbar vertebrae were obtained from 15 human cadavers available for anatomical dissecting practice at the Department of Anatomy of Akita University School of Medicine. The specimens were preserved in a 1% phenol solution after dissection. The average age was 70 years at death (range 49–95 years). The vertebrae with metastatic changes or remarkable deformities as shown on the radiograms, were excluded from this study.

Measurement of Bone Mineral Density Using Quantitative Computed Tomography

Specimens were immersed in water and degassed for 12 h before measuring BMD. Quantitative computed tomography (QCT) was performed with the Toshiba E 400 CT Scanner (Toshiba Co., Tokyo, Japan). To simulate clinical subjects, the specimens were placed in the bottom of a water bath 16 cm deep. A 10-mm thick transverse slice was scanned in the mid-line of the pedicle (Fig. 1). The region of interest (ROI) was defined by using a cursor placed just inside the cortical shell, excluding the vein entrance in each vertebra.

According to the calibration method, scanning was done with urethane-fiber phantoms containing chambers of $CaCO_3$ solutions.

Mechanical Test

During dissection, all adhering soft tissue was removed from the specimen and the vertebrae were disarticulated after measuring BMD. Then each vertebra was embedded in methylmethacrylate up to the base of the pedicles for testing.

The screw used in this study was an Akita Device Screw, modified by ourselves (outer diameter, 7.0 mm; core diameter, 4.0 mm; thread length, 40 mm; self-tapping type, SUS 316, Mizuho Co. Niigata City, Japan). During screw insertion, the maximum torque was measured by a screwdriver (Nakamura Co. Tokyo, Japan). The vertebrae that showed incorrect screw placement or pedicle breakage on the radiogram were excluded.

Each embedded vertebra was mounted on the Electrohydraulic Materials Testing System (Shimadzu Autograph I-10T, Shimadzu Manufacturing Co. Tokyo, Japan) in which the maximum capacity of the load cell was limited to 4500 N, and the following mechanical tests were performed: (1) The pull-out test: To determine the load needed to pull the screw out along its axial direction; (2) The tilting test: To determine to load needed at the screw-plate junction to tilt the screw approximately 4° in the cranial direction. The force was applied paralell to the axial direction. The end of a 3-cm length plate was pivoted 2 mm through a universal joint. It was confirmed by a special gauge

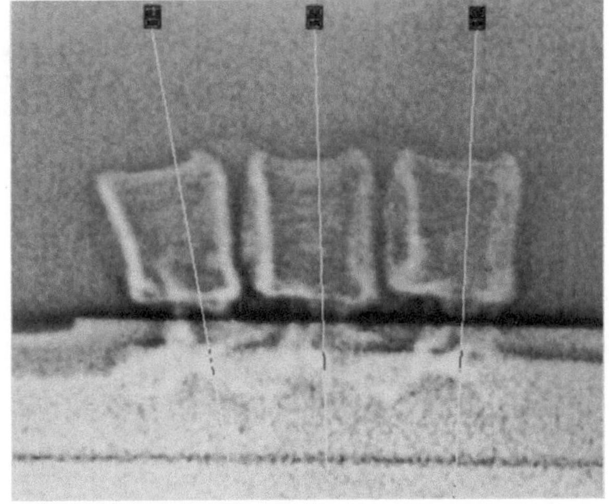

Fig. 1. Measurement of the bone mineral density (BMD) using quantitative computed tomography (QCT). A 10 mm thick transverse slice was scanned in the mid-line of the pedicle

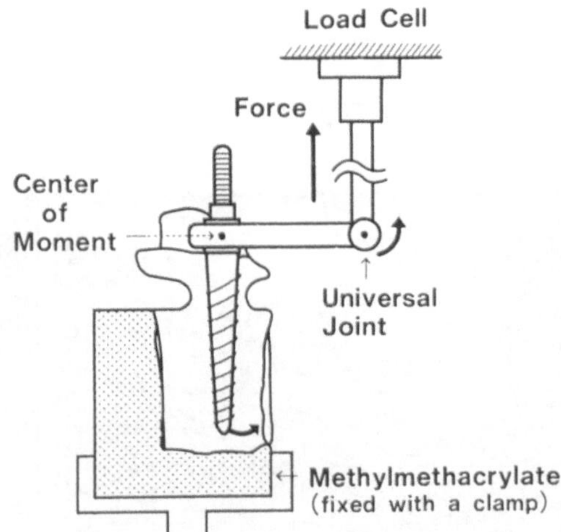

Fig. 2. Apparatus for the tilting and cut-up tests. The end of the 3 cm long plate was connected to the load cell through the univerval joint

that the screw did not displace in its axial direction (Fig. 2); (3) The cut-up test: To determine the load needed to tip the superior end-plate up. For this test, the superior end-plate was not embedded in methylmethacrylate.

The speed of the cross-head was set at 1 mm/min.

Results

The pull-out load was defined as the maximum load observed just before an abrupt decrease on a load-displacement curve. A typical load-displacement curve for the tilting and cut-up tests is shown in the Fig. 3. The line is nearly

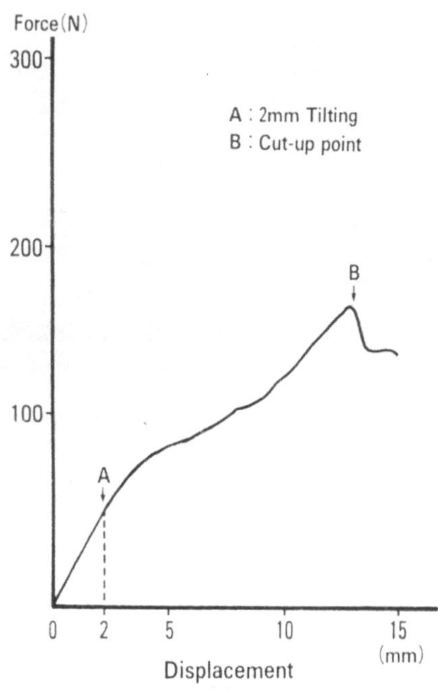

Fig. 3. The typical load-displacement curve in the tilting and cut-up tests. It was almost a linear line up to the 2 mm point (*A*) after which it gradually curved. The cut-up by the screw was detected by a big dip (*B*)

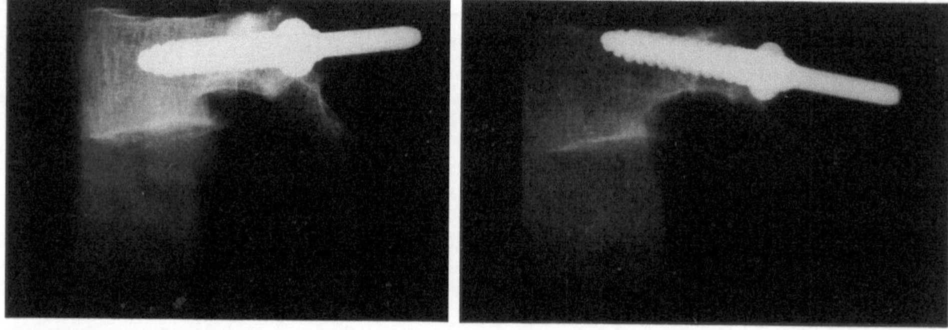

Fig. 4. The radiograms of pre-load vertebra (*right*), and post-load vertebra (*left*), showing the screw tilted and cut the end-plate after loading

linear line up to the 2-mm (elastic limit) point. After the 2-mm point, it gradually curved. The cut-up of the end plate was defined as a decrease of force followed immediately by an increase of force, thereby creating a dip on the curve, and this was confirmed on the radiograms (Fig. 4).

The mean BMD of all the third, fourth, and fifth lumbar vertebrae was 130 ± 53.2 mg/ml (mean ± SD, $n = 30$). The average maximum insertion torque was 0.4 ± 0.25 Nm. A positive correlation between the maximum insertion torque and BMD was found (Fig. 5).

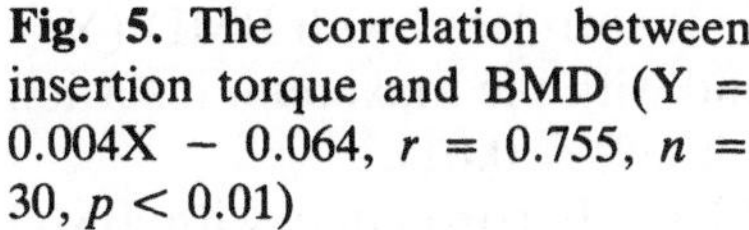

Fig. 5. The correlation between insertion torque and BMD (Y = 0.004X − 0.064, r = 0.755, n = 30, p < 0.01)

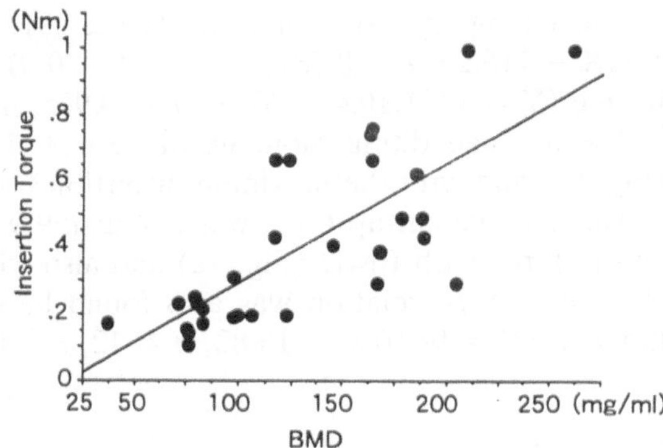

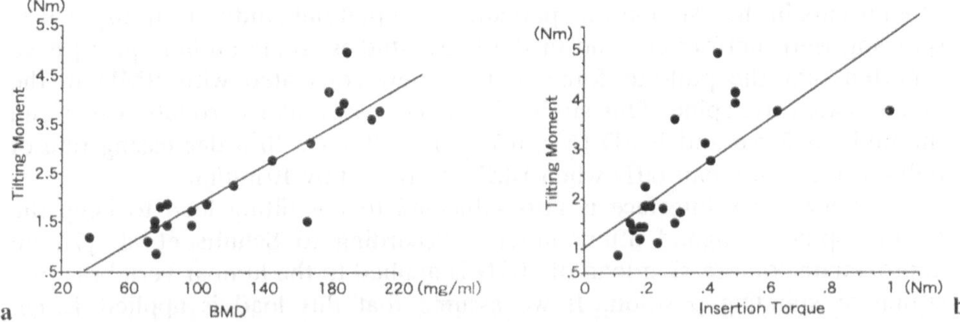

Fig. 6. a The correlation between tilting moment and BMD (Y = 0.020X − 0.090, r = 0.882, n = 21, p < 0.01). **b** The correlation between tilting moment and insertion torque (Y = 4.30X + 1.02, r = 0.732, n = 21, p < 0.01)

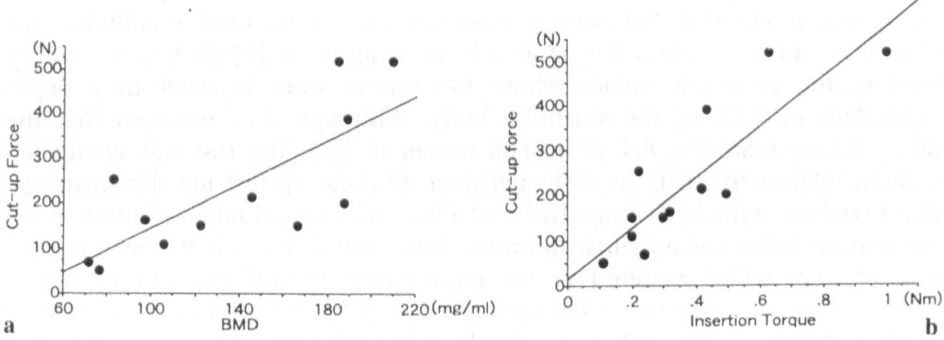

Fig. 7. a The correlation between cut-up force and BMD (Y = 2.44X − 97.61, r = 0.76, n = 15, p < 0.01). **b** The correlation between cut-up force and insertion torque (Y = 558.80X + 24.08, r = 0.857, n = 12, p < 0.01)

The average pull-out force was 582 ± 431.2 N. It correlated with BMD (Y = 5.71X − 115.23, $r = 0.737$, $n = 15$, $P < 0.01$) and with the maximum insertion torque (Y = 1431.10X − 67.09, $r = 0.925$, $n = 15$, $P < 0.01$).

The average tilting moment was 2.4 ± 1.21 Nm. It correlated with BMD (Fig. 6a) and with the maximum insertion torque (Fig. 6b).

The average cut-up force was 234 ± 159.9 N. There was a correlation of the cut-up force with BMD (Fig. 7a) and also with the maximum insertion torque (Fig. 7b). A correlation was also found between the cut-up force and tilting moment (Y = 98.07X − 16.82, $n = 12$, $r = 0.797$, $P < 0.05$).

Discussion

One of the complications of transpedicle screwing is that the pull-out of a screw often occurs in the osteoporotic patient. Many pull-out studies of transpeedicle screwing were performed, and in the latest studies, some authors [4–6] have reported that the pull-out force of the screw correlated with BMD in the human cadaveric spine. Our study also showed a similar correlation between the pull-out force and BMD ($r = 0.737$, $P < 0.01$) with a decreasing rate of pull-out force of about 60 N when BMD decreased by 10 mg/ml.

The bone-screw interface is also subjected to the tilting load to keep the lumbar spine realigned after surgery. According to Schults et al. [7], an approximate compression load of 400 N is applied to the lumbar vertebrae in a sitting or standing position. If we assume that this load is applied 1.5 cm anteriorly from the center of tilting or rotation in the functional spinal unit, at least 3.0 Nm [(400 N × 1.5 cm = 6 Nm) divided by two screws] is necessary to sustain the load. Our tilting test also showed that alignment of vertebrae with an average BMD of 95 ± 33.3 mg/ml could not be maintained under the 3.0 Nm tilting moment.

The cut-up of the screw through the vertebral end-plate is also a serious complication when the distraction maneuver is attempted in surgery or when the flexion moment in the lumbar spine is great. Under these conditions, the vertebrae can not sustain the applied load. Krag et al. [8] studied the cut-up load in the cadaveric spines where the screws were inserted to a depth equivalent to 80% of the vertebral body. Although they reported that the mean cut-up load was 8.4 ± 0.8 Nm (mean ± SE), the test was conducted without respect to BMD in each specimen. Our cut-up test has demonstrated that vertebrae with an average BMD of 130 ± 53.2 mg/ml failed to prevent the screw from being cut up when the mean force was 234 ± 159.9 N with a lever arm of 3 cm which resulted in an approximate flexion moment of 7.0 ± 4.80 Nm. Also, a correlation between the cut-up force and BMD ($r = 0.76$, $n = 12$, $P < 0.01$) was found. These results suggest that there is a possibility that the osteoporotic vertebra may be cut up, if a flexion moment of 7.5 Nm (15 Nm divided by two screws) is physiologically applied to the lumbar spine [9].

The insertion torque of a screw is primarily generated by the shearing force and friction between the screw threads and the cancellous bone. We revealed that the maximum insertion torque correlated with BMD ($r = 0.755$, $P < 0.01$), pull-out load ($r = 0.925$, $P < 0.01$), tilting moment ($r = 0.732$, $P < 0.01$), and cut-up force ($r = 0.875$, $P < 0.01$). Our measurement of the insertion torque was based on somewhat subjectively defined end points, but no other techniques have been reported that predict the stability of the transpedicle screwing in surgery. Therefore, our results suggest that measurement of the insertion torque of transpedicle screwing could be a useful predictor of the mechanical stability of screws.

Conclusions

1. It was confirmed that the pull-out load of transpedicle screws (the stability along its axial direction) was significantly affected by BMD.
2. There is a possibility for the vertebrae with a mean BMD of 130 ± 53.2 mg/ml to be cut up even in the physiological circumstances.
3. The maximum torque while inserting a screw can predict its mechanical stability.

References

1. Blauth M, Tscherne H, Haas N (1987) Therapeutic concept and results of operative treatment in acute trauma of the thoracic and lumbar spine: The Hannover experience. J Orthop Trauma 1:240–252
2. Dick W, Kluger P, Magerl F, Woersdöfer O, Zäch G (1985) A new device for internal fixation of thoracolumbar and lumbar spine fractures: The "Fixateur Interna". Paraplegia 23:225–232
3. Kinnard P, Ghibely A, Gordon D, Trias A, Basora J (1986) Roy-Camille plates in unstable spinal conditions: A preliminary report. Spine 11:131–135
4. Coe JD, Warden KE, Herzig MA, McAfee PC (1990) Influence of bone mineral density on the fixation of thoracolumbar implants: A comparative study of transpedicular screws, laminar hooks, and spinous process wires. Spine 15:902–907
5. Soshi S, Shiba R, Kondo H, Murota K (1991) An experimental study on transpedicular screw fixation in relation to osteoporosis of the lumbar spine. Spine 16:1335–1341
6. Wittenberg RH, Shea M, Swartz DE, Lee KS, White AA, Hayes WC (1991) Importance of bone mineral density in instrumented spine fusions. Spine 16:647–652
7. Schults A, Andersson G, Örtengren R, Haderspeck K, Nachemson A (1982) Loads on the lumbar spine: Validation of a biomechanical analysis by measurements of intradiscal pressures and myoelectric signals. J Bone Joint Surg 64A:713–720
8. Krag MH, Beynnon BD, Pope MH, Frymoyer JW, Haugh LD, Weaver DL (1986) An internal fixator for posterior application to short segments of the thoracic, lumbar, or lumbosacral spine: Design and testing. Clin Orthop 203:75–98
9. Allan DG, Russel GG, Moreau MJ, Raso VJ, Budney David (1990) Vertebral end-plate failure in porcine and bovine models of spinal fracture instrumentation. J Orthop Res 8:154–156

The Most Specific Skeletal Site for DEXA Measurement in Diagnosis of Established Osteoporosis

HIROMICHI NORIMATSU, SHIGEKI SEKIYA, and JUN KAWANISHI[1]

Key Words. Established osteoporosis, diagnosis, dual-energy X-ray absorptiometry (DEXA), lumbar spine, appendicular bones

Introduction

Dual-energy X-ray absorptiometry (DEXA) has been widely accepted for the diagnosis of osteoporosis, evaluation of therapeutic effects, and identification of people at risk for osteoporosis. Several skeletal sites have been selected for bone mineral density (BMD) measurement, such as lumbar A-P, lumbar lateral, femoral neck, distal 1/3 of the forearm, ultradistal of the forearm, calcaneus, and total body, but each skeletal site has a small difference in BMD value because each site has its own specific composition of cortical and trabecular bones, as well as its own mechanical metabolic properties. The purpose of this study was to determine the most sensitive skeletal site of bone mineral measurement by DEXA for the diagnosis of established osteoporosis.

Materials and Methods

The patients in the control group consisted of 65 postmenopausal women and the study group consisted of 86 patients with postmenopausal or senile osteoporosis. The mean age was significantly different between the control (63.9 years) and study (67.7 years) groups. Mean weight and body mass index (BMI) for patients with osteoporosis were lower than the control group (Table 1). The control group consisted of healthy postmenopausal women who had no metabolic disease. Patients with osteoporosis were identified by the symptoms

[1] Department of Orthopedic Surgery, Kagawa Medical School, 1750-1 Ikenobe, Miki-cho, Kagawa, 761-07 Japan

Table 1. Body size of two groups.

	Cases	Age (years)	height (cm)	weight (kg)	BMI (kg/cm^2)
Control	65	63.9 ± 8.2	149.0 ± 5.9	52.5 ± 9.2	23.6 ±3.7
Osteoporosis	86	67.7 ± 9.1	147.6 ± 5.9*	47.9 ± 8.0	22.0 ± 3.2**

* $P < 0.002$, ** $P < 0.01$

Table 2. Daily calcium intake and activity score measured by Yoshikawa's scoring system.

	Calcium intake (mg/day)	Activity score (patients)
Control	542.0 ± 216.1 (21)	3.0 ± 1.1 (23)
Osteoporosis	555.7 ± 246.4 (24)	2.7 ± 1.2 (28)

of low back pain and loss of trabecular pattern in the vertebral bodies under lumbar X-ray films.

Daily calcium intake was measured over a 3-day period and activity of daily living (ADL) were examined by questionnaire using Yoshikawa's scoring system [1]. BMD was measured by Lunar DPX-α machine (USA) at four skeletal sites: The anteroposterior projection of L2–4, lateral projection of L2–3, femoral neck, and distal 1/3 of the forearm.

Results

Average daily calcium intake of the control group was 542 ± 216 mg. There was no difference in the daily calcium intake between the two groups. Also, no difference was observed in ADL between the two groups (Table 2).

In vivo precision errors of the Lunar DPX-α at the (47–72 years) at our institute were 1.6% for lumbar A-P, 3.6% for lumbar lateral, 2.3% for the femoral neck, and 1.9% for the forearm.

Slopes of the regression lines in the control group was −0.0069 for lumbar A-P and −0.002 for lumbar lateral BMD (Fig. 1). Otherwise the slopes of the regression line for the appendicular skeletons were much steeper than two lumbar projections: −0.0059 for the femoral neck and −0.011 for the distal forearm (Fig. 2). Annual decrease of control BMD after 50 years was greater in the distal forearm than other three skeletal sites. Lumbar lateral BMD decreased much slower than lumbar A-P and appendicular bone BMDs (Fig. 3).

The BMD of patients with osteoporosis at each skeletal site showed significantly lower value than the BMD of controls both in the 50–60 years range and above 70 years (Fig. 4). Discrimination (Z-score) of BMD between the two groups was significantly enhanced at each skeletal site and the Z-score

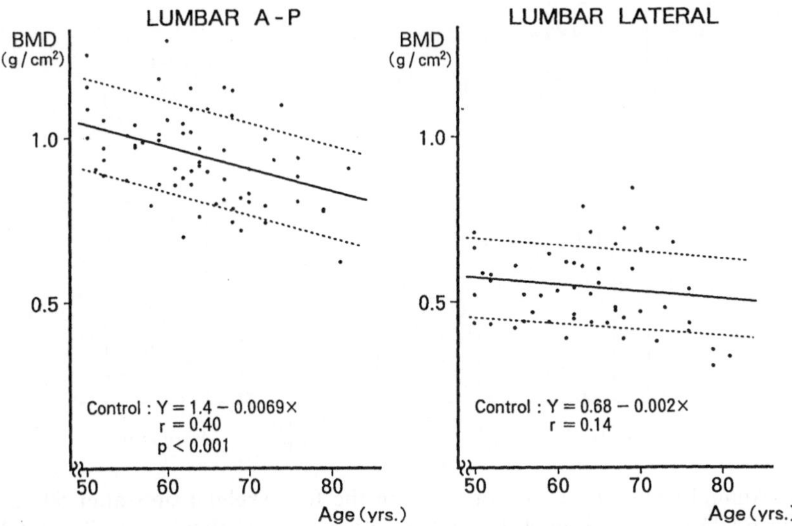

Fig. 1. Control bone mineral density (BMD) for lumbar A-P and lumbar lateral views. The slope of the regression line for lumbar A-P was −0.0069 ($P < 0.001$), and that for lumbar lateral was −0.002 ($P < 0.1$)

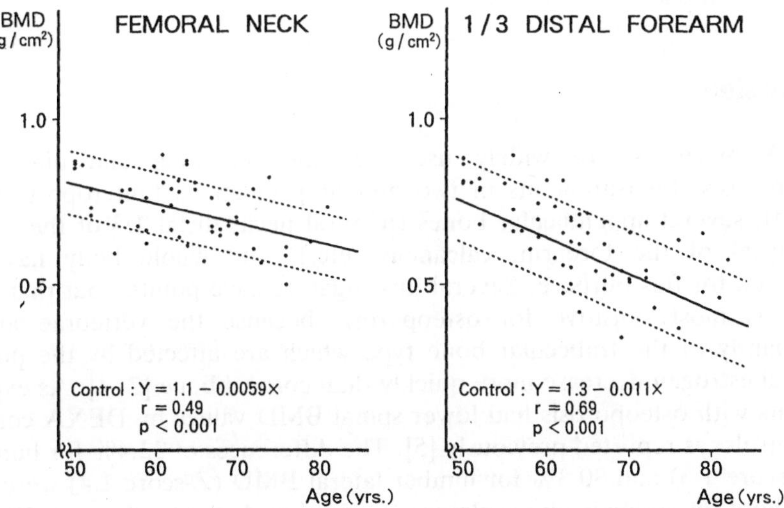

Fig. 2. Control BMD for the femoral neck and distal 1/3 of the forearm. The slope of the regression line for the femoral neck was −0.0059 ($P < 0.001$) and that for the forearm was −0.011 ($P < 0.001$)

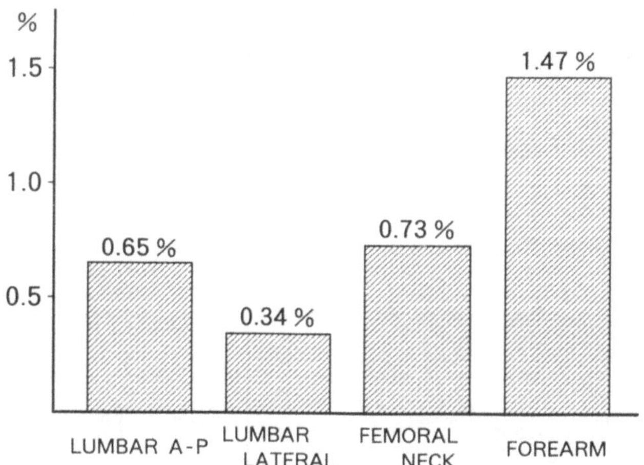

Fig. 3. Annual decrease of control BMD in the four skeletal sites after 50 years. The forearm BMD decreased much faster than other three skeletal sites ($P < 0.001$). The lumbar lateral BMD decreased slower than lumbar A-P and two appendicular skeletal sites ($P < 0.001$)

for patients aged 50–69 years was greater in the two lumbar projections than in the two appendicular skeletons. The Z-score for the subjects above 70 years decreased at each site (Table 3).

Discussion

DEXA machines are widely used for the screening and diagnosis of osteoporosis. Measurements in two lumbar projections (anteroposterior and lateral), several appendicular bones (femoral neck, distal 1/3 of the forearm, ultradistal of the forearm, calcaneus, etc.), and whole body have been evaluated for this purpose. Several investigators have pointed out that lumbar BMD is most sensitive for osteoporosis because the vertebrae are predominantly of the trabecular bone type which are affected by the postmenopausal estrogen decrease more quickly than cortical bone [2–4]. As expected, patients with osteoporosis had lower spinal BMD values by DEXA compared to controls, as reported previously [5]. The differences of 22.4% for lumbar A-P (Z-score 1.5) and 30.3% for lumbar lateral BMD (Z-score 1.4) were higher than those for appendicular skeletons (femoral neck 10.6%, forearm 17.9%) in patients aged 50–69 years.

Sometimes, however, the BMD by lumbar A-P projection is overestimated in subjects who have spondylotic changes at the lumbar spinal bodies or the posterior elements, and ossification of the abdominal aorta. To eliminate this overestimation, lateral projection of the lumbar spine has been investigated. Even though advances in DEXA technology allow the use of a higher current

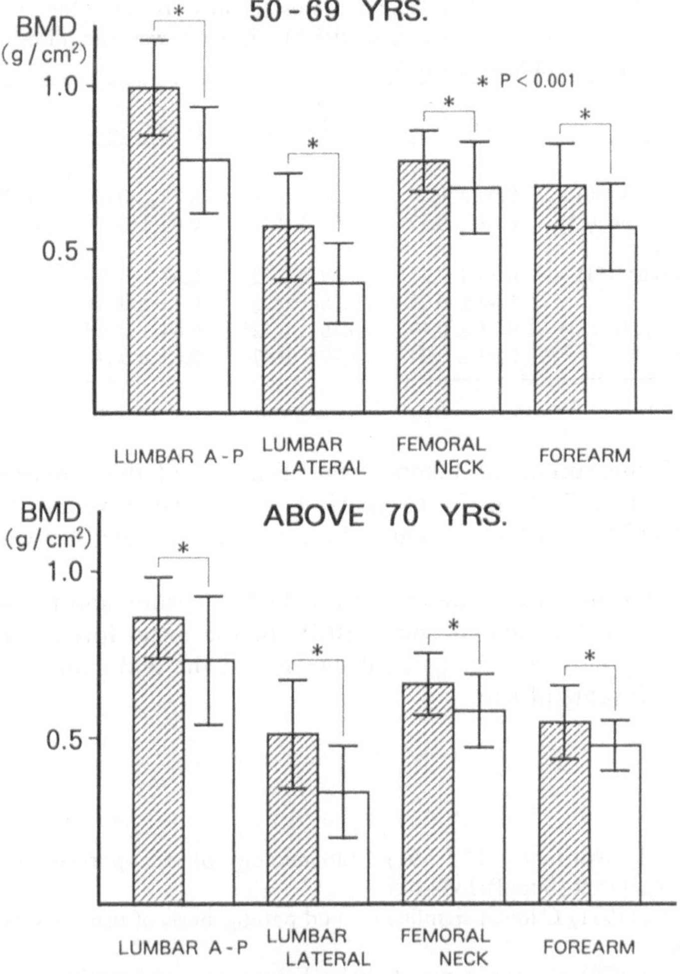

Fig. 4. Mean BMD of four skeletal sites for the control (*hatched bars*) and study (*open bars*) groups for 50–69 years and above 70 years of age. BMD in patients with osteoporosis was significantly lower than that in controls

and a narrower beam, in vivo precision errors in lateral BMD measurement are still greater (2%–3%) than in lumbar A-P BMD measurement (less than 1.0%) in young adults [6–7].

Even though sensitivity of peripheral BMD measurement is not better than spinal projections, several peripheral bone sites (calcaneus, distal 1/3 of the radius) are useful in the identification of osteoporosis patients with a high risk for fracture or diagnosis of osteoporosis in subjects over 70 years [8]. In this

Table 3. BMD value at four skeletal sites (g/cm^2). BMD values for osteoporosis were adjusted by age and weight. Z-score was the discrimination between control and osteoporosis.

	Lumber A-P	Lumbar lateral	Femoral neck	Forearm
Control				
50–69 years (50)	0.98 ± 0.14	0.56 ± 0.16	0.75 ± 0.09	0.67 ± 0.13
Over 70 years (15)	0.87 ± 0.12	0.52 ± 0.16	0.66 ± 0.10	0.55 ± 0.10
Osteoporosis				
50–69 years (51)	0.76 ± 0.16*	0.39 ± 0.12*	0.67 ± 0.13*	0.55 ± 0.13*
Z-score	1.49 ± 0.29	1.38 ± 0.23	0.75 ± 0.21	0.95 ± 0.26
Over 70 years (35)	0.73 ± 0.19*	0.36 ± 0.12*	0.60 ± 0.10*	0.48 ± 0.08*
Z-score	0.79 ± 0.34	1.19 ± 0.27	0.65 ± 0.20	0.78 ± 0.17

* $P < 0.001$

study, BMD measurements taken at the distal 1⁄3 of the forearm showed a larger difference (17.9% in 50–69 years, 12.7% above 70 years) than femoral neck BMD (10.6% in 50–69 years, 9.1% above 70 years) between the two groups.

In conclusion, the most suitable site for BMD measurement in the diagnosis of osteoporosis is the lumbar spine. BMD of the distal forearm is useful in subjects with spondylotic change, calcification of the abdominal aorta, or for those above 70 years of age.

References

1. Yoshikawa T, Norimatsu H (1991) Epidemiology of osteoporosis in Okinawa. J Bone Min Metab 9 (Suppl):135–145
2. Nordin BEC (1971) Clinical significance and pathogenesis of osteoporosis. Br Med J 1:571–576
3. Mazess RB (1979) Measurement of skeletal status by non-invasive methods. Calcif Tissue Inf 28:89–92
4. Wahner HW, Riggs BL, Beabout JW (1977) Diagnosis of osteoporosis: Usefulness of photon absorptiometry of radius. J Nucl Med 18:432–437
5. Duboeuf F, Meunier PL, Delmas PD (1991) Lateral measurement of the bone mineral density (BMD) of the lumbar spine measured with a Lunar DPX L: Preliminary results. Calcif Tissue Int 48 (Suppl):A76
6. Souza ACA, Nakamura T, Stergiopoulos (1990) Measurement of vertebral body using dual energy x-ray absorptiometry in lateral projection. In: Overgaard C, et al. (eds) Third international symposium on osteoporosis, Handelstrykkeriet, Aalborg, pp 640–642
7. Pouilles JM, Tremollieres F, Todorovsky N, Ribot C (1991) Precision and sensitivity of dual-energy x-ray absorptiometry in spinal osteoporosis. J Bone Miner Res 6:997–1002
8. Wasnich RD, Ross PD, Heilbrun LK, Vogel JM (1987) Selection of the optimal skeletal site for fracture risk prediction. Clin Orthop 216:262–269

Bone Volume Measurement of Lumbar Spine by DEXA in One-Bound Volleyball Players

HIDETAKA SEKIGUCHI[1], HIDEAKI E. TAKAHASHI[1], YOSHIO KOGA[1], TATSUHIKO TANIZAWA[1], and IKUKO EZAWA[2]

Key Words. Sports activity in elderly people, prevention of osteoporosis, bone volume, DEXA

Introduction

Participation in sports activity by elderly people seems to be effective in preventing osteoporosis. We analyzed the efficacy of light sports for maintaining the bone volume of the lumbar spine in elderly people.

Materials and Methods

Group A: 127 one-bound volleyball players (45 males, 82 females). The males were between 62 and 95 years of age (av 73.9 years). The females were between 51 and 81 years (av 67.6 years). Group B: 59 non-sports players (17 males, 42 females). The males were between 64 and 81 years. (av 68.7 years). The females were between 58 and 83 years (av 68.3 years). Males in group A were significantly ($P < 0.05$) older than those in group B. Subjects in both groups lived in the same city.

One-bound volleyball is 6-person team volleyball in which the ball is permitted "one bound" before hitting. Males in group A trained between 1 year 10 months and 18 years 7 months (av 11 years). Females in group A trained between 9 months and 16 years 10 months (av 8 years 11 months). They trained twice a week, and one training session takes 2 h. We had previously

[1] Department of Orthopedic Surgery, Niigata University School of Medicine, Asahimachi-dori 1-757, Niigata, 951 Japan
[2] Japan Women's College, 2-8-1 Mejirodai, Bunkyo-ku, Tokyo, 112 Japan

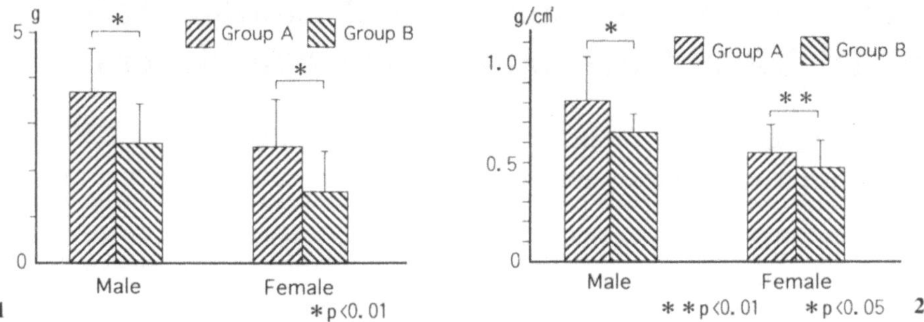

Fig. 1. Bone mineral content (BMC) on the L3 lateral view. $^*P < 0.01$

Fig. 2. Bone mineral density (BMD) on the L3 lateral view. $^*P < 0.05$; $^{**}P < 0.01$

demonstrated that energy consumption in 2 h training is approximately the same as that in 1 h walking.

In this study, we investigated bone mineral content (BMC) and bone mineral density (BMD) on the L2–4 AP view and the L3 lateral view by dual-energy X-ray absorptiometry (DEXA) using the Hologic QDR-1000 (Waltham, Mass.). Body height, body weight, serum calcium (Ca), inorganic phosphate (P), and alkaline phosphatase (Alp) were measured. Oral calcium intake was also investigated. Student's *t*-test was used to assess differences between the two groups.

Results

In both sexes, BMC on the L3 lateral view in group A was greater than that in group B ($P < 0.01$, Fig. 1), and BMD on the L3 lateral view in group A was also greater than that in group B (in males $P < 0.05$, in females $P < 0.01$, Fig. 2). BMC and BMD on the L2–4 AP view did not differ between the two groups. It was reported that bone volume increases in proportion to body mass index (BMI) [1]. In this study, BMI did not differ between the two groups (Fig. 3). Oral calcium intake did not differ between the two groups (Fig. 4). Serum Ca, P, and Alp were normal in all subjects and did not differ between the two groups.

Discussion

It has previously been reported that bone volume (BMC or BMD) of the lumbar spine on the L2–4 AP view is influenced by spondylotic change and that on the L3 lateral view reflects cancellous bone volume [2,3]. This explains why our results indicated that bone volume on the L3 lateral view in group A

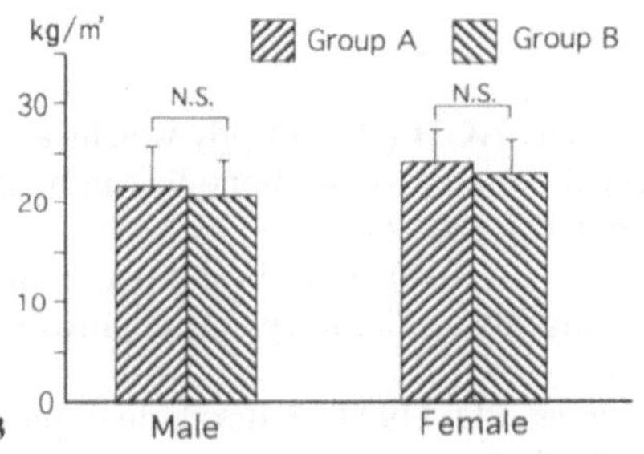

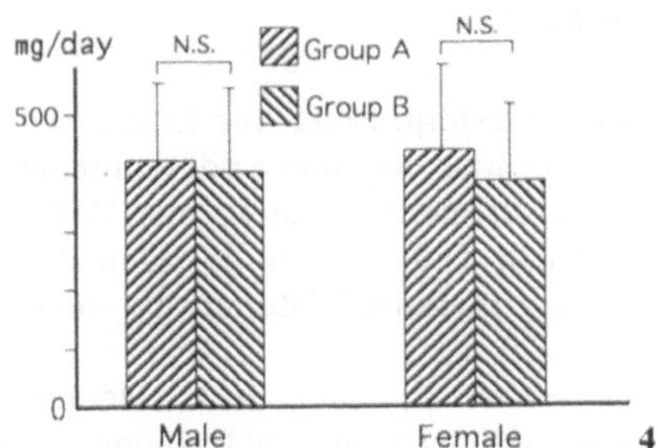

Fig. 3. Body mass index. *N.S.*, not significant

Fig. 4. Oral Ca intake. *N.S.*, not significant

was greater than that in group B, while that on the L2–4 AP view did not differ between the two groups. BMI and oral calcium intake did not differ between the two groups. Light sports, such as one-bound volleyball, therefore seem to be effective in maintaining bone volume in the lumbar spine in elderly people.

Walking or playing gateball for 1 h a day are encouraged for elderly people to maintain bone volume. Energy consumption in 2 h of one-bound volleyball playing is the same as that in 1 h of walking. Therefore, walking 1 h only twice a week may maintain bone volume.

However, subjects in group A may have been active in their younger days and initial peak bone mass in group A may have been higher than that in group B. To more precisely determine the efficacy of light sports for maintaining bone volume in elderly people, a prospective study is needed using groups with no difference in bone volume.

Summary

1. We analyzed the efficacy of light sports for maintaining bone volume of the lumbar spine in elderly people.
2. BMC and BMD of the L3 lateral view in one-bound volleyball players were greater than those in non-players of both sexes.
3. BMI and oral calcium intake did not differ between the two groups.
4. Light sports, such as one-bound volleyball, seem to be effective for maintaining bone volume in elderly people.

References

1. van Beresteijn ECH, van Laarhoven JPRM, Smals AGH (1992) Body weight and/or endogenous estradiol as determinants of cortical bone mass and bone loss in healthy early postmenopausal woman. Acta Endocrinol 127:226–230
2. Slosman DO, Rizzoli R, Donath A, Bonjour J (1990) Vertebral bone mineral density measured laterally by dual-energy X-ray absorptiometry. Osteoporosis Int 1:23–29
3. Uebelhart D, Duboeuf F, Meunier PJ, Delmas PD (1990) Lateral dual photon apsorptiometry. A new technique to measure the bone mineral density at the lumber spine. J Bone Miner Res 5:525–531

Changes of Bone Mineral Content of Lumbar Spine in Osteoporotic Patients Treated with Vitamin D and Calcitonin

TATSUHIKO TANIZAWA[1], SABURO NISHIDA[1], NORIAKI YAMAMOTO[1], SHINOBU ASAI[2], and HIDEAKI E. TAKAHASHI[1]

Key Words. Osteoporosis, dual-energy X-ray absorptiometry, vitamin D, calcitonin, lumbar spine

Introduction

Recently, bone mineral measurement using dual-energy X-ray absorptiometry (DEXA) has become more widespread while the results after treatment for osteoporosis have not been sufficiently reported. The aim of the present study was to demonstrate the changes in bone mineral density of the lumbar spine after treatment with vitamin D or calcitonin or combination of both in osteoporotic patients.

Subjects and Methods

Subjects

Twenty-eight female patients with primary osteoporosis (age range 54–93 years, mean 71.1 years) and 15 female patients with secondary osteoporosis treated with glucocorticoid due to various diseases (5 systemic lupus erythematosus, 2 dermatomyositis, 1 rheumatoid arthritis, 1 bronchial asthma, 1 idiopathic thrombocytopenic purpura, 1 pemphigus, 1 nephrotic syndrome, 1 progressive systemic sclerosis, and 2 other causes. They ranged in age from 22 to 76 years, mean 52.9 years) were included in this study.

The patients were classified into 3 groups according to the treatment of osteoporosis. In group 1, oral alphacalcidol was administered continuously

[1] Department of Orthopedic Surgery, Niigata University School of Medicine, Asahimachi-dori 1-757, Niigata, 951 Japan
[2] Department of Orthopedic Surgery, Nekoyama-Miyao Hospital, Niigata, Japan

(0.5–0.75 μg daily); in group 2, 10 units of eel calcitonin was injected into the patients subcutaneously once or twice per week; in group 3, combination therapy of alphacalcidol and eel calcitonin was given simultaneously at the same dosage described for groups 1 and 2.

Group 1 included 25 cases of osteoporosis (15 primary and 9 secondary); group 2 included 8 cases (6 primary and 2 secondary); and group 3 included 10 cases (7 primary and 3 secondary).

The mean dosage of prednisolone given to the patients with secondary osteoporosis was 12.3 mg/day (range 5–17.5 mg/day) and the mean duration of administration was 3.8 years (range 1.5–7 years).

Methods

The bone mineral content (BMC) of the 2nd to 4th lumbar vertebrae, in A-P projection, was measured by DEXA using a Hologic QDR 1000 W system (Toyo Medic, Tokyo, Japan) and expressed as a percent. The measurement was performed at 0, 6, and 12 months after the treatment.

Serum biochemical markers, bone Gla protein (BGP) and M-PTH, were collected before the treatment and at 3 months after the treatment.

Statistics

The statistical analysis used in this study was Student's paired *t*-test.

Results

At 6 and 12 months after the treatment, there was no significant change in BMC, in both primary and secondary osteoporotic patients, although the mean value was slightly higher at 12 months in both groups (Table 1).

Serum level of M-PTH showed no differences between pretreatment and posttreatment in both groups, while the serum level of BGP was significantly reduced ($P < 0.05$) in the patients with primary osteoporosis (Table 2).

In relation to the subgroups classified by the treatment, there were no significant changes of BMC in groups 1 and 2. On the contrary, a significant increase ($P < 0.05$) of lumbar BMC was found at 12 months after the treatment in group 3 (Table 3). Serum level of BGP was significantly reduced ($P < 0.05$) after the treatment in group 2 treated with calcitonin.

Discussion

Canniggia et al. [1] reported the long-term treatment with 1 alpha, 25 dihydroxyvitamin D_3 in postmenopausal osteoporosis. Although none of these patients received calcium supplementation, the results showed not only an

Table 1. Percent change of lumbar bone mineral content (BMC) (L2–4) 6 and 12 months after the treatment.

	6 months	12 months
Primary osteoporosis	+1.3% (±0.04)	+3.0 (±0.09)
Secondary osteoporosis	−0.1% (±0.04)	+2.8 (±0.14)

Mean ± SD

Table 2. Changes in serum parameters before and after 3 months of treatment.

	Pretreatment	Posttreatment
Primary osteoporosis		
M-PTH	342.6 ± 119.9	318.8 ± 141.6 pg/ml
BGP	8.8 ± 3.2	6.9 ± 2.7* ng/ml
Secondary ostcoporosis		
M-PTH	322.6 ± 134.5	318.0 ± 193.1 pg/ml
BGP	13.3 ± 14.6	13.0 ± 13.3 ng/ml
Group 1		
M-PTH	403.5 ± 152.6	372.5 ± 161.4 pg/ml
BGP	8.4 ± 3.3	6.6 ± 3.6 ng/ml
Group 2		
M-PTH	330.6 ± 68.7	380.0 ± 166.2 pg/ml
BGP	15.6 ± 13.4	13.1 ± 13.1* ng/ml
Group 3		
M-PTH	273.3 ± 84.0	224.3 ± 87.7 pg/ml
BGP	7.3 ± 3.2	7.8 ± 2.1 ng/ml

Mean ± SD
BGP, Bone Gla protein
$^*P < 0.05$

Table 3. Percent change of lumbar BMC (L2–4) in patients with different types of treatment.

	6 months	12 months
Group 1	+0.9% (±0.03)	+2.5% (±0.10)
Group 2	+0.9% (±0.03)	+2.0% (±0.05)
Group 3	+0.8% (±0.04)	+9.4% (±0.76)*

Mean ± SD
$^*P < 0.05$

increase of calcium absorption in the intestine but also that the increment of total body calcium increased by +1.20%, while it was −1.7% in the control group after 1 year of follow-up. Moreover, nontraumatic vertebral fractures apparently decreased after the treatment.

In old age, the enzymatic activity of 25-hydroxyvitamin D_1 hydroxylase, which produces the active vitamin D, diminishes [2]. Furthermore, the function or number of vitamin D-binding receptors in the gut is decreased in senile ostoeporosis [3]. This results in decreased intestinal absorption of calcium which leads to an increase in parathormone (PTH) secretion. Treatment of osteoporosis with vitamin D analogues normalizes and improves calcium absorption and balance. A reduced fracture rate of the vertebrae has been achieved by treatment with alphacalcidol for 1 year [4]. In the present study, the BMD of the lumbar spine (L2–4) was preserved with vitamin D therapy. The duration of treatment was 1 year, which was not long enough to clarify the effect of this agent on osteoporosis. While further investigation is necessary, it should be emphasized that vitamin D is physiological and quite safe as an agent for bone metabolism since there were no adverse effects during the treatment.

In a controlled double-blind study using salmon calcitonin, Mazzuoli et al. [5] demonstrated an increase in BMC of the distal radius in association with a decrease in total urinary hydroxyproline excretion. Civitelli et al. [6] also reported the positive effect of salmon calcitonin on postmenopausal osteoporosis; not only did the vertebral bone mineral content increase, but this increase was more pronounced in high turnover osteoporosis. Thus, calcitonin appears to be indicated for patients with high turnover osteoporosis [7], inhibiting osteoclastic bone resorption and subsequently lowering the bone turnover. We have not measured the biochemical markers of bone resorption, but it is likely that the eel calcitonin reduced osteoclastic bone resorption.

Combination therapy with vitamin D and calcitonin has not been well understood. Palmieri et al. [8] demonstrated beneficial effects following treatment with calcitonin and vitamin D for over 3 years. There was no significant change in cortical bone mass measured by single-photon bone densitometry but a 43% increase of trabecular bone mass was observed by histomorphometry. With this therapy, the fracture rate of the spine was three times lower. A significant increase in the BMC of the lumbar spine was also obtained in this study. Although the number of patients is small and the duration of treatment is short in this study, the present results suggest that there may be some beneficial effect of combining these drugs on osteoporosis. As previously mentioned, vitamin D administration may supplement decreased calcium absorption in the gut, which is prevalent among elderly patients, thus improving the balance of calcium to a positive value. Calcitonin seems to be more beneficial when the turnover of bone is high, as is mostly seen in postmenopausal women. The combination of these agents may cause the calcium balance to become positive in osteoporosis regardless of the degree of bone turnover.

References

1. Caniggia A, Nuti R, Lore F, Martini G, Turchetti V, Righi G (1990) Long-term treatment with calcitriol in postmenopausal osteoporosis. Metabolism 39:43–49

2. Deluca HF (1990) Osteoporosis and the metabolites of vitamin D. Metabolism 39:3–9
3. Gallagher JC (1990) The pathogenesis of osteoporosis. Bone Miner 9:215–227
4. Fujita T (1990) Studies of osteoporosis in Japan. Metabolism 39:39–42
5. Mazzuoli GF, Passeri M, Gennari C, Minisola R, Antonelli R, Valtorta C, Palummeri E, Cervellin GF, Gonnelli S, Francini G (1986) Effects of salmon calcitonin in postmenopausal osteoporosis: A controlled double blind study. Calcif Tissue Int 38:3–8
6. Civitelli R, Gonnelli S, Zacchei F, Bigazzi S, Vattimo A, Avioli LV, Gennari C (1988) Bone turnover in postmenopausal osteoporosis. J Clin Invest 82:1268–1274
7. Gennari C: Salmon calcitonin (Miacalcic) nasal spray in prevention and treatment of osteoporosis. Clin Rheum 8:61–65
8. Palmieri GMA, Pitcock JA, Brown P, Karas JG, Roen LJ (1989) Effect of calcitonin and vitamin D in osteoporosis. Calcif Tissue Int 45:137–141

Part IV.

Pathogenesis, Diagnosis and Treatment of Ossification and Degenerative Spine

Ossification of the Posterior Longitudinal Ligament —Hereditary Investigations

TAKASHI SAKOU, EIJI TAKETOMI, SHUNJI MATSUNAGA, MASAO YAMAGUCHI, and KYOUJI HAYASHI[1]

Abstract. Ossification of the posterior longitudinal ligament (OPLL) in the cervical spine is not uncommon in Japan, but is rarely reported in other countries. The etiology of this disease has not yet been clarified. Meanwhile, systematic factors or regional factors have been mentioned as the cause of ossification. Systematic factors include: (1) race, (2) hormonal abnormality, (3) metabolic disturbances, (4) infection, (5) ankylosing spinal hyperostosis, (6) fluorine intoxication, (7) genetic factors, and others. Regional factors include: (1) mechanical stress to the cervical spine and, (2) disc degeneration. Recently, the possibility of familial predisposition has been suggested. In our familial study, OPLL was found in 30 out of 65 OPLL patient's families (47 of 224 siblings). Two patients were identical twins and the investigation revealed that the twins had the same type of ossification. The human leukocyte antigen (HLA)-haplotype was analyzed in 33 of the families in which any of the siblings were proven to have OPLL. The study showed that HLA-haplotypes formed certain types of clusters. Very interestingly, in each of these siblings with ossification both HLA-haplotypes were identical with those of the proband, and ossification was not found in any siblings with one HLA-haplotype different from that of the proband. These findings strongly suggest the involvement of genetic factors in the pathogenesis of OPLL. We believe that ossification occurs as a result of the interaction between various factors including regressive degeneration due to aging and environmental factors on the basis of genetic predisposition. The pathogenesis of the ossification is discussed in relation to the findings of a series of our studies concerning genetic factors.

Key Words. Ossification of the posterior longitudinal ligament (OPLL), genetic background, human leukocyte antigen, HLA haplotype

[1]Department of Orthopaedic Surgery, Faculty of Medicine, Kagoshima University, 8-35-1 Sakuragaoka, Kagoshima, 890 Japan

Introduction

Ossification of the posterior longitudinal ligament (OPLL) was unheard of before Dr. Tsukimoto's report of an autopsy case in 1960 [1]. Although rarely reported in other countries, OPLL in the cervical spine has been found to be rather common in Japan from the many reports of OPLL patients and through the national survey made by a research team of the Health and Welfare Ministry [2,3]. Although various systemic and local pathogenic factors have been suggested to explain the etiology of OPLL, the pathogenic mechanism has not been elucidated [4]. However, genetic investigations have revealed familial predisposition to OPLL, suggesting the involvement of genetic factors.

Herein, we discuss the findings of our recent studies on the etiology of this disease.

Clinical Features and Pathology

Clinical Features

The age at onset of OPLL is most often over 40 years and it occurs predominantly in males. The initial symptoms are usually complaints of neck pain and tingling sensation in the extremities, and later spastic paralysis development which eventually becomes chronic.

Pathological Findings

Histologically, the ossification of the ligament is mostly enchondral. In the posterior margin of the disc fibrocartilage, tissue proliferation is marked, but disc degeneration is not (Fig. 1). The spinal cord is flattened and atrophied because of compression, but there are no significant destructive changes within the cord (Fig. 2).

Etiology

Although various systemic and local pathogenic factors have been suggested to explain the etiology of OPLL, the etiology of the disease has not been clarified (Table 1). OPLL is often accompanied by marked vertebral hyperostotic changes, ossification in the thoracic and lumbar spines, ossification of the ligamentum flavum, and ossification around the joint, hip joints, ankle joints, and shoulder joints which occurs at a high frequency. Some doctors believe that this ossification should be classified as a disease of the spinal ligaments.

There seems to be a racial difference in its incidence. OPLL has been reported to be peculiar to the Japanese population, and is rare among Caucasians [2,3]. The incidence of OPLL in the general Japanese population

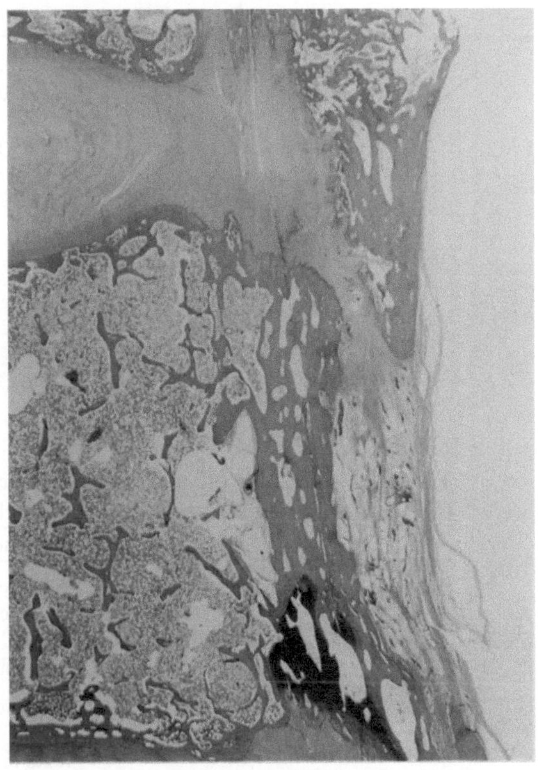

Fig. 1. Histological specimen of ossification of the posterior longitudinal ligament (OPLL) obtained from autopsy. H&E, ×5

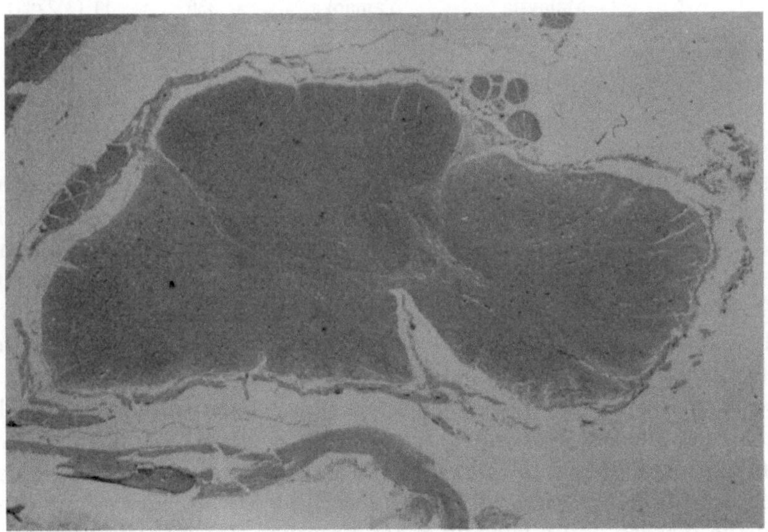

Fig. 2. Pathological changes of spinal cord in an OPLL patient. H&E, ×3

Table 1. Etiology.

Systemic factors	Regional factors
Race	Mechanical stress to the cervical spine
Hormonal abnormality	Disc degeneration
Metabolic disorders	
Infection	
Ankylosing spinal hyperostosis	
Fluorosis	
Heredity	
Hypervitaminosis A	
Diabetes mellitus	

Table 2. Incidence of ossification of posterior longitudinal ligament (OPLL) in foreign countries (outpatient clinic).

	Country	Reporter	Subjects (n)	OPLL (+)
Europe & USA	USA (Hawaii)	Yamauchi	490	3 (0.61%)
	USA (Mayo)	Yamauchi	854	2 (0.23%)
	West Germany	Sasaki	1060	1 (0.09%)
	Italy	Terayama	1258	22 (1.74%)
Asia	Singapore	Kurokawa	496	2 (0.40%)
	Korea	Sakou	726	13 (1.79%)
	Korea	Tezuka	891	7 (0.79%)
	Hong Kong	Kurokawa	498	9 (1.81%)
	Taiwan	Kurokawa	500	12 (2.41%)
	Philippines	Yamaura	332	5 (1.51%)
	Malaysia	Yamaoka	336	11 (3.27%)

has been reported to be 1.9%–4.3% among people over 30 years of age [5]. The ossification was radiographically found in 0.1%–1.7% of the outpatients with cervical spine disorders in USA and Europe and as much as 3.3% in Asia (Table 2). However, no epidemiological overseas studies have been conducted on the general population except for our studies in Taiwan on 1004 Chinese, and 529 Takasago tribes-people over 30 years of age, in which the incidence was only 0.2% [6]. These values are evidently lower than the 1.9% incidence in our study on the Japanese population (Table 3).

Recently, many doctors have suggested a genetic involvement in this disease. In general, genetic involvement in a disease can often be confirmed by: (1) a high familial incidence of the disease, (2) a significantly higher coincidence of the disease in monozygotic twins than in dizygotic twins, and (3) a correlation between the disease and a specific genetic marker (HLA). We examined each of these items.

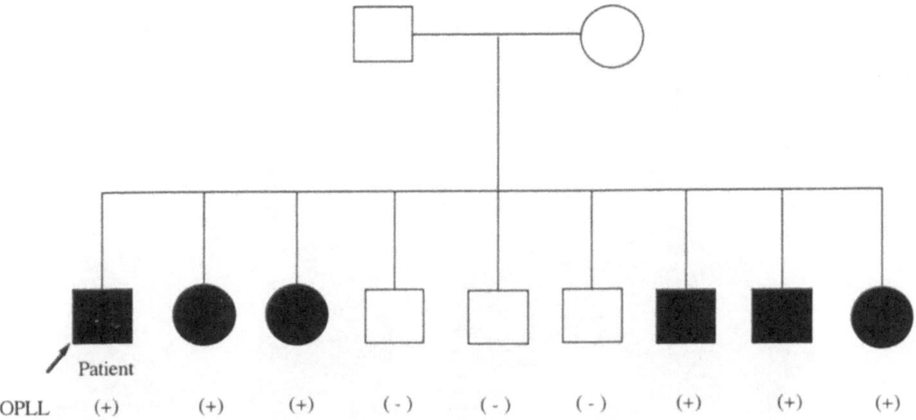

Fig. 3. OPLL patient (proband) and his family

Table 3. Incidence of OPLL in Japan (general population).

Area	Reporter	Subjects			OPLL (+)
Tokushima	Ikata	Male	339	705	18 (2.6%)
		Female	366		
Yaeyama	Otani	Male	578	1046	21 (2.0%)
		Female	468		
Kagoshima	Sakou	Male	195	585	11 (1.9%)
		Female	390		
Yachiho	Otsuka	Male	404	973	33 (3.4%)
		Female	569		
Tokushima	Ikata	Male	122	415	18 (4.3%)
		Female	293		

Family Study

We examined the familial incidence. The subjects were mostly the parents and siblings of the patients. Among the 72 families we studied, OPLL was confirmed in 45 out of 125 relatives [7]. This incidence is nearly the same as that obtained in a nationwide survey (30%).

Case Report. In one patient, a 64-year-old male, continuous-type ossification was found in the whole cervical spine. He had five brothers and three sisters. OPLL was found in two brothers and in all three sisters (Fig. 3). The genotype of this disease was suggestive of recessive inheritance, using the proband method and *A-priori* method.

Study of Monozygotic Twins with OPLL

It is important to examine identical twins to prove the involvement of genetic factors in a disease, but there have been few such reports in the study of

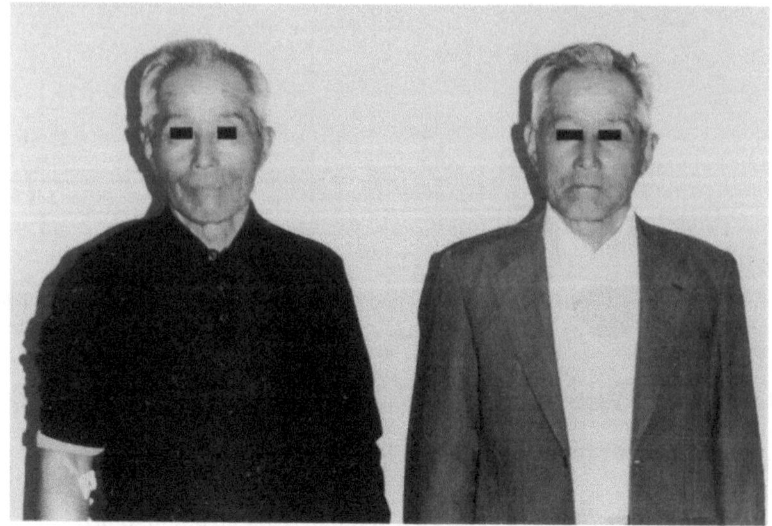

Fig. 4. OPLL twins

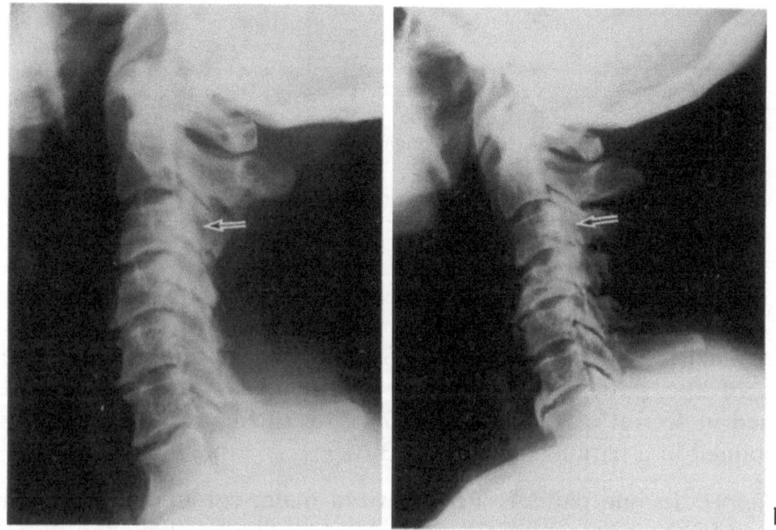

Fig. 5a,b. Lateral X-ray films of cervical spine of OPLL twins. **a** Patient. **b** Twin brother

OPLL. We had one case of OPLL in twins [8]. They were 74-year-old twin brothers. The blood-type examination revealed that they were identical twins (Fig. 4). In the cervical spine, the proband had continuous type OPLL in C2–C4, and his twin brother had the same condition in C3–C6. Analogous types of ossification in the cervical spine are often observed in monozygotic twins (Fig. 5); this also suggests the involvement of genetic factors in OPLL.

HLA Haplotype Analysis

Human leukocyte antigen (HLA) analysis is useful for the determination of the presence or absence of genetic causation. Human leukocyte antigen genes are located on the short arm of the sixth chromosome in humans, and are serologically classified into six antigenic types, namely, HLA-A, B, C, DR, DQ, and DP [9]. In the orthopedic field, the B27 antigen was found in about 90% of patients with ankylosing spondilitis [10]. B27 was also relatively risky for Reiter's disease, and DR4 for rheumatoid arthritis. Studies of HLA phenotypes in OPLL have shown the frequent appearance of Aw24, A11, Bw40, and Cw7, but none of the results were statistically significant. Antigens (HLA) have been studied by a number of investigators in relation to the genetic predisposition to OPLL, but all these studies dealt with phenotype rather than HLA haplotype [11–13]. However, considering the clear tendency of inheritance disclosed by family surveys, the genes responsible for OPLL should be detectable by the HLA haplotype analyses.

The HLA haplotype, which represents the sequence of HLA genes on a chromosome, can be determined by studying HLAs in the family. Four combinations were present among the siblings. Haplotypes differ with the individual and there are a great variety of combinations. Children inheret one allele from each of their parents.

We examined the correlation between HLA haplotype and OPLL in the patients and their kin [14]. Families of 37 patients, 171 family members in all, were studied. Most of the family members lived in the Kagoshima area. Several HLA cluster formations were recognized in 25 of the 37 patients. In the remaining 12 patients, the phenotype was different (Table 4). This fact suggests that the HLA haplotype itself dose not play a major role in ossification. However, the disorder occurred in 60% of the family members with two haplotypes identical to those of the patients. If only one haplotype corresponded to one of the patient's, the incidence of OPLL was lower. If the haplotype did not correspond at all, the risk was much less (Fig. 6).

Case Report. One patient studied has a brother and a sister. The brother, with two identical haplotypes to those of the patient, has OPLL. The sister, with no haplotypes in common, does not have OPLL (Fig. 7).

Discussion

OPLL is an intractable disease which can lead to severe spinal cord impairment resulting from chronic compression of the spinal cord by the ossified ligament. Despite many years of studies on a nationwide scale, the etiology of this

Table 4. Human leukocyte antigen haplotypes of OPLL probands.

Proband	Age	OPLL type	Haplotype		
1	54	mix.	A2 Bw52Cw-DR2 DQw1	/	A24 Bw60Cw3DRw8DQ-
22	57	seg.	A2 Bw52Cw-DR2 DQw1	/	A24 Bw61Cw-DR4 DQw4
2	73	seg.	A26 Bw52Cw-DR2 DQw1	/	A2 B37 Cw7DRw8DQ-
3	65	mix.	A24 Bw52Cw-DR2 DQw1	/	A24 B39 Cw3DR4 DQw3
4	59	seg.	A24 Bw52Cw-DR2 DQw1	/	A24 Bw59Cw-DR4 DQw4
26	56	seg.	A24 Bw52Cw-DR2 DQw1	/	A11 Bw60Cw3DRw8DQ-
32	69	seg.	A24 Bw52Cw-DR2 DQw1	/	A31 Bw62Cw3DRw8DQw4
34	45	seg.	A24 Bw52Cw-DR2 DQw1	/	A24 Bw61Cw-DR- DQ-
38	60	mix.	A24 Bw52Cw-DR2 DQw1	/	A- B35 Cw-DR- DQ-
5	53	mix.	A24 Bw52Cw-DR2 DQw1	/	A26 Bw62Cw3DR2 DQw1
18	54	seg.	A2 Bw55Cw1DR- DQw4	/	A26 Bw62Cw3DR2 DQw1
19	64	seg.	A11 Bw54Cw1DRw8DQw3	/	A26 Bw62Cw3DR2 DQw1
39	64	seg.	A2 B- Cw-DR- DQ-	/	A26 Bw62Cw3DR2 DQw1
7	71	seg.	A2 Bw62Cw3DR9 DQw3	/	A26 Bw62Cw3DR5 DQw3
6	72	mix.	A2 Bw- Cw-DR9 DQw3	/	A26 Bw62Cw3DR5 DQw3
8	64	cont.	A2 B35 Cw7DR- DQ-	/	A26 Bw62Cw3DR5 DQw3
10	63	seg.	A24 B35 Cw1DR2 DQw1	/	A26 Bw62Cw3DR4 DQw3
9	67	mix.	A26 B35 Cw-DR2 DQw1	/	A24 Bw62Cw3DR4 DQw3
27	49	seg.	A24 Bw60Cw4DR9 DQw3	/	A24 Bw62Cw3DR4 DQw3
17	59	cont.	A31 Bw60Cw3DR- DQw3	/	A24 Bw62Cw4DR4 DQw3
24	60	seg.	A- B- Cw-DR2 DQw1	/	A24 Bw62Cw4DR4 DQw3
31	48	seg.	A2 Bw59Cw1DR4 DQw4	/	A11 Bw62Cw4DR4 DQw3
35	67	seg.	A26 B- Cw7DR4 DQw3	/	A24 B7 Cw7DR1 DQw1
20	60	seg.	Aw33B44 Cw-DRw6DQw1	/	A24 B7 Cw7DR1 DQw1
11	53	seg.	Aw33B44 Cw-DRw6DQw1	/	A24 Bw- Cw7DRw8DQ-
25	74	mix.	Aw33B44 Cw-DRw6DQw1	/	A31 Bw60Cw3DR2 DQw1
23	50	seg.	Aw33B44 Cw-DR2 DQw1	/	A31 B51 Cw-DR1 DQw1
12	63	cont.	A24 Bw54Cw1DR4 DQw4	/	A2 Bw60Cw3DRw8DQ-
13	58	mix.	A24 Bw54Cw1DR4 DQw4	/	A24 B51 Cw-DR9 DQw3
14	68	seg.	A2 Bw61Cw-DR2 DQw1	/	A- B- Cw-DR4 DQw3
15	62	mix.	A24 Bw59Cw1DR4 DQw4	/	A24 B51 Cw1DR9 DQw3
16	44	mix.	A26 Bw60Cw7DRw8DQ-	/	A2 B35 Cw3DR9 DQw3
21	60	seg.	A24 Bw52Cw-DR9 DQw3	/	A- B51 Cw-DR5 DQ-
37	66	mix.	A26 Bw52Cw-DR9 DQw3	/	A- Bw61Cw3DR9 DQ-
28	63	mix.	A2 Bw54Cw-DR4 DQw3	/	A11 B39 Cw-DR2 DQw1
29	62	mix.	A26 Bw61Cw3DR4 DQw3	/	A2 Bw60Cw-DR2 DQw1
30	66	seg.	A2 B51 Cw3DR2 DQw1	/	Aw33Bw61Cw-DR3 DQw1
33	71	cont.	A- Bw61Cw3DRw6DQw1	/	A2 Bw60Cw-DR4 DQw3
36	73	cont.	A24 B- Cw-DR- DQw4	/	A31 Bw54Cw1DR4 DQw3

mix., Mixed type; *cont.*, continuous type; *seg.*, segmented type

disease has not yet been clarified [4]. However, since about 40% of the patients with OPLL are from OPLL-susceptible families and because twins with this disease are sometimes encountered, many investigators agree in that some genetic factors are closely related to the etiology of this disease [2,3,5,14]. Our survey of HLA haplotypes in the families of OPLL patients revealed several clusters of HLA haplotypes. However, since those haplotypes found are also seen among the general Japanese population, and because OPLL also occurs even when HLA haplotypes form no clusters known to be associated with OPLL, it seems unlikely that HLA haplotypes are directly related to the etiology of OPLL.

In view of the genetic background suggested by surveys of families and twins, and considering the finding from an analysis of patient family haplotypes showing that the incidence of OPLL was high for members of a family sharing

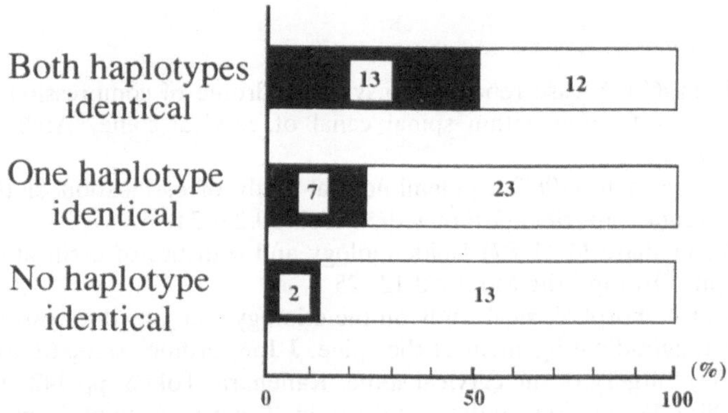

Fig. 6. Relationship between OPLL and identity of haplotypes in the proband and relatives. The *closed bar* represents OPLL(+), and *open bar* OPLL(−)

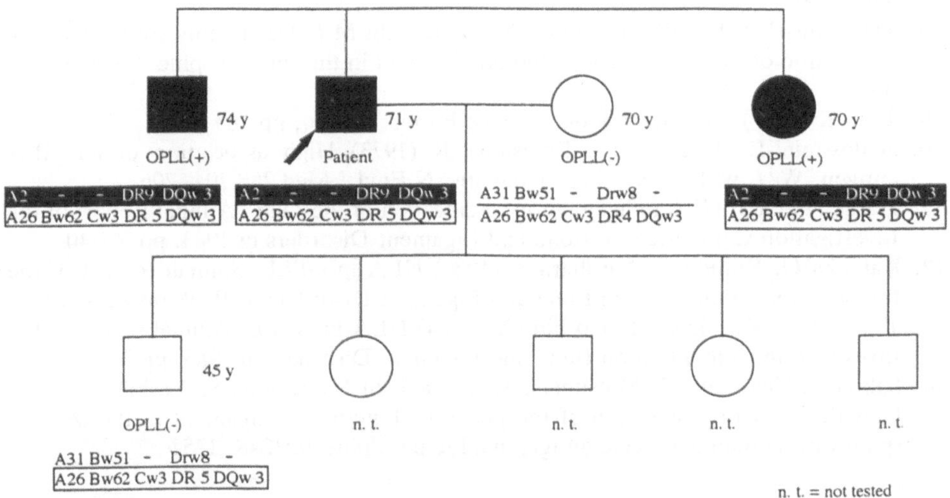

Fig. 7. HLA haplotype analysis in OPLL patient family

two haplotypes with an OPLL-affected member of the same family, it is likely that there is an unknown pathogenic gene which is closely related to the onset of OPLL which confers a predisposition, or increased susceptibility, to certain individuals. It is also likely that this gene is associated with HLA genes. Regarding the etiology of OPLL, we speculate that the posterior longitudinal ligament ossifies when genetic abnormalities are combined with environmental factors such as aging-related degeneration and mechanical trauma. Based on this assumption, we are now attempting to identify the pathogenic gene by isolating lymphocytes from peripheral blood of patient's family members and extracting DNA from these lymphocytes for restriction fragment analysis.

References

1. Tsukimoto H (1960) A case report-autopsy of syndrome of compression of spinal cord owing to ossification within spinal canal of cervical spine. Arch Jpn Chir 239:1003–1007
2. Yamauchi H, Izawa K (1987) Epidemiological study of ossification of the spinal ligament in foreign countries. Orthopaedic Mook 50:26–34
3. Otsuka K, Yanagihara M (1987) Epidemiology and statistics of ossification of the spinal ligament. Orthopaedic Mook 50:12–25
4. Saika M (1987) A morphological study on the etiology and growth of ossification of the posterior longitudinal ligament of the spine. J Jpn Orthop Assoc 61:1059–1072
5. Sakou T (1989) Surgery of the cervical spine. Kanehara, Tokyo, pp 142–144
6. Sakou T (1985) Population study of OPLL in Taiwan. Annual Report of the Investigation Committee on Bone and Ligament Disorders in 1984. pp 66–70
7. Uehara H, Sakou T, Morimoto N, Morizono Y, Nakagawa M, Utino K (1988) Family study of ossification of posterior longitudinal ligament. Orthoped Traumatol 36:800–802
8. Taketomi E, Sakou T, Matsunaga S, Yamaguchi M (1992) Family study of a twin ossification of the posterior longitudinal ligament in the cervical spine. Spine 33:55–56
9. Tsuji K (1987) HLA handbook. Science Forum, Tokyo, pp 163–167
10. Schlosstein L, Terasaki PI, Bluestone R (1973) High association of an HLA antigen, W27, with ankylosing spondylitis. N Engl J Med 288:704–706
11. Hasue H (1983) HLA in ligamentous ossification of the spine. Annual Report of the Investigation Committee on Bone and Ligament Disorders in 1983. pp 37–40
12. Kataoka O, Kimura H, Kurihara A (1980) HLA in OPLL. Annual Report of the Investigation Committee on Bone and Ligament Disorders in 1979. pp 124–125
13. Tsuyama N, Kurokawa T, Hoshino Y (1984) HLA in OPLL. Annual report of the Investigation Committee on Bone and Ligament Disorders in 1983. pp 37–40
14. Sakou T, Taketomi E, Matsunaga S, Yamaguchi M, Sonoda S, Yashiki S (1991) Genetic study of ossification of the posterior longitudinal ligament in the cervical spine with human leukocyte antigen haplotype. Spine 16:1248–1252

Role of Type XI Collagen in Development of Ossification of Posterior Longitudinal Ligament of the Spine

Masashi Yamazaki[1], Sumio Goto[1], Hiroaki Yamakoshi[1], Atsushi Terakado[1], Katsuhiko Arai[2], Yutaka Nagai[2], and Hideshige Moriya[1]

Key Words. Ossification of the posterior longitudinal ligament (OPLL), hyperostosis, anticollagen antibody, type XI collagen, immunohistochemistry

Introduction

Ossification of the posterior longitudinal ligament (OPLL) of the cervical spine is characterized by a heterotopic bone formation advancing in the spinal ligament. OPLL sometimes develops into a huge mass inside the spinal canal, causing severe compression myelopathy. In the developmental process of OPLL, cartilage-specific type II collagen was shown to appear in the pre-ossifying ligament [1], indicating that the expression of cartilage-type collagen is closely related to the onset and progression of OPLL.

Recently, the presence of minor collagen types IX, X, and XI was confirmed in cartilage tissue together with type II collagen [2]. Among these collagens, type XI collagen was composed of 1α, 2α, and 3α chains in which 1α(XI) and 2α(XI) chains behave similarly to α1(V) and α2(V) chains of type V collagen in electrophoretic mobility, and it was shown to be distributed around chondrocyte lacunae and the cell surface region, as shown by immunohistochemical examinations [2,3]. The function of type XI collagen is not well understood, but based on its tissue distribution it seems to play a role in the interaction between cell and the extracellular matrix [2]. Our previous study on the spinal hyperostotic mouse (twy/twy) demonstrated that cartilaginous metaplasia of ligament cells accompanied by type XI collagen expression seems to be closely related to the onset and progression of spinal hyperostosis [3].

[1] Department of Orthopaedic Surgery, Chiba University School of Medicine, 1-8-1 Inohana, Chuo-ku, Chiba, 260 Japan
[2] Department of Tissue Physiology, Medical Research Institute, Tokyo Medical and Dental University, 2-3-10 Kandasurugadai, Chiyoda-ku, Tokyo, 101 Japan

Table 1. Radiologic and clinical data of patients with ossification of the posterior longitudinal ligament.

Case	Sex	Age (years)	Distribution of the lesion	Type of ossification	Type of operation
1	M	50	C4–C6	Segmental	Ant
2	F	38	C5–C6	Continuous	Ant
3	F	61	C4–C7	Mixed	Ant
4	M	61	C4–C6	Mixed	Ant
5	M	54	C1–C5	Continuous	Post
6	M	67	C2–C7	Mixed	Post
7	M	43	C2–C4	Continuous	Post
8	M	55	C4–C6	Mixed	Post

Ant, Anterior decompression and interbody fusion; *Post*, cervical enlargement laminoplasty

In this study, the distribution patterns of collagen types, especially type XI, in the developmental process of OPLL are described, with special reference to a possible mechanism of OPLL pathogenesis.

Materials and Methods

The radiologic findings of eight patients with OPLL who were examined are summarized in Table 1. OPLL, including the non-ossified posterior longitudinal ligament, was obtained in one piece from four patients during anterior surgery, and the C7 spinous process, including the supra and interspinous ligaments was also taken from four patients during laminoplasty. Specimens obtained surgically from five patients with cervical spondylotic myelopathy, in whom no hyperostotic change was seen radiologically, were examined as controls.

The tissue specimens were fixed in 10% buffered formaldehyde, decalcified in 0.3 M EDTA/0.05 M Tris-HCl buffer, pH 7.6, at 4°C, and then bisected sagittally. Paraffin sections were stained with hematoxylin-eosin (H-E), and immunohistochemically stained with monoclonal antibody to human type I or human type II collagen (Cosmo Biochemicals, Tokyo, Japan) and with polyclonal antibodies to canine type XI collagen [2] according to the peroxidase-antiperoxidase method [3]. The antibodies to type XI collagen used in this study recognized only the 1α(XI) chain, showing no cross-reaction with type II collagen [2].

Results

Posterior Longitudinal Ligament

Marked thickening of the posterior longitudinal ligament was observed in OPLL-affected patients. H-E staining showed the growth of fibrocartilage-like

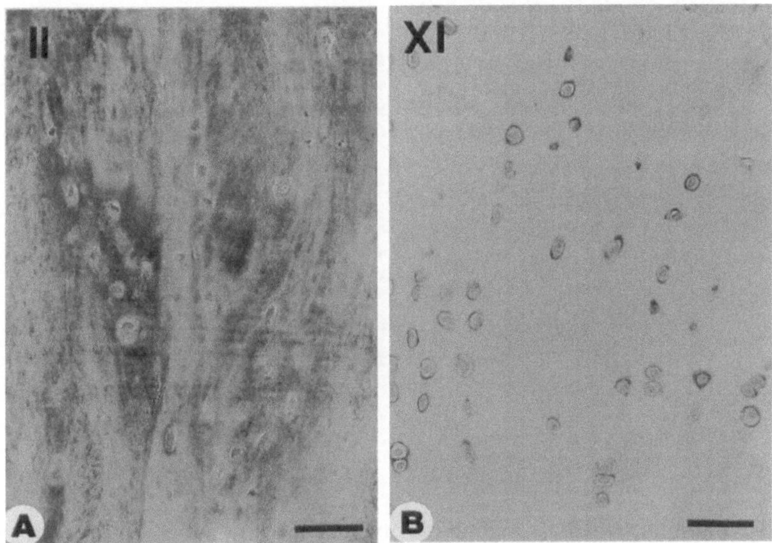

Fig. 1A,B. Immunoperoxidase staining for type II and type XI collagen at the fibrocartilage-like tissue proliferating at the transitional area from ossified to normal posterior longitudinal ligament tissue. **A** Stained with anti-type II and **B** anti-type XI collagen antibodies. *Bars*, 50 μm

tissue at the transitional area from OPLL to the ligaments. In this pre-ossifying tissue, the hyperplastic matrix was well stained with antibody to type II collagen (Fig. 1A), and the pericellular region of the fibrocartilage-like cells was specifically stained with antibodies to type XI collagen (Fig. 1B).

In the ligaments a litte farther from OPLL, proliferation of the round-shaped cells was also observed. Of particular interest was the expression of cartilaginous types of collagen in this area, where matrices only reacted with anti-type XI collagen antibodies, but not with anti-type II collagen antibody (Fig. 2A,B). This finding was very much in contrast with the controls in which ligament cells were fibroblastic and no cartilaginous type of collagen except type I collagen was detected.

Supra and Interspinous Ligaments

Although no hyperostotic change was seen around the spinous process by radiologic examination (Fig. 3A), marked growth of fibrocartilage-like tissue occurred at the ligament insertion in OPLL-affected patients (Fig. 3B). In this fibrocartilage-like tissue, the intercellular matrix was well stained with anti-type II collagen antibody (Fig. 4A), and the pericellular region was stained with anti-type XI collagen antibodies (Fig. 4B).

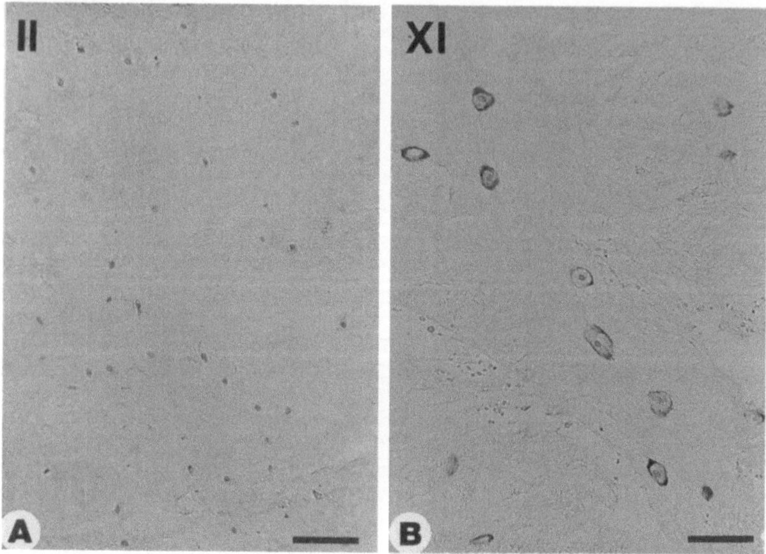

Fig. 2A,B. Immunoperoxidase staining for type II and type XI collagen at the posterior longitudinal ligament farther from ossified ligament tissue. **A** Stained with anti-type II and **B** anti-type XI collagen antibodies. *Bars*, 50 μm

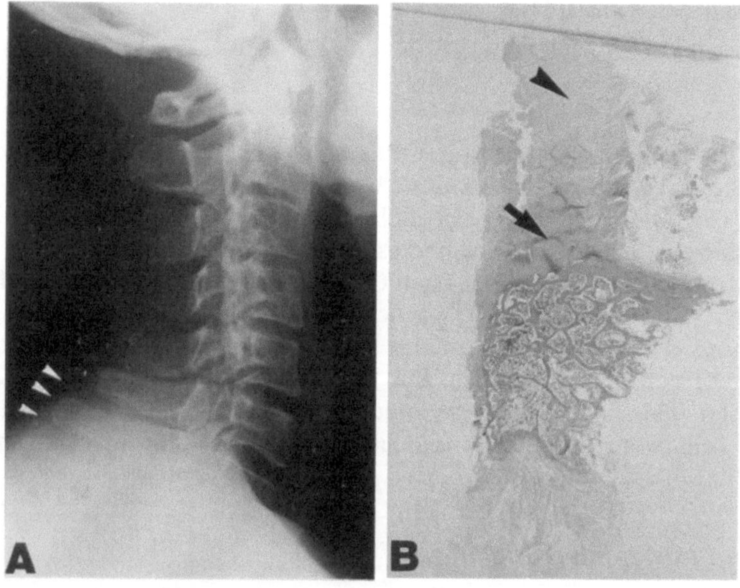

Fig. 3A,B. Case 5: A 54-year-old man with ossification of the posterior longitudinal ligament (OPLL). **A** Plain lateral roentgenogram showing continuous OPLL between C1 and C5. Area depicted in **B** is indicated by *arrowheads*. **B** Hematoxylin-eosin staining of the C7 spinous process and the supra and interspinous ligaments showing proliferation of fibrocartilage-like tissue at the ligament insertion. The *arrow* indicates the area of Fig. 4A,B, and the *arrowhead* the area of Fig. 4C,D

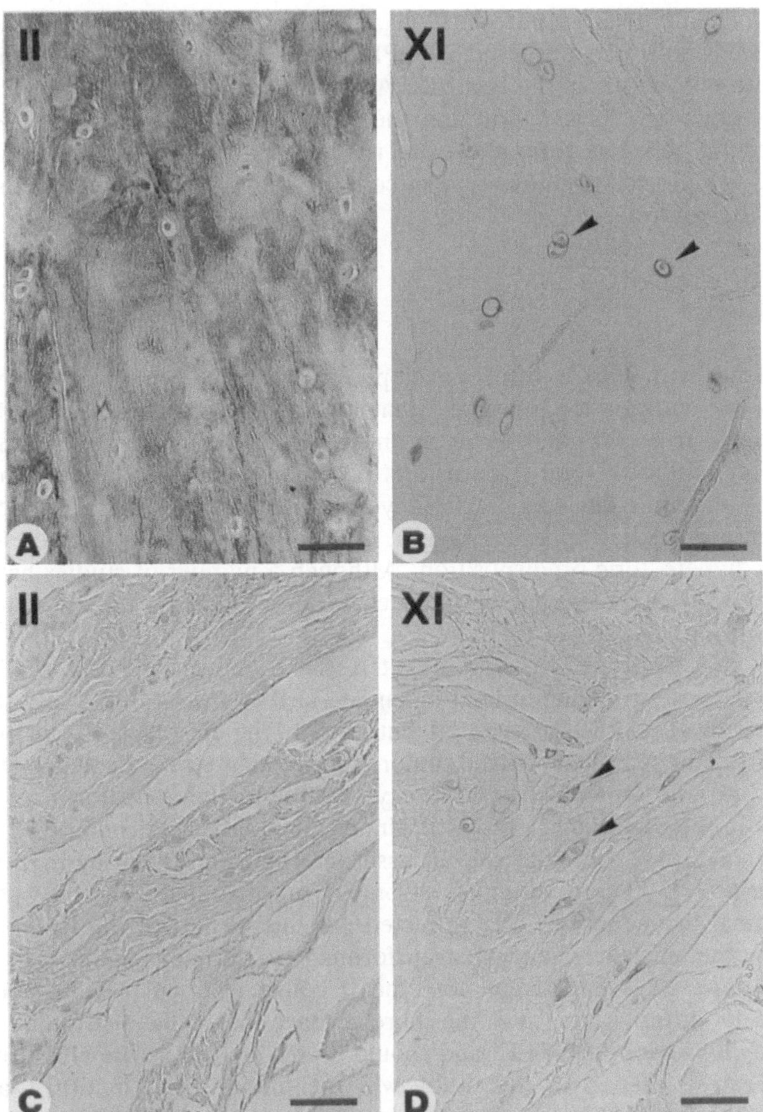

Fig. 4A–D. Immunoperoxidase staining for type II and type XI collagen at the fibrocartilage-like tissue proliferating at the ligament insertion to the spinous process **A,B** and at the supra and interspinous ligaments farther from the insertion **C,D**. **A** Stained with anti-type II, **B** anti-type XI, **C** anti-type II, and **D** anti-type XI collagen antibodies. *Bars*, 50 μm. Pericellular regions reacting with anti-type XI collagen antibodies are indicated by *arrowheads* **B,D**

In the ligaments farther from the ligament insertion, proliferation of round-shaped cells was also observed in OPLL-affected patients, whereas ligament cells were fibroblastic in the controls. As for the expression of the cartilaginous types of collagen, matrices around the round-shaped cells reacted only with anti-type XI collagen antibodies, but not with anti-type II collagen antibody (Fig. 4C,D). No cartilaginous type of collagen was present around the ligament cells in the controls.

Discussion

As patients with OPLL often develop ossification of other spinal ligaments such as the anterior longitudinal ligament and ligamentum flavum, OPLL is now thought to be the same entity as ankylosing spinal hyperostosis (ASH) and diffuse idiopathic skeletal hyperostosis (DISH) [4]. Genetic studies on OPLL indicated that this disorder is possibly controlled by an autosomal dominant inheritance [4]. These findings suggest that OPLL occurs in the presence of a systemic hyperostotic predisposition. Although a number of studies have been performed on the developmental mechanisms of OPLL, the details of this predisposition are not yet clear.

In the present study, we demonstrated that round-shaped cells proliferated among the posterior longitudinal ligaments farther from OPLL, and the cells reacted with antibodies to type XI but not to type II collagen. Our previous study on canine mammary mixed tumors showed that type XI collagen was well detected around metaplastic chondrocytes prior to the appearance of type II collagen in the earlier stage of cartilaginous metaplasia, indicating that type XI collagen may play a crucial role in tissue morphogenesis during cartilaginous metaplasia [2]. These findings strongly suggest that, in the posterior longitudinal ligaments in OPLL-affected patients, a part of the ligament cells undergo metaplastic changes, transforming to round-shaped cells which produce type XI collagen but not type II collagen. Such round-shaped cells may easily differentiate into the fibrocartilage-like cells distributed in the pre-ossifying region of OPLL, and should be referred to as pre-chondrocytes.

Of greatest interest in this study was the finding that, in OPLL-affected patients, the round-shaped cells which produce only type XI collagen were also present among the supra and interspinous ligaments where no hyperostotic change was seen. This finding suggests that the spinal ligament cells in patients with OPLL have acquired the potential to transform into pre-chondrocytes not only in the posterior longitudinal ligaments but also in other spinal ligaments including the supra and interspinous ligaments. This unusual phenotypic expression of the spinal ligament cells may be closely related to the systemic hyperostotic predisposition in this disease. In the presence of this predisposition, OPLL is thought to occur due to the interaction of other factors including local physical stress.

Our previous study showed that inhibin, which is one of the members of the TGF-β family, was expressed during the process of cartilaginous metaplasia [5]. In addition, recent reports have shown that TGF-β induces the transformation of undifferentiated mesenchymal cells to chondrocytes in vitro [6], and that TGF-β was present in the cytoplasm of chondrocytes adjacent to OPLL [7]. Taking the findings described above into account, it is suggested that, in the earlier stage of ligamentous ossification in OPLL, type XI collagen may induce the ligament cells to differentiate into metaplastic chondrocytes in conjunction with some endogenous factor(s) including the TGF-β family.

Acknowledgments. This study was supported in part by a grant from the Division of Intractable Diseases, Public Health Bureau, The Ministry of Health and Welfare of Japan (Investigation Committee on Ossification of Spinal Ligaments).

References

1. Yasui N, Ono K, Yamaura I, Konomi H, Nagai Y (1983) Immunohistochemical localization of types I, II, and III collagens in the ossified posterior longitudinal ligament of the human cervical spine. Calcif Tissue Int 35:159–163
2. Arai K, Uehara K, Nagai Y (1989) Expression of type II and type XI collagens in canine mammary mixed tumors and demonstration of collagen production by tumor cells in collagen gel culture. Jpn J Cancer Res 80:840–847
3. Yamazaki M, Moriya H, Goto S, Saitoh Y, Arai K, Nagai Y (1991) Increased type XI collagen expression in the spinal hyperostotic mouse (twy/twy). Calcif Tissue Int 48:182–189
4. Terayama K (1989) Genetic studies on ossification of the posterior longitudinal ligament of the spine. Spine 14:1184–1191
5. Arai K, Uehara K, Nagai Y (1989) Expression of type II, IX, and XI collagen in mammary mixed tumor. Abstracts of Pan-Pacific Connective Tissue Societies Symposium, POS-001-022, Cairns, Australia
6. Seyden S, Segarini PR, Rosen DM, Thompson AY, Bentz H, Graycar J (1987) Cartilage-inducing factor B is a unique protein structure and functionally related to transforming growth factor β. J Biol Chem 262:1946–1949
7. Kawaguchi H, Kurokawa T, Hoshino Y, Kawahara H, Ogata E, Matsumoto T (1992) Immunohistochemical demonstration of bone morphogenetic protein-2 and transforming growth factor-β in the ossification of the posterior longitudinal ligament of the cervical spine. Spine 17:s33–s36

Evaluation of Bone Mineral Densities in Ossification of Posterior Longitudinal Ligament Using Dual-Energy X-Ray Absorptiometry

Satoshi Mori[1], Yukio Kinjo[1], Fuminori Kanaya[1], Sakae Sato[1], Kunio Ibaraki[1,2], and Hiroaki Takara[3]

Key Words. Ossification of posterior longitudinal ligament (OPLL), bone mineral density (BMD), dual-energy X-ray absorptiometry (DEXA), hyperostotic inclination, diffuse idiopathic skeletal hyperostosis (DISH)

Introduction

Ossification of posterior longitudinal ligament (OPLL) is an abnormal ossification of the spinal ligament and sometimes causes severe compressive myelopathy. Because of frequent association with ossification of other spinal and skeletal ligaments, OPLL has been classified as a type of ankylosing spinal hyperostosis (ASH) [1], or diffuse idiopathic skeletal hyperostosis (DISH) [2,3]. Pathological chondral ossification and bone remodeling were observed following the thickening of the ligaments [4], but the etiology remains unknown. It is considered that both local factors, such as mechanical stress or bone morphogenic factors, and generalized factors such as heredity or hormones may play a role in ossification. The purpose of this study is to determine whether bone mineral densities of OPLL patients can be used as an indicator of generalized hyperostotic inclination. This was done by comparing their bone mineral densities (BMDs) with those of normal subjects.

Patients and Methods

Ninety-two OPLL patients, 58 males (30–88 years old) and 34 females (25–77 years old) who visited our clinics between 1986 and 1991 were compared to 208 healthy volunteers collected in our institute, 104 males (20–76 years old) and

[1]Department of Orthopedic Surgery, [2]Research Center of Comprehensive Medicine, and [3]Health Administration, University of the Ryukyus, 207 Uehara, Nishihara, Okinawa, 903-01 Japan

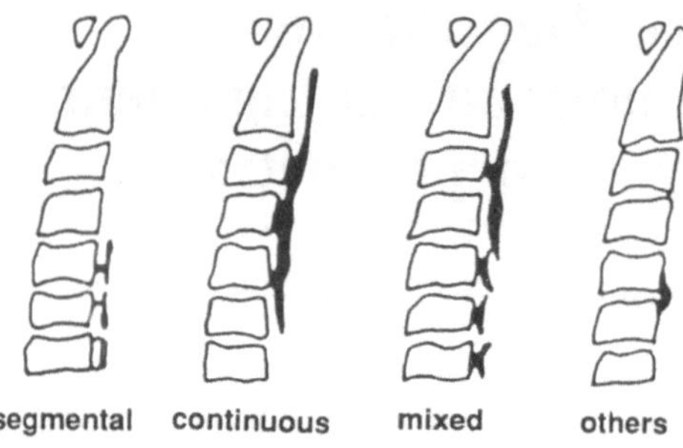

Fig. 1. Types of ossification of the posterior longitudinal ligament (OPLL)

104 females (20–85 years old). Neurological function was evaluated and scored with Japanese Orthopedic Association (JOA) cervical myelopathy scoring system, in which total 17 points are assigned according to the following indices: Motor (8 points), sensory (6 points), and bladder (3 points) [5]. A JOA score of more than 16 was classified as excellent, 10–14 as good, 5–9 as fair, and less than 4 as poor. X-ray examinations for cervical, thoracic, and lumbar spines were performed on all OPLLs. The OPLLs were classified according to ossification patterns such as segmental, continuous, mixed, or other (Fig. 1) [6]. Association of ossifications in other spinal ligaments such as ossification of anterior longitudinal ligament (OALL) or ossification of yellow ligament (OYL) was also determined. Bone mineral densities were measured by dual-energy X-ray absorptiometry (DEXA) using either Lunar DP3 or DPX. L2–4 and the femoral neck were scanned for all patients with OPLL and total body was scanned for 49 patients with OPLL using DPX. In vivo cross calibration previously done between DP3 and DPX showed excellent correlation (L2–4: $r^2 = 0.99$, femoral neck: $r^2 = 0.97$). Bone mineral was assessed either by bone mineral density (BMD: g/cm^2) or by percent of age-matched control value. Either the Mann-Whitney U-test or Student's *t*-test were used for statistical analysis.

Results

Incidence

Most OPLL patients were over 40 years old at the time of examination and the highest incidence were found among patients in their 50's in both sexes (29 of 58 males, 14 of 37 females; Fig. 2). In male OPLL patients, two were in their 30's, none in their 20's, while one female patient was in her 20's, and none in their 30's. The overall incidence of OPLL patients younger than 40 was rare (3%).

Neurological Function

In male OPLL patients, neurologic function was excellent in 33 cases (57%), good in 13 cases (22%), fair in 4 cases (7%), and not evaluated in 8 cases

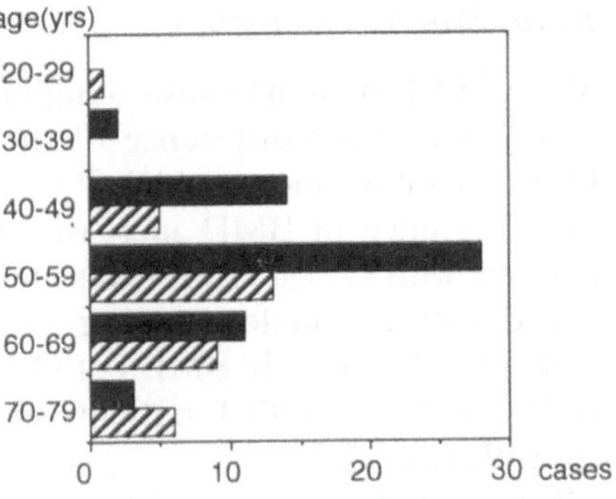

Fig. 2. Age distribution of OPLL. *Solid bars*, male; *hatched bars*, female

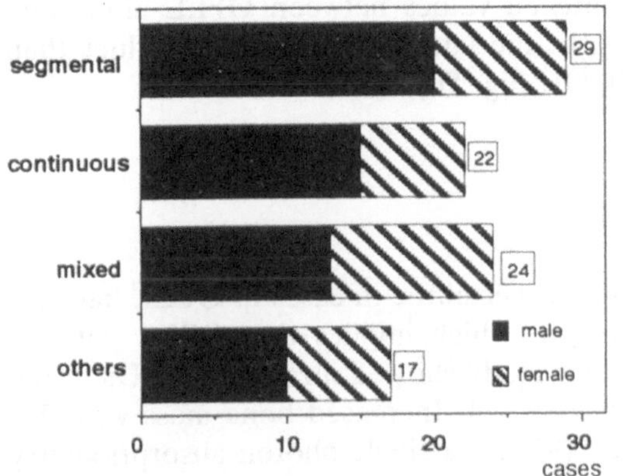

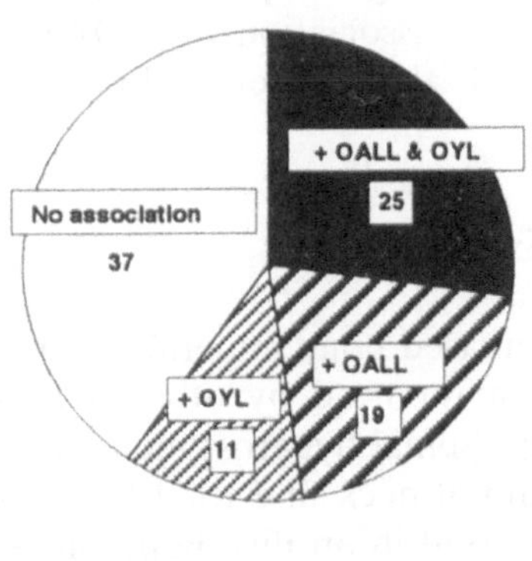

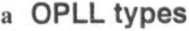

Fig. 3a,b. X-ray findings of OPLL. *Solid bars*, male; *hatched bars*, female; *OALL*, ossification of the anterior longitudinal ligament; *OYL*, ossification of the yellow ligament

(14%). In female OPLL patients, it was excellent in 22 cases (64%), good in 8 cases (24%), and not examined in 4 cases (12%). No correlation was found between JOA scores and bone mineral densities.

X-Ray Findings

Determination of the ossification patterns of OPPL revealed segmental type in 29 cases (32%; 20/9: male/female), continuous type in 22 cases (24%; 15/7: male/female), mixed type in 24 cases (26%; 13/11: male/female) (Fig. 3a). Twenty-five OPLL patients (27%) also demonstrated both OALL and OYL, 19 (21%) with OALL only, 11 (12%) with OYL only, and 37 (40%) had OPLL only. More than half of the patients with OPLL (60%) showed association with either OALL or OYL, in which OALL showed the highest association rate (44 cases, 48%) with OPLL (Fig. 3b).

Bone Mineral Densities

Male OPLL patients showed higher L2–4 BMD than the controls in their 30's and 40's and the difference of the BMDs diminished with age, while female OPLL patients showed higher L2–4 BMD than controls after their 50's, and the difference in BMD increased with age (Fig. 4a). In the femoral neck of patients with OPLL, BMD was higher than the controls in both sexes and in all decades except males in their 70's, but no statistical significance was found (Fig. 4b). Total body BMDs of OPLL patients were plotted against the control BMDs and most OPLL patients showed relatively higher BMD values than the controls (Fig. 4c).

Comparing the percent of age-matched values between segmental, continuous, and mixed types, continuous and mixed types showed significantly higher values than the segmental type in L2–4 ($P < 0.001$, Fig. 5a). Comparing the percentage of age-matched values between OPLL alone and that in association with OALL or OYL, the latter showed higher values than OPLL alone in femoral neck ($P < 0.001$, Fig. 5b).

Discussion

Increased bone mineral density of lumbar vertebrae in cases of OPLL has also been reported by other investigators [8], which implies that OPLL patients have spinal hyperostotic tendencies. Our study showed increased BMDs in the femoral neck and total body, as well as L2–4. Increased bone mass was also reported in an iliac bone biopsy study [9] and a single-photon absorptiometry study of the radius [10]. These findings support the idea that OPLL is associated with not only spinal but also generalized hyperostotic inclination.

Male and female OPLL patients showed different patterns of change in bone mineral densities with age. In males, the difference of BMDs between OPLL patients and normal subjects diminished with age, which suggests that the hyperostotic inclination of OPLL is more active at a young age. Among females with OPLL, L2–4 BMD showed less acceleration of postmenopausal bone loss. It was reported that estrogen levels (E_1, E_2) were high in males with OPLL and in severe OPLL cases, relatively high in females with OPLL comparing to sex- and age-matched controls [11]. It is therefore possible that estrogen metabolism might play a role in ossification of the ligaments.

The onset of the disease is after 20 years of age. The highest incidence was found among patients in their 50's. More than half OPLL patients had associated ossification of other spinal ligaments. Continuous and mixed types showed higher L2–4 BMD than did the segmental type. These findings raise a few questions as to whether: (1) Aging is related to onset and development of the disease, and (2) whether segmental type develops into mixed or continuous type later in life. Most OPLL patients remain subclinical, unless they develop neurological disturbance. The large population of silent OPLL makes it

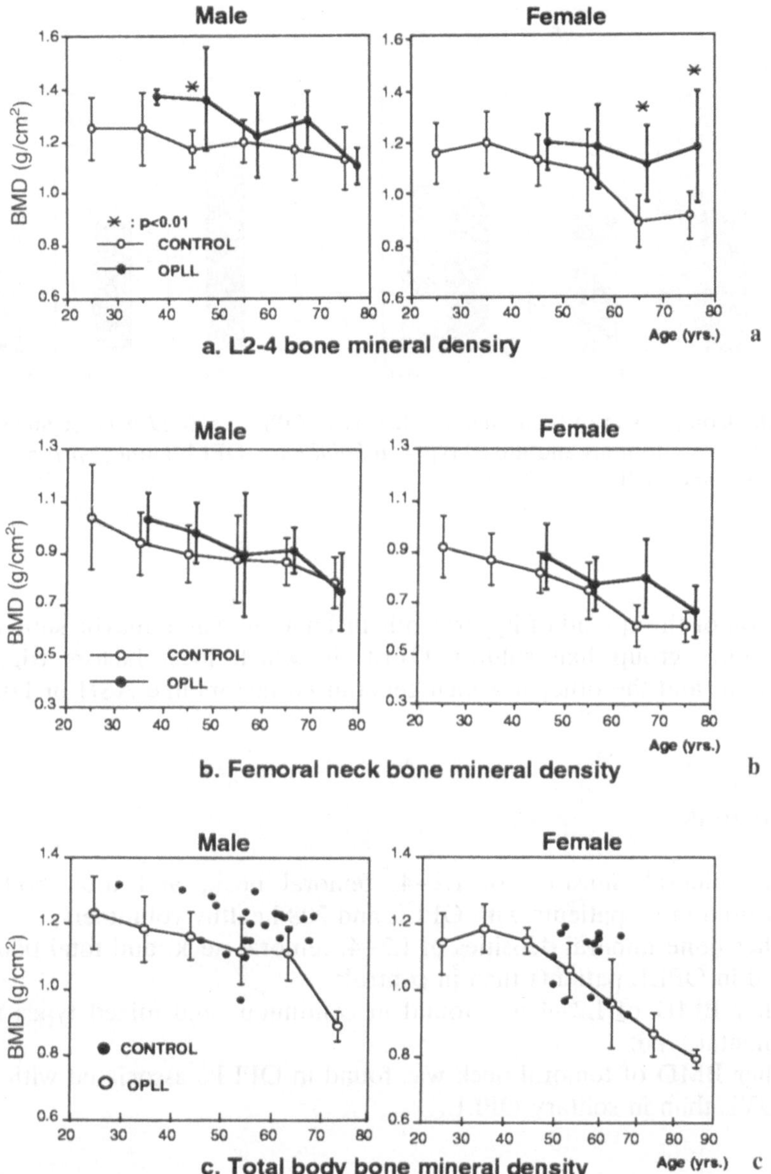

Fig. 4a–c. Bone mineral density (OPLL vs. control)

difficult to determine the nature of the disease. In the future, well organized populational studies must be done to answer these questions. OPLL associated with OALL and OYL showed higher femoral neck BMD than did OPLL alone, which suggests that different factors may be related to the severity of

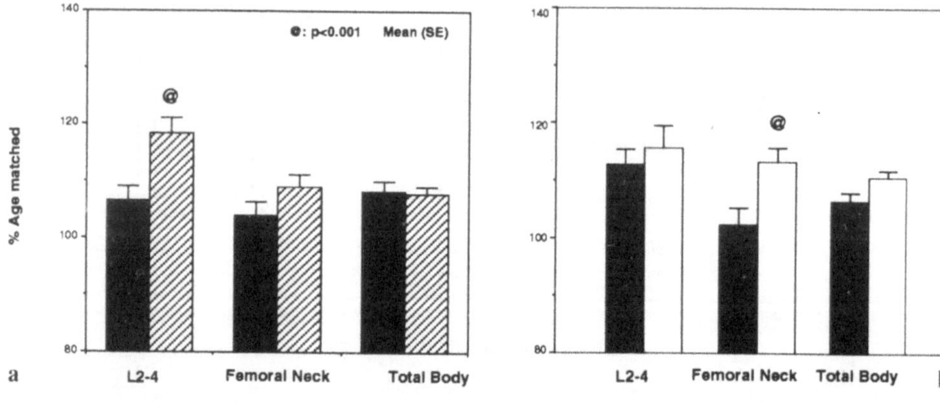

Fig. 5a,b. Comparison of bone mineral density in OPLL. **a** *Solid bars*, segmental type; *hatched bars*, continuous and mixed types. **b** *Solid bars*, OPLL alone; *open bars*, OPLL with OALL and OYL

expression or the spread of hyperostotic inclination. There maybe subgroups in OPLL: One group like solitary OPLL in which local factors trigger the ossification, and the other in which generalized factors like ASH or DISH are related.

Conclusions

1. Bone mineral densities of L2–4, femoral neck, and total body were measured in 92 patients with OPLL and 208 healthy volunteers.
2. Higher bone mineral densities of L2–4, femoral neck, and total body were found in OPLL patients than in controls.
3. Higher BMD of L2–4 was found in continuous and mixed types than in segmental type.
4. Higher BMD of femoral neck was found in OPLLs associated with OALL or OYL than in solitary OPLL.

Acknowledgments. This study was sponsored by the investigation committee on the ossification of the spinal ligaments of the Japanese Ministry of Health and Welfare and the content was presented at the 1991 annual meeting of the committee.

References

1. Forestier J, Lagier R (1971) Ankylosing spinal hyperostosis of the spine. Clin Orthop 74:65–83
2. Forestier J, Rotes-Querol J (1950) Senile ankylosing hyperostosis of the spine. Ann Rheum 9:321–330
3. Resnick D, Shaul SR, Robin JM (1975) Diffuse idiopathic skeletal hyperostosis (DISH): Forestier's disease with extraspinal manifestation. Radiology 115:513–524
4. Goto S (1981) Studies of ossification of the posterior longitudinal ligament in the cervical spine using microradiography and histochemistry. J Jpn Orthop Assoc 55: 451–466
5. Tsuyama N (1951) Japanese Orthopedic Association cervical myelopathy scoring system. J Jpn Orthop Assoc 50(5)
6. Tsuyama N (1975) Editorial In: Investigation committee reports on ossification of spinal ligaments of Japanese Ministry of Health and Welfare 1–3
7. Mori S, Kinjo Y, Ibaraki K, Takara H (1992) Bone mineral density in ossification of posterior longitudinal ligament. Investigation committee reports on ossification of spinal ligaments of Japanese Ministry of Health and Welfare 279–283
8. Mamada T, Kurokawa T, Hoshino Y, Ohnishi I, Seichi A, Saita K (1992) Bone mineral measurement using QDR-1000 in ossification of cervical posterior longitudinal ligament. Investigation committee reports on ossification of spinal ligaments of Japanese Ministry of Health and Welfare 288–293
9. Tei JS (1985) Roentogenological and quantitative microradiographic study on ossification of posterior longitudinal ligament. J Jpn Orthop Assoc 59:153–166
10. Hoshino Y (1982) Study of calcium metabolism in ossification of spinal ligaments. Investigation committee reports on ossification of spinal ligaments of Japanese Ministry of Health and Welfare 97–99
11. Okada M, Motegi M, Fujita R, Ikeda M, Tabe S, Umeda Y (1981) Measurement of sex steroid in ossification of posterior longitudinal ligament of cervical spine (in Japanese). Rinsho Seikei Geka 16:846–854

Ossification of the Ligamentum Flavum and Disc Degeneration

Akiyoshi Yamazaki, Takao Homma, Seiji Uchiyama, and Hideaki E. Takahashi[1]

Key Words. Ossification, ligamentum flavum, disc degeneration, disc hernia, hyperostosis

Introduction

Ossification of the ligamentum flavum (OLF) has been recognized as a definite clinical entity as is ossification of the posterior longitudinal ligament (OPLL). The incidence of both are reported to be high especially in Japan. OLF develops mostly in the lower thoracic spine in middle-aged persons and causes compression myelopathy which generates numbness and motor weakness in the lower limbs, urinary disturbance, and even bedridden status (Fig. 1).

On the genesis of OLF; aging, tendency of hyperostosis, anatomical peculiarity, and dynamic factors represented by disc degeneration have been mentioned, but the etiology of OLF, like OPLL, is still unknown. We investigated the relationship between OLF and disc degeneration and the relation between OLF and OPLL.

Patients and Methods

Twenty cases (male 8, female 12) operated for OLF in Niigata University Hospital since 1975 were studied. Age at operation ranged from 34–71, (average 57 years). The total number of levels operated on for OLF was 41. The lesions existed from T3/4 to L4/5. T10/11 was the most common level (39%), followed by T11/12 (24%). Eight cases (40%) had OPLL in the cervical or thoracic spine.

---

[1]Department of Orthopedic Surgery, Niigata University School of Medicine, Asahimachi-dori 1-757, Niigata, 951 Japan

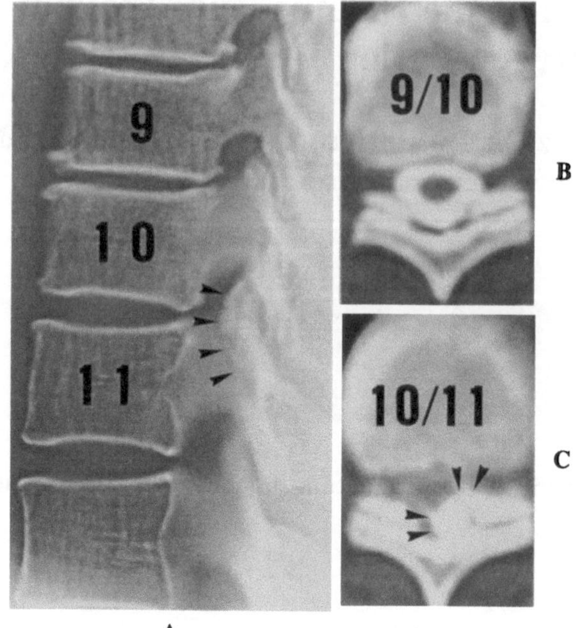

Fig. 1. *A*: X-P shows ossification of the ligamentum flavum (OLF) at T10/11 level. *B*: CTM (T9/10) shows no OLF. *C*: OLF (T10/11) compresses the spinal cord markedly

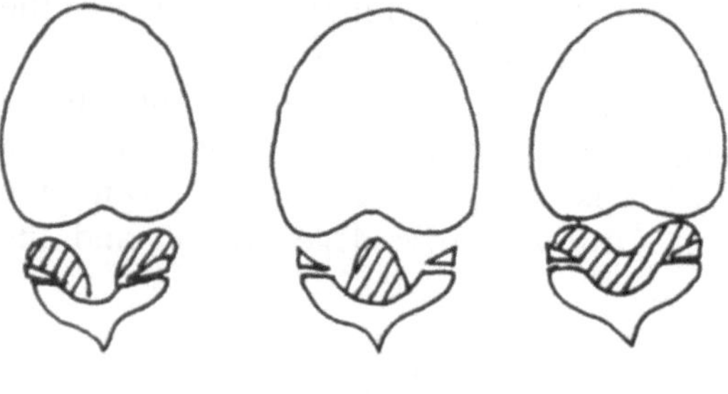

Fig. 2. Classification of OLF by Shimazaki et al. [2]

Disc degeneration was divided into 3 grades; non, moderate and high. From lateral radiographs based on the classification by Tsuji [1], the degree of disc narrowing and the size of the osteophyte was used in classification. Posterior bulging of the disc was evaluated by computerized axial tomography myelogram (CTM) and magnetic resonance imaging (MRI). Morphological types of OLF by CT scanning were divided into lateral, median, and a mixture of both (mixed type) according to the classification by Shimazaki et al. [2] (Fig. 2).

Results and Discussion

In 41 levels of OLF, moderate disc degeneration was found in 29 (71%) and high degeneration was found in 12 (29%). No disc showed normal findings.

In five patients, discs at the level of OLF were more degenerated than adjacent cranial and caudal 3 discs.

Posterior disc bulging was seen in 8 out of 23 discs (35%) and 7 out of 14 patients (50%) (Fig. 3).

Up to this time there have been various views on the relationship between OLF and disc degeneration. Yanagi et al. [3] reported that there was not any significant relationship between them. On the other hand, Kurakami et al. [4] said there was a significant relationship. Furthermore, Shimazaki et al. [2] also mentioned that it remained unclear whether there was a relationship or not.

These results suggest that intervertebral instability accompanied with disc degeneration have relationship to the genesis of OLF.

The lateral type OLF was seen in 68% of disc levels, and the mixed type was found in 32%, the median type was not seen in our series. Shimazaki et al. [2] reported OLF of the lateral type was seen in 45% of disc levels, of mixed type in 41%, and of median type in 14%, similar to our report.

Disc degeneration was seen in all patients with lateral and mixed types of OLF. Forty-eight percent of patients with lateral OLF and 20% with mixed

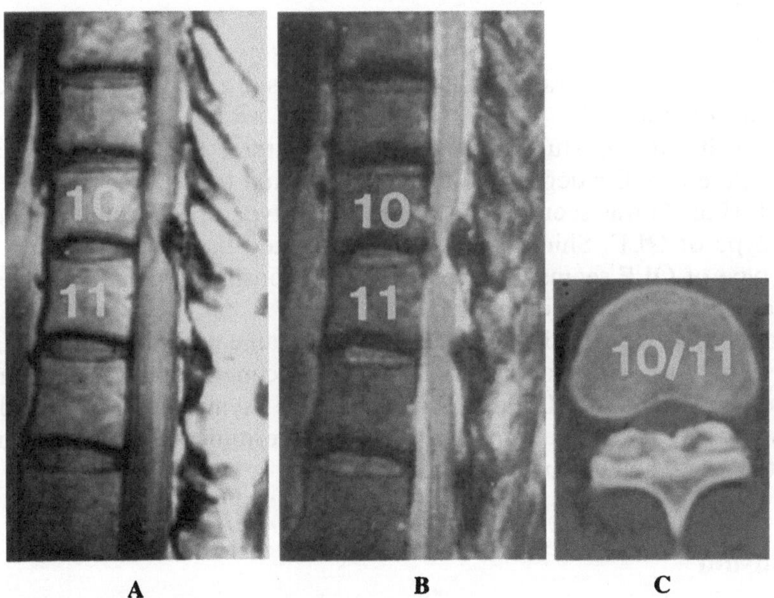

Fig. 3. Posterior disc bulging combined with OLF. *A*: MRI (T1 weighted image). *B*: MRI (T2 weighted image). *C*: CTM (T10/11)

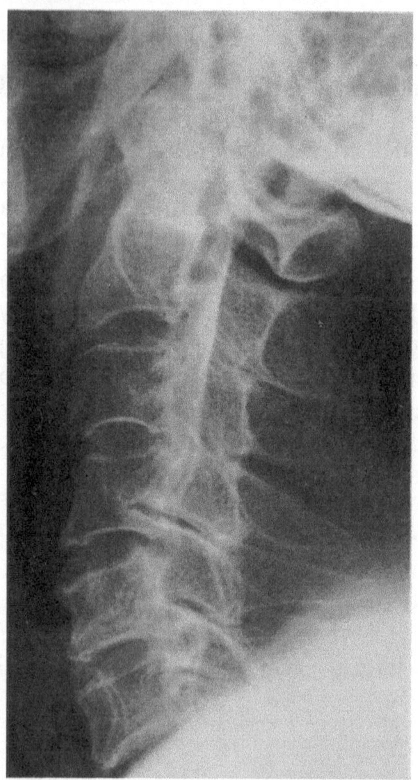

Fig. 4. Ossification of the posterior longitudinal ligament (OPLL) (cervical)

OLF had highly degenerated discs. These results are similar to those reported by Shimazaki et al. [2].

The results of our study suggest that the lateral type of OLF was more closely related to disc degeneration than the mixed type.

OPLL (Fig. 4) was seen in 90% of the mixed type of OLF and in 10% of the lateral type of OLF. Shimazaki et al. [2] reported the same tendency. So the mixed type of OLF seems to have a close relationship to generalized tendency of hyperostosis represented by OPLL.

Hiraoka [5] reported that one-third of 128 frame specimens had OLF, and Sakou et al. [6] said that all of 49 frame specimens had OLF. From their studies, many cases of OLF are considered to be asymptomatic. Local dynamic factors may be one of the important keys to determine whether OLF grows to a size that causes neurological deficit.

Conclusion

1. Disc degeneration and OPLL were investigated in twenty patients operated for OLF.

2. OLF was related to the disc degeneration and posterior bulging of disc.
3. The lateral type of OLF was more closely related to the disc degeneration and the mixed type was more closely related to the tendency of hyperostosis.

References

1. Tsuji H (1972) Pathology of lumber disc lesions (in Japanese). Kanehara Shuppan, Tokyo, pp 27–38
2. Shimazaki K, Kimura S, Hirohata K, Shou T, Kataoka O (1989) The relation between the ossification of yellow ligament and the disc degeneration (in Japanese). Cent Jpn J Orthp Traumat 32:122–124
3. Yanagi T, Kato H, Yamamura Y, Sobue I (1972) Ossification of spinal ligaments (in Japanese). Clin Neurol 12:571–577
4. Kurakami C, Kaneda K, Abumi K, Hashimoto T, Shirado O, Takahashi H, Takeda N, Fujiya M (1988) Study on pathology of ossification of the ligamentum flavum of the thoracolumbar spine (in Japanese). Rinsho Seikei Geka 23:441–448
5. Hiraoka S (1955) Ossification of the ligamentum flavum in the intervertebral foramen (in Japanese). Geka no Ryouiki 3:6–11
6. Sakou T, Tomimura K, Maehara T, Morimoto T, Yano Y, Ohsako S, Kawamura H, Kouji T, Shibuya E, Morizono Y, Itoh T (1977) Pathology of ossification of the flavum (in Japanese). Rinsho Seikei Geka 12:368–376

Relationship Between Magnetic Resonance Imaging and Clinical Results of Decompression Surgery for Cervical Myelopathy

Hiroshi Okumura and Takao Homma[1]

Key Words. Magnetic resonance imaging, decompression surgery, cervical myelopathy, spinal cord, intramedullary lesion

Introduction

Magnetic resonance imaging (MRI) has been widely applied to the diagnosis of diseases of the spine and the spinal cord, and there are many reports that it is a very useful tool in the diagnosis of spinal disorders [1–3]. MRI has been shown to be especially valuable not only for compressive lesions, but also for intramedullary lesions [4,5]. In this study of about 60 patients with cervical myelopathy, we studied the relationship between MRI and the clinical results of decompression surgery. The prediction of surgical results based MRI is also discussed.

Patients and Methods

Pre- and postsurgical MRI in 60 patients with cervical myelopathy were investigated. Thirty-six patients were diagnosed with cervical spondylotic myelopathy, 18 with cervical ossification of the posterior longitudinal ligament (OPLL), and 6 with cervical disc herniation. The average age of the 40 males and 20 females at surgery was 52 years, and the average morbidity period was 2 years and 3 months. Japanese Orthopaedic Association (JOA) score was 12 points preoperatively, and 14 points postoperatively. The overall recovery ratio determined by Hirabayashi's method was 43%. The surgical procedure

[1] Department of Orthopedic Surgery, Niigata University School of Medicine, Asahimachi-dori 1-757, Niigata, 951 Japan

consisted of anterior decompression in 27 patients, posterior decompression in 26, and both anterior and posterior decompression in 7.

MRI was performed using a Siemens Magnetom (1.5 T) with SE sequences with short and long repetition times in the sagittal and axial planes. Slice thickness was 3 mm, and the imaging matrix was 256 × 256.

Evaluation of MR Imaging

On T1-weighted MRI in the sagittal plane, cord compression, atrophy, and cystic cavity in the spinal cord were investigated. In the axial plain, flat ratio was calculated. On T2 weighted images in the sagittal plane, high-signal-intensity areas (HSIA) in the spinal cord were investigated. Size was determined in relation to the vertebral height; a small HSIA was defined as one-half or less of the vertebral height, and a large HSIA as more than one-half.

Classification Based on Magnetic Resonance Imaging

In patients with severe cord compression, the intramedullary condition could not be observed on preoperative magnetic resonance (MR) images, and the spinal cord atrophy status was obscure. Postoperative MR images which visualized the spinal cord clearly, were therefore used to classify the patients into the following five groups: Group A, normal spinal cord; group B, no atrophy of the spinal cord, but an obvious HSIA in the spinal cord; group C, normal signal intensity, but with atrophy of the spinal cord; group D, spinal cord atrophy and an obvious HSIA; and group E, residual spinal cord compression.

The relationship of each MRI to each of the four preoperative clinical parameters of morbidity period, clinical severity, degree of cord compression, and HSIA was statistically evaluated. In addition, the relationship of recovery ratio to preoperative HSIA, each postoperative MR image, and transition of HSIA status was examined.

Results

On the basis of analysis of postoperative MRI, 16 cases were classified as group A, 25 as group B, 5 as group C, 6 as group D, and 8 as group E. Table 1 shows the relationship between a morbidity period and postoperative MRI. Morbidity period was not correlated with HSIA, but was correlated with spinal cord atrophy ($\chi^2 = 24.231$, $P < 0.01$). Table 2 shows the relationship between clinical severity and postoperative MRI. Preoperative clinical severity was not correlated with HSIA, but was correlated with spinal cord atrophy ($\chi^2 = 12.643$, $P < 0.01$). Table 3 shows the relationship between cord compression and postoperative MRI. The degree of preoperative cord compression was not

Table 1. Relationship between morbidity period and postoperative magnetic resonance imaging (MRI).

Group	Morbidity group			
	<1 year	⩾1 year < 2 years	⩾2 years	
A	12	4	0	16
B	9	8	8	25
C	0	0	5	5
D	0	0	6	6
Total	21	12	19	52

Table 2. Relationship between preoperative neurological severity and postoperative MRI.

Group	Preoperative severity (JOA score)			
	17~13	12~10	9~0	
A	13	1	2	16
B	14	6	5	25
C	0	2	3	5
D	1	1	4	6
Total	28	10	14	52

Table 3. Relationship between the degree of preoperative cord compression and postoperative MRI.

Group	Preoperative cord compression (%)[a]			
	~40	39~30	29~	
A	2	11	3	16
B	0	17	8	25
C	0	1	4	5
D	0	0	6	6
Total	2	29	21	52

[a] $\frac{\text{AP diameter}}{\text{transverse diameter}} \times 100$ (%)
(in MRI T1 axial view)

correlated with HSIA, but was correlated with spinal cord atrophy ($\chi^2 = 14.806$, $P < 0.01$). Table 4 shows the relationship between preoperative HSIA and postoperative MRI. There was a significant correlation between preoperative HSIA and postoperative HSIA ($\chi^2 = 28.636$, $P < 0.01$).

The recovery ratio was calculated for the 36 patients in whom HSIA status could be determined before operation. As shown in Fig. 1, the mean recovery

Table 4. Relationship between preoperative intramedullary high intensity area and postoperative MRI.

Group	Preoperative intramedullary high intensity area			
	Negative	Positive	Obscure (severe cord compression)	
A	14	2	0	16
B	0	18	7	25
C	0	0	5	5
D	0	2	4	6
Total	14	22	16	52

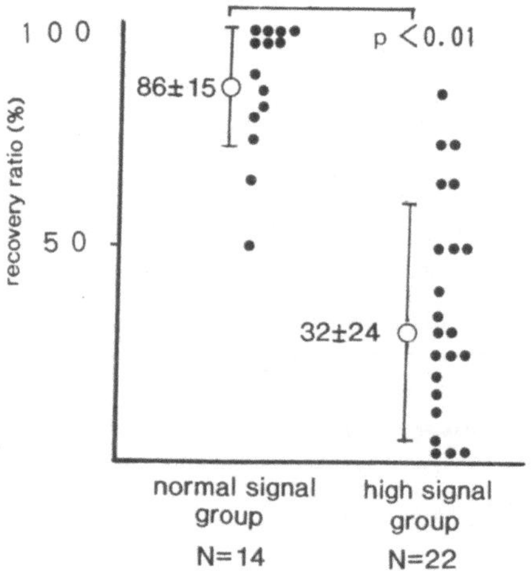

Fig. 1. Comparison between preoperative normal signal group and high signal group in a recovery ratio

ratio in the 22 patients with HSIA before operation (32 ± 24%) was significantly lower than that in the 14 patients with normal signal before operation (86 ± 15%). The recovery ratio in each group is shown in Fig. 2. Group A (normal MRI) showed the highest recovery ratio, followed by group B (HSIA), group C (cord atrophy), and group D (HSIA and cord atrophy), respectively. The mean recovery ratio in group A (87 ± 12%) was significantly higher than that in each of the other groups ($P < 0.01$).

We evaluated pre- and postoperative HSIA status in 36 patients in whom intramedullary condition could be determined preoperatively. Figure 3 indicated that the recovery ratio in the normal signal group (89 ± 13%) and that in which HSIA disappeared following surgery (75 ± 0%) was higher than that of other patients ($P < 0.01$). The latter included patients in whom HSIA of any height relative to the vertebral body remained unchanged, and in whom HSIA (with or without cystic necrosis in the spinal cord) extended to more than half the height of the vertebral body postoperatively.

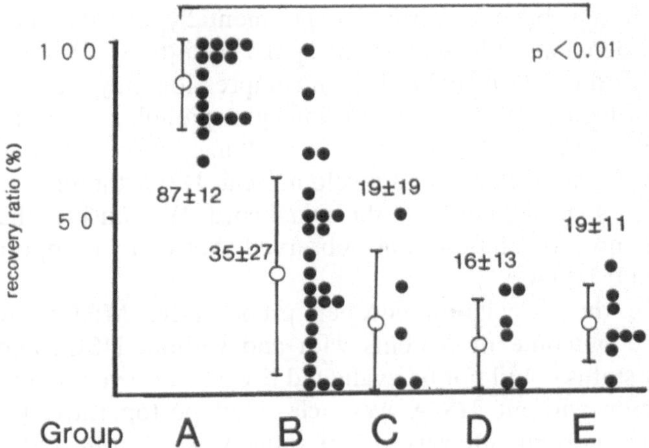

Fig. 2. Recovery ratio in each group

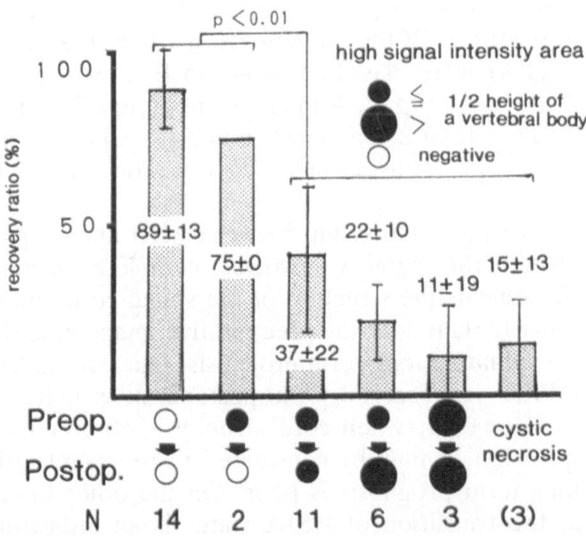

Fig. 3. Comparison of the transition of the high signal intensity area

Discussion and Conclusion

Our analysis of the relationship between preoperative clinical parameters and postoperative MRI indicated that, while spinal cord atrophy frequently showed a relationship to the morbidity period, preoperative severity, and degree of cord compression, there was no correlation of these factors with postoperative HSIA. HSIA is reported to frequently accompany cervical cord injury (45–

80%), and it has been confirmed experimentally in rats that HSIA is an indicator of edema and bleeding in the spinal cord [6–8]. Thus, even when the morbidity period is relatively brief, high compression may induce HSIA similar to that found in cases of cervical cord injury or pathology. On the other hand, even if compression is relatively mild, a prolonged morbidity period may give rise to HSIA due to ischemia and myelomalacia. HSIA therefore can indicate a variety of pathological changes in the spinal cord. We consider that it is for this reason that no correlation was observed between preoperative clinical parameters and HSIA.

To analyze the association between preoperative MRI to prognosis, we evaluated the outcome of patients with and without HSIA and of those in whom HSIA status could not be evaluated because of severe cord compression. All 14 patients without HSIA were classified postoperatively as group A, indicating that normal intensity preoperatively is a strong indicator of good outcome. On the other hand, of the 22 patients with HSIA, 2 (9%) were classified as group A, 18 (82%) as group B, and 2 (9%) as group D. The probability that HSIA will disappear after operation is thus very low, while that of postoperative HSIA is high. A high recovery ratio can therefore not be expected in these patients. Of the 16 patients in whom HSIA status could not be evaluated, 7 (44%) were classified as group B after surgery, 5 (31%) as group C, and 4 (25%) as group D. All patients in groups C and D had had long morbidity period (more than 2 years), while in 5 (71%) of 7 patients in Group B it was less than 2 years. Thus, a high recovery ratio can not be expected in this group either.

Our examination of the relationship between MRI and long-term prognosis indicates that, when the surgery involves complete decompression, the postoperative MRI reveals the structure of the spinal cord and intramedullary conditions more clearly than does the preoperative imaging, and may therefore be more useful in evaluating long-term prognosis. Our data indicate that, when no atrophy or HSIA is observed with postoperative MRI, the long-term prognosis is good. However, when cord atrophy is observed with MRI after complete decompression, it may be considered to represent a deficit of nerve fibers, and the long-term prognosis is poor. On the other hand, when HSIA can be observed, the transition of HSIA status is an indicator of long-term prognosis. Postoperative decrease of the size of the HSIA may be considered to reflect largely reversible pathological changes. Conversely, postoperative increase or unchanged status indicates that long-term prognosis is poor, since this HSIA status may reflect largely irreversible pathological changes.

In summary, in the assessment of the prognosis of patients with cervical myelopathy, preoperative MRI can be useful in the evaluation of overall postoperative prognosis, and postoperative MRI can be used to more accurately assess long-term prognosis.

References

1. Al-Mefty O, Harkey LH, Middleton TH, Smith RR, Fox JL (1988) Myelopathic cervical spondylotic lesions demonstrated by magnetic resonance imaging. J Neurosurg 68:217–222
2. Brown BM, Schwarts RH, Frank E, Blank NK (1988) Preoperative evaluation of cervical radiculopathy and myelopathy by surface-coil MR imaging. AJNR 91:859–866
3. Mehalic TF, Pezzuti RT, Applebaum BI (1990) Magnetic resonance imaging and cervical spondylotic myelopathy. Neurosurgery 26:217–225
4. Ramanauskas WL, Wilner HI, Metes JJ, Lazo A, Kelly JK (1989) MR imaging of compressive myelomalacia. J Comput Assist Tomogr 13:399–404
5. Takahashi M, Yamashita Y, Sakamoto Y, Kojima R (1989) Chronic cervical cord compression: Clinical significance of increased signal intensity on MR images. Radiology 173:219–224
6. Kulkarni MV, McArdle CB, Kopanicky D, Miner M, Cotler HB, Lee KF, Harris JH (1987) Acute spinal cord injury: MR imaging at 1.5 T. Radiology 164:837–843
7. Mirvis SE, Geisler FH, Jelinek JJ, Joslyn JN, Gellad F (1988) Acute cervical spine trauma: Evaluation with 1.5 T MR imaging. Radiology 166:807–816
8. Hachney DB, D MeD Sci RA, Joseph PM, Carvlin MJ, McGrath JT, Grossman RI, Kassab EA, DeSimone D (1986) Hemorrhage and edema in acute spinal cord compression: Demonstration by MR Imaging. Radiology 161:387–390

Expansive Open-Door Laminoplasty with Reconstruction of Spinous Process

Yoshihiko Ohshima, Yoshio Ohta, Hiroshi Sato, Masahiro Hayashi, Noritoshi Hiramoto, Minoru Yokota, Michio Mori, Tomokazu Ito, Taro Nagashima, Nobuhiko Sato, Hiroshi Takei, and Younosuke Arii[1]

Key Words. Cervical spine, cervical myelopathy, laminoplasty, spinous process, decompression

Introduction

Kirita devised a safer procedure of cervical laminectomy in 1968 [1]. Since that time, extensive cervical laminectomy has been widely employed in the treatment of patients with compression myelopathy.

Long-term follow-up studies of laminectomized patients, however, revealed that the improved neurological symptoms sometimes worsen again in the postoperative course. Laminoplastic cervical canal enlargement for compressive myelopathy has been developed to prevent postoperative cervical deformity and instability which are responsible for neurological deterioration [2,3]. Oyama et al. introduced "expansive lamina-Z plasty" in 1972 [4], and many kinds of laminoplastic procedures have been reported since then [5–11].

The authors devised a new surgical procedure of expansive laminoplasty in 1984 [9], which preserves the spinous processes with unilateral paravertebral muscles and reattaching to the opened laminas. The purpose of this paper is to introduce this procedure and its effectiveness with regard to the prevention of cervical deformity and instability.

Patients and Methods

Eighty-seven patients with a follow-up ranging from 6 months to 5 years are the subjects for this investigation. These cases consist of 63 with cervical spondylotic myelopathy, 15 with ossification of the posterior longitudinal

[1] Department of Orthopaedic Surgery, Yamagata University School of Medicine, Iida Nishi 2-2-3, Yamagata, 990-23 Japan

ligament (OPLL), and 9 with central cord injury with a narrowed canal. The range of laminoplasty extended from C2 to T2, and was the most frequent between C3 and C6 in this series. The upper- and lower-most laminas were operated on using dome-like expansive laminoplasty, as described by Matsuzaki [8]. Neurological recoveries were estimated by the criteria for evaluating the results of surgery for cervical myelopathy established by the Japanese Orthopaedic Association (JOA) score. Radiological examinations were conducted to determine the anteroposterior diameter of the osseous canal, range of motion, alignment, and listhesis of the cervical spine.

Operative Procedure

The procedure of opening the lamina is the same as the expansive open-door laminoplasty developed by Hirabayashi, but different in the approach and manner of dealing with the spinous process [12,13]. The access to the spinous process is done by incising the lateral margin of the nuchal ligament which is left with the spinous processes and unilateral paravertebral extensor muscles. Exposing one side of laminas, the spinous processes are severed at the base by a right angle bone saw. The opposite side of the lamina is exposed by retracting the spinous processes with the corresponding paravertebral muscle pedicle. The exposed side of the lamina is cut, and two wires are passed through the cuts in the lamina. Using the wires, the severed spinous processes are fixed tightly on the center of the opened lamina. Paravertebral extensor muscles on the open side are then reattached to the spinous processes. Longer spinous processes, e.g. the sixth and seventh cervical and first thoracic, should be shortened at the base by 2–3 mm to strengthen the suspension effect of the spinomuscular complex (Fig. 1).

Postoperative Management

Patients undergoing laminoplasty are usually confined to bed for several days after surgery and allowed to stand and walk with a soft cervical brace, which should be used for 3 months after the operation. The cervical spine is maintained a little dorsiflexed so that the spinal cord can move posteriorly. Isometric exercise of the neck muscles is recommended to begin gradually from 6 weeks after surgery.

Results

Neurological Improvement

The average JOA score of the patients preoperatively was 8.9, and postoperatively 12.6. Evaluating according to the Kurokawa method, clinical results indicated 21% excellent, 55% good (Table 1).

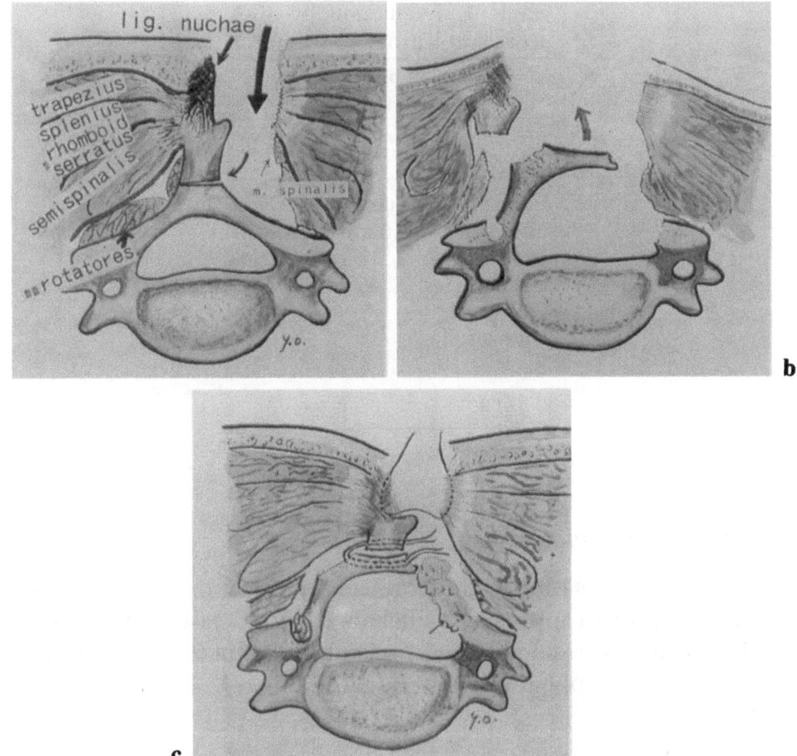

Fig. 1. a Access to the spinous process is done by incising the lateral margin of the nuchal ligament which is left with the spinous processes and unilateral paravertebral extensor muscles. Exposing one side of the laminas, the spinous processes are severed at the base by a right angle bone saw. **b** Prior to opening the lamina two wires are passed through the open side of the lamina. Opening the lamina is done a little at a time, as the hinge is bent like a green stick fracuture. **c** The pedicles spinous processes are fixed tightly on the center of the opened lamina by the wires. Paravertebral extensor muscles of the open side are reattached to the spinous processes. *lig*, ligament; *m*, muscularis

Anteroposterior Diameter Widening of Osseous Spinal Canal

The width of the osseous canals of the cervical spine were evaluated by the canal-to-body ratio in AP diameter. The average canal-to-body ratio improved from 0.76 preoperatively to 1.03 postoperatively.

Range of Motion of the Cervical Spine

After surgery range of motion (ROM) of the cervical spine decreased in every case. The average ROM changed from 32.9° to 15.1°, as measured 12 months after surgery.

Table 1. Evaluation by JOA score and Kurokawa's criteria.

Evaluation by JOA Score (average)		
Preoperative	Postoperative	
8.9	12.6	
Evaluation by Kurokawa's criteria using motor function of JOA score		
Excellent	17 cases	21%
Good	48	55
Fair	2	2
Unchanged	14	16
Worse	6	7
Total	87 cases	

Alignment of the Cervical Spine

Kyphotic deformity was observed before surgery in 20 cases. After surgery, the kyphosis was improved in 3 cases, unchanged in 10 cases, and increased in 3 cases of this group. Normal alignment was observed in 67 cases before surgery. Only one these cases appeared kyphotic after surgery.

Retrolisthesis

Retrolisthesis of more than 3 mm was observed in 37 vertebrae of 35 cases before surgery. After surgery, it disappeared in 7 cases, decreased in 17 cases, was unchanged in 13 cases, and did not increase in any case. No cases of newly developed listhesis was observed.

Discussion

Many kinds of laminoplastic enlargement operations of the cervical canal have been reported [5–12]. Many authors pay little attention to the role of the spinous processes and the extensor muscles attached to the spinous processes [10,13,14]. Kurokawa emphasizes the role of myoplasty to achieve good alignment after surgery [7]. It should be considered that when the extensor musculature and the posterior ligaments work, the spinous processes act as a lever. The advantages of the authors' method are as follows: (1) Reconstructed spinous processes give full play to extensor muscle function which helps keep good alignment and stability of the cervical spine; (2) unilateralextensor muscles remain intact as the pedicle of the spinous processes; and (3) the laminar door is kept open by the reconstructed spinomuscular complex without reclosing.

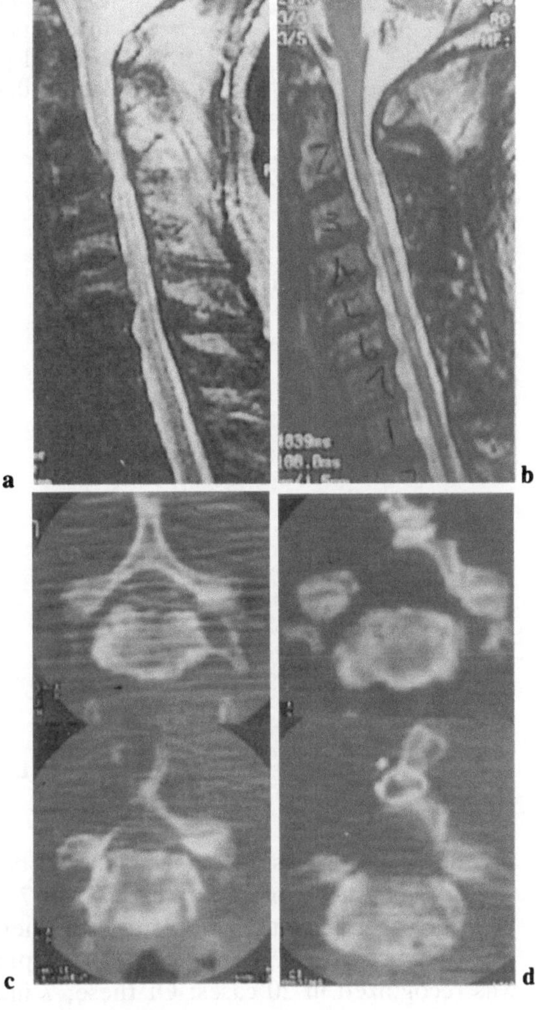

Fig. 2a–d. A 63-year-old male with cervical spondylotic myctopathy (CSM) has laminoplasty of the cervical spine. **a** MRI shows multisegmental cord compression before surgery. **b** The spinal cord shifted posteriorly and is decompressed after surgery. Total JOA score recovered from 7 to 14. **c** Preoperative CT. **d** Cervical canal is sufficiently enlarged

Postoperative AP diameter of the canal was stabilized about 4 weeks after surgery by bony union of the hinge. The rate of widening seems sufficient for obtaining good operative results (Fig. 2), but it is not always determined correctly in this operation. For younger patients or patients with athetotic movement due to cerebral palsy, iliac bone block is grafted to the defect at the open side of the lamina. The floating lamina is stabilized by this procedure. The lamina is reconstructed entirely (Fig. 3). These cases are not included in this series.

In laminectomy and expansive laminoplasty, a spinal cord compressed anteriorly is decompressed by means of posterior shifting of the spinal cord. When the cervical alignment is kyphotic, its effect becomes less.

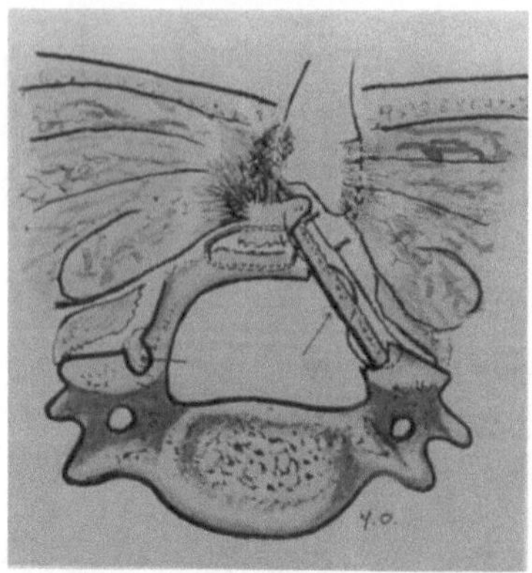

Fig. 3. For younger patients or patients with involuntary movement of the cervical spine as in cerebral palsy, iliac bone block is grafted to the lamina defect

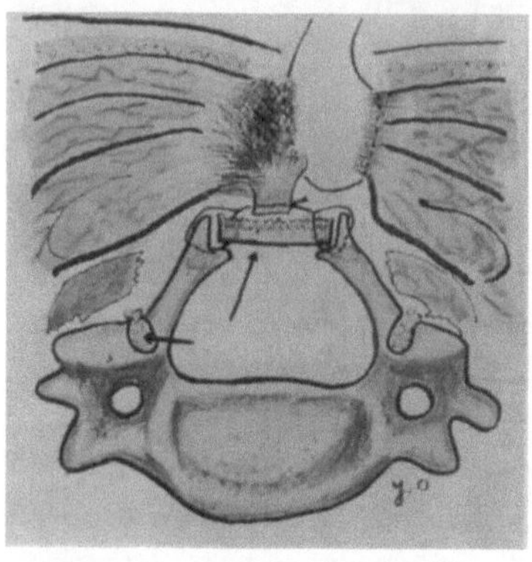

Fig. 4. Laminoplasty by sagittal splitting

Mono- and polysegmental kyphotic deformities were recognized before surgery. These deformities increased in 7 cases, were unchanged in 10 cases, and decreased in 3 cases after surgery. There was no newly developed kyphotic deformity after surgery in this series except in one case, but kyphotic deformity was recognized in 20 cases: Of these, 7 increased, 10 were unchanged, and 3 decreased after surgery. Postoperative kyphotic deformity may be improved by extensor muscle training, but in this aspect was not studied in the present series.

The range of motion of the cervical spine was variable within 12 months after surgery. The neutral alignment of the cervical spine may be influenced mostly by the alignment during postoperative immobilization. It is recommended that patients maintain cervical lordosis with a cervical brace for the immobilizing period. This is very important, expecially for cases with cervical kyphosis or a straight cervical spine.

In the early stage, the authors did laminoplasty by sagittal splitting of the lamina and opened the French window, bridging iliac bone block between two windows and reattaching pedicled spinous process on the iliac bone block (Fig. 4). Later, the authors noticed that this method is too complicated and needs many bony unions. Furthermore, laminar splitting along the lateral side is safer than along the mid-dorsal line of the lamina. For these reasons, the authors adopted Hirabayashi's method for laminoplasty as a general rule.

Conclusion

It is concluded that reconstructed spinous processes with muscle pedicle prevents cervical deformity and instability after expansive laminoplasty.

Acknowledgments. The authors are grateful to Professor Watanabe for his helpful suggestions.

References

1. Kirita Y (1976) Posterior decompression for cervical myelopathy due to ossified posterior longitudinal ligament (in Japanese). Shujutsu 30:287–302
2. Cattell HS, Clark GL Jr (1967) Cervical kyphosis and instability following multiple laminectomies in children. J Bone Joint Surg[Am] 49:713–720
3. Sim FH, Svien JH, Bickel WH, Janes JM (1974) Swan-neck deformity following extensive cervical laminectomy. J Bone Joint Surg[Am] 56:564–580
4. Oyama M, Hattori S, Moriwaki N (1973) A new method of cervical laminectomy (in Japanese). Cent Jpn J Orthop Traumatol 16:792–794
5. Hirabayashi K (1978) Expansive open-door laminoplasty for cervical spondylotic myelopathy (in Japanese). Shujutsu 32:1159–1163
6. Tsuji H (1978) En bloc laminectomy. Orthopaedic Surgery (in Japanese) (Seikeigeka) 29:1755–1761
7. Kurokawa T, Tsuyama N, Tanaki H (1982) Enlargement of spinal canal by sagittal splitting of spinal processes (in Japanese). Bessatsu Seikeigeka 2:234–240
8. Matsuzaki H, Toriyama S (1986) Dome enlargement of the spinal canal of the second cervical spine (in Japanese). Shujutsu 40:1875–1881
9. Tomooka K, Ohshima Y, Samoto T, Ohta Y, Asahina I, Sato M, Yamahara S (1984) Spinal canal enlargement for multilevel cervical spondylosis (in Japanese). Ann Touhoku Seisai 27:114–117
10. Itoh T, Tsuji H (1985) Technical improvements and results of laminoplasty for compressive myelopathy in the cervical spine. Spine 10:729–746
11. Ohmori K, Ishida Y, Suzuki K (1987) Suspension laminotomy: A new surgical technique for compression myelopathy. Neurosurgery 21:950–957
12. Ohshima Y, Sato H, Hayashi M, Yokota M, Hiramoto N (1991) A technique of laminoplasty: Expansive open-door laminoplasty reattaching pedicled spinous process (in Japanese). Spine and Spinal Cord 4:577–583
13. Hirabayashi K, Watanabe K, Wakano K, Suzuki N, Satomi K, Ishii Y (1983) Expansive open-door laminoplasty for cervical spinal stenotic myelopathy. Spine 8:693–699
14. Tsuji H (1982) Laminoplasty for patients with compressive myelopathy due to so-called spinal canal stenosis in cervical and thoracic regions. Spine 7:2–34

Diagnostic Validity of MRI in Lumbar Herniated Intervertebral Disc

KEY-YONG KIM, YUNG-TAE KIM, CHOON-SUNG LEE, and JUNG-JAE KIM[1]

Key Words. MRI, classification, lumbar HIVD

Introduction

In addition to the impressive quality of its images, the negligible risk and multiplanar capabilities of magnetic resonance imaging (MRI) have led to its widespread use for studying the spine. It is now the primary imaging study for most spinal evaluations. Recently, with the development of high-resolution surface-coil MRI, it became possible to characterize and differentiate various subgroups of lumbar disc disease.

Preoperative typing of lumbar herniated intervertebral discs (HIVD) can provide appropriate planning for management of the disease. However, few studies have been reported on the diagnostic accuracy of MRI in typing in lumbar HIVD. The purpose of this study was to evaluate the diagnostic accuracy of MRI in typing lumbar HIVD compared with operative findings.

Patients and Methods

The patients of this prospective study were previously unoperated patients with symptoms suggestive of disc disruption or herniation. MRI of 242 lumbar discs in 211 patients (29 patients had two levels and one patient three levels) were analyzed preoperatively. The operative findings were then compared with the MRI films to determine its predictive ability. Age ranged from 13 to 73 years (mean age 36.6 years).

[1]Department of Orthopedic Surgery, Asan Medical Center, University of Ulsan, Medical College, 388-1 Poongnap-dong Songpa-gu, Seoul, 138-040, Korea

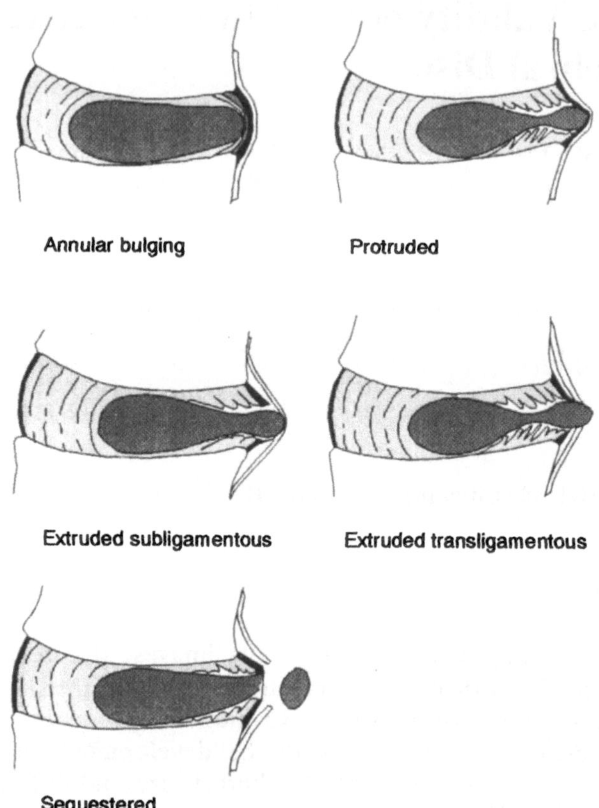

Fig. 1. Schematic illustration of the MRI classification of herniated intervertebral discs

Examinations were performed on 1.0T (Shimadzu SMT-100X, Kyoto, Japan) and 1.5T (Signa, GE, Milwaukee, Wis.) units. The authors' imaging protocol was sagittal T1-weighted, proton density, T2-weighted, axial T1-weighted spin echo images, and axial fast gradient echo images. Gadolinium-DTPA (Gd-DTPA) enhancement was done in 77 patients for which the image was obscure or when a ruptured or sequestered disc was suspected preoperatively. The type of each herniated disc was determined preoperatively using the classification modified from that of Burton [1], Macnab and McCulloch [2,3], Masaryk et al. [4], Schellinger et al. [5], and Thomas and Wiltse [6] (Fig. 1).

Results

Of 71 suspected protruded discs on MRI, 56 proved to be protruded; 10, extruded subligamentous; and 5, extruded transligamentous. Of 84 suspected

Table 1. Comparison of the four groups of herniated discs.

	Sensitivity	Specificity	Accuracy
Protruded	92%	91%	92%
ESL	71%	82%	79%
ETL	52%	92%	81%
Sequestered	92%	99%	97%
Total			85%

ESL, Extruded subligamentous; *ETL*, extruded transligamentous

extruded subligamentous discs, 54 proved to be subligamentous; 24, transligamentous; 5, protruded; and 1, sequestered. Of 50 suspected extruded transligamentous discs, 36 were transligamentous; 12, subligamentous; and 2, sequestered. Of 37 suspected sequestered discs, 33 proved to be sequestered; and 4, extruded transligamentous. Therefore, the overall accuracy of MRI in predicting the type of HIVD is 86.3% (correct in 179 of 242 discs) and somewhat higher in protruded and sequestered than in extruded discs (Table 1).

We analyzed MRI findings of 179 discs for which preoperative typing was proved correct, and tried to identify the images on which annulus rupture was most clearly recognizable. Among 56 protruded discs, the sagittal proton density image was most helpful in 40 and the T2-weighted image in 16 discs in recognizing intact annulus. For 123 extruded or sequestered discs in which the annulus was ruptured, the proton density image was the most helpful in 108 and the T2-weighted image in 15 (Fig. 2). The intactness of posterior longitudinal ligament is clearly defined on T2-weighted image in 84 of 90 extruded discs (Fig. 3).

The Gd-DTPA enhanced axial T1-weighted image was particularly helpful in differentiating a sequestered disc. The anterior rim of the free fragment was enhanced in 28 of 33 sequestered discs and the sequestered disc material was separated from the posterior margin of the mother disc by a white enhanced rim, in contrast to non-enhancement of simple extruded discs in which enhancement was done (Fig. 4). Disc migration was found in 43 among the 181 cases of extruded and sequestered discs. Thirty-one cases showed migration in an inferior direction. Of 28 cases of anterior rim enhancement, 3 showed subligamentous sequestered type.

Discussion

Preoperative determination of type of herniation is advantageous in planning the management of HIVD. Among the present diagnostic modalities, MRI delineates not only the extent and pattern of herniation but also changes in anatomical structures of the disc. If criteria can be established based on

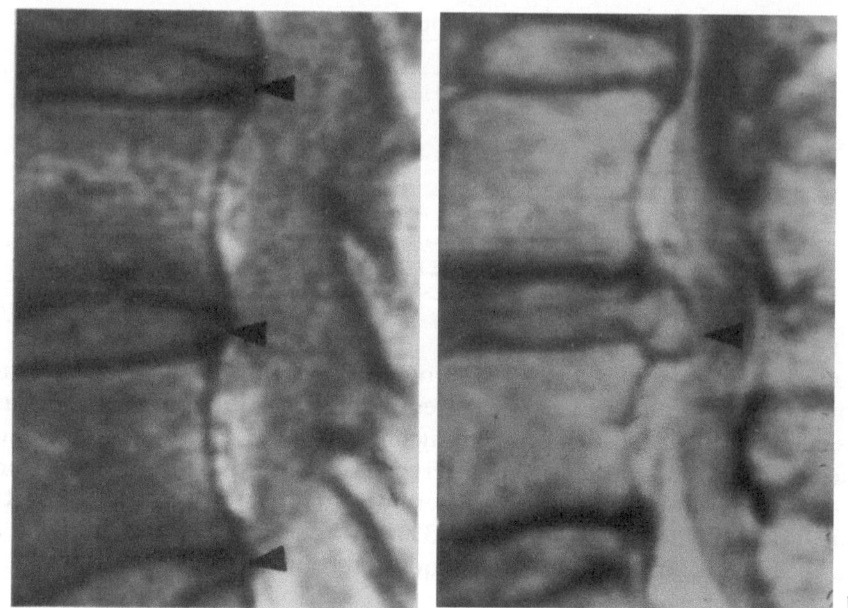

Fig. 2a,b. Annulus fibrosus on proton density imaging **a** Intact annulus fibrosus (*arrowheads*) and **b** ruptured annulus fibrosus (*arrowhead*)

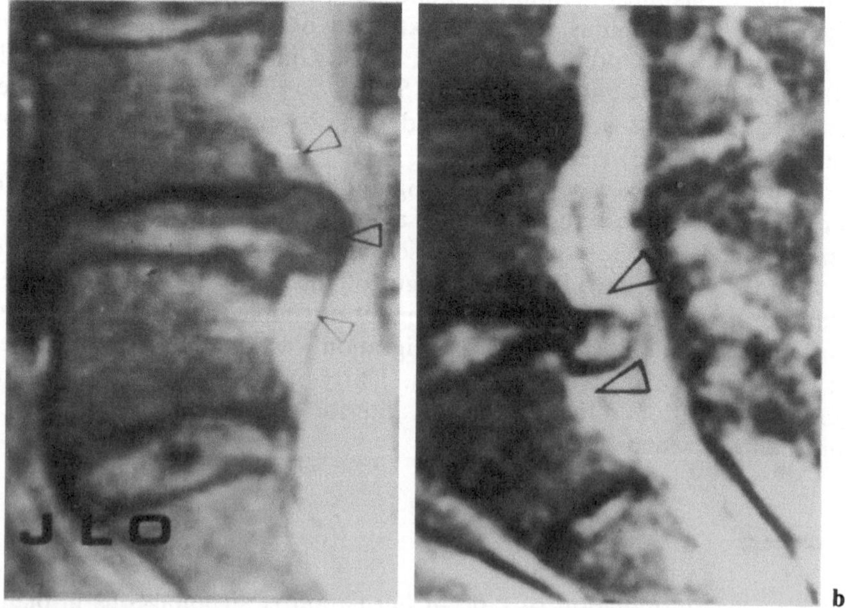

Fig. 3a,b. Posterior longitudinal ligament (PLL) line on T2-weighted image. **a** Intact PLL line in extruded subligamentous type (*open arrowheads*). **b** Disrupted PLL line in extruded transligamentous type (*open arrowheads*)

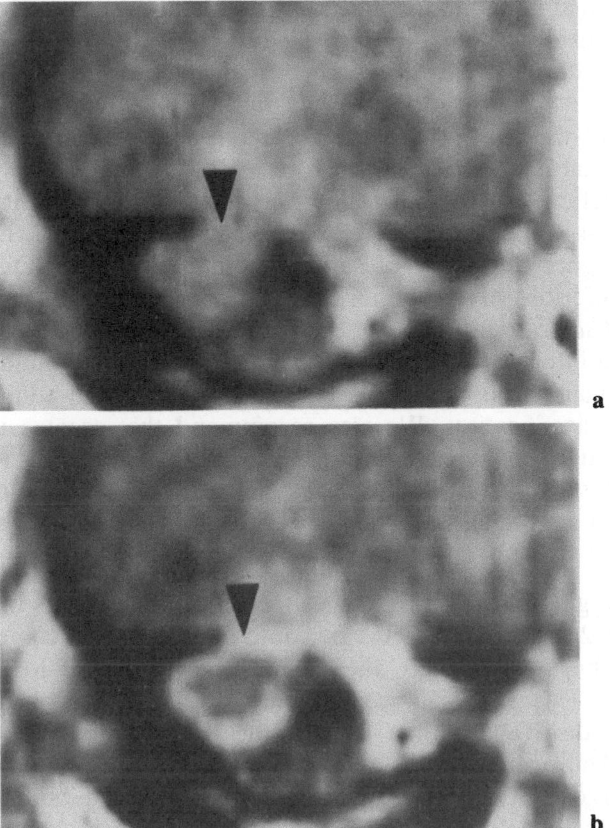

Fig. 4a,b. Gd-DTPA-enhanced axial T1-weighted image in a sequestered disc. **a** Preenhanced image shows herniated disc fragment (*arrowhead*). **b** Anterior rim enhancement of free fragment in postenhanced image (*arrowhead*)

preoperative MRI findings, the best treatment can be selected earlier. From the viewpoint of planning and management, it is widely accepted that percutaneous methods such as chemonucleolysis or percutaneous discectomy are not indicated for herniated discs with a ruptured annulus [2,5,7]. Therefore, identifying the condition of the annulus fibrosus is important in deciding the management. Proton density image showed the condition of the annulus fibrosus well and it was the most meaningful in differentiating protruded discs from extruded ones [8,9]. The extruded disc showed relatively lower diagnostic accuracy (80%) than that of protruded (92%) or sequestered (97%) discs, and it could be explained by the difficulty in defining the small posterior longitudinal ligament slit even on Gd-DTPA-enhanced images. It is important to identify extruded transligamentous and sequestered discs because they are resistant to conservative treatment and the percutaneous methods such as chemonucleolysis or percutaneous discectomy are contraindicated [6,10,11].

Sequestered discs can be more accurately diagnosed with Gadolinium-DTPA enhancement, which showed anterior rim enhancement of the sequestered portion on T1-weighted axial images and round rim enhancement on T1-weighted sagittal images [1,4,8,12,13].

Clear depiction of disc migration on MRI could prevent negative disc exploration [14–16] and a more extensive surgical approach. Fries et al. [15] observed a higher frequency of superior migration (78%), Dillon et al. [17] found 50% inferior, 40% superior, and 10% bidirectional motion. We found disc fragment migration in 24% of the extruded and sequestered discs, most of which showed inferior migration (71%). In this series, we found three peculiar cases of subligamentous sequestered disc, so we propose adding this type to our previous classification. We also recommend that great caution be taken during explorations of this type not to dislodge the fragment.

Through this study, we found that MRI is a very important and reliable diagnostic tool for the classification of HIVD, for the planning adequate treatment modality, and for minimizing the frequency of negative disc exploration.

Summary. Magnetic resonance images (MRI) of 211 patients with lumbar disc herniation at 242 levels were divided into 5 groups and compared with the operative findings to evaluate the diagnostic accuracy of MRI classification prospectively. This study showed a relatively lower diagnostic accuracy of the extruded disc (80%) than that of the protuded (92%) or sequestered (97%) disc. The overall accuracy of MRI in predicting the types of herniated intervertebral disc was 86.3%. Sequestered disc could be more accurately diagnosed with Gadolinium-DTPA enhancement, which showed anterior rim enhancement of the sequestered portion on T1-weighted axial imaging. We concluded that high-resolution MRI is sensitive in detecting disc disease and specific in characterizing various subgroups of disc herniation, especially sequestered discs.

References

1. Burton CV (1988) Gravity lumbar reduction. In: Kirkaldy-Willis WH (ed) Managing low back pain. Churchill Livingstone, New York, pp 307–314
2. Macnab I, McCulloch JA (1990) Disc Ruptures, In: Macnab I (ed) Backache, Williams and Wilkins, Baltimore, pp 130–134
3. McCulloch JA (1989) Pathogenesis of sciatica. In: McCulloch (ed) Principles of microsurgery for lumbar disc disease. Raven, New York, pp 43–45
4. Masaryk TJ, Ross JS, Modic MT, Boumphrey F, Bohlman H, Wilber G (1988) High-resolution MR imaging of sequestered lumbar intervertebral disks. Am J Roentgenol 150:1155–1162
5. Schellinger D, Manz HJ, Vidic B, Patronas NJ, Deveikis JP, Muraki AS, Abdullah DC (1990) Disc fragment migration. Radiology 175:831–836

6. Thomas JC, Wiltse LL (1988) Patient selection for automated percutaneous discectomy. In: Wiltse LL (ed) Automated percutaneous lumbar discectomy, University of California, San Francisco, pp 9–14
7. Suk SI, Lee CK, Lee CS, Kim WJ, Jang BS (1990) Clinical experience of automated percutaneous lumbar discectomy. J Korean Orthop Assoc 25:500–509
8. Hueftle MG, Modic MT, Ross JS, Masaryk TJ, Carter JR, Wilber RG, Bohlman HH, Steinberg PM, Delamarter RB (1988) Lumbar spine postoperative MR imaging with Gd-DTPA. Radiology 167:817–824
9. Ross JS, Modic MT, Masaryk TJ (1989) Tears of the anulus fibrosus: Assessment with Gd-DTPA enhanced MR imaging. Am J Neuroradiol 10:1251–1254
10. Nordy EJ, Lucas L (1973) A comparative analysis of lumbar disc disease treated by laminectomy or chemonucleolysis. Clin Orthop 90:110–129
11. Smith L (1975) Failure with chemonucleolysis. Orthop Clin N Am 6:255–258
12. Kim KY, Kim YT, Lee CS, Shin MJ (1992) MRI classification of lumbar herniated intervertebral disc. Orthopaedics 15:499–454
13. Ross JS, Modic MT, Masaryk TJ, Carter J, Marcus RE, Bohlman H (1990) Assessment of extradural degenerative disease with Gd-DTPA enhanced MR imaging correlation with surgical and pathologic findings. Am J Neuroradiol 10: 1243–1249
14. Burton CV, Kirkaldy-Willis WH, Yong-Hing K, Heithoff KB (1981) Causes of failure of surgery on the lumbar spine. Clin Orthop 157:191–199
15. Fries JW, Abodeely DAK, Vijungco JG, Yeager VL, Gaffey WR (1982) Computed tomography of herniated and extruded nucleus pulposus. J Comput Assist Tomogr 6:874–887
16. Macnab I (1971) Negative disc exploration. An analysis of the causes of nerve-root involvement in sixty-eight patients. J Bone Joint Surg [Am] 53:891–903
17. Dillon WP, Kaseff LG, Knackstedt VE, Osborn AG (1983) Computed tomography and differential diagnosis of the extruded lumbar disk. J Comput Assist Tomogr 7:699–975

Anterior Interbody Fusion for Lumbar Spondylolisthesis

Sen-Yuen Lin and Chun-Kwang Wu[1]

Abstract. We reviewed 88 cases of lumbar spondylolisthesis, including isthmic and degenerative types, which were treated with anterior interbody fusion using an iliac bone strut. The surgery was done between 1973 and 1990, with a minimum follow-up of 1 year and 6 months. The mean follow-up period was 7 years. The age distribution was from 13 to 74 years old, with a mean of 46.8 years. Female patients were predominant. Most of our cases of spondylolisthesis were L4 on L5 or L5 on S1 with a Meyerding's classification of grade I to grade II. Our clinical results revealed that the mean Japanese Orthopedic Association (JOA) score was 15.0 preoperatively and improved to 24.3 postoperatively. There was significant improvement in leg pain, claudication, and sensory disturbances. A roentgenographic study by Dabbs measurement [1] in our study showed a 27.7% increase in the disc height and a 24% correction of slippage during follow-up. By the insertion of an adequate iliac graft, we could rearrange a deformity, such as scoliosis, hyperlordosis, or hypolordosis. Under the definition of relieving clinical symptoms and signs, we had an 86% satisfaction rate. This corresponds well to our 85% fusion rate, although we realized that in other series the results were not so positive. During follow-up, 90% of patients returned to work, but 35% of them changed lighter jobs. Although some complications occurred, such as vascular injury during operation, abdominal hernia, and donor site infection or paresthesia, we did not encounter such severe conditions as pulmonary embolisms, impotence, or retrograde ejaculation. We believe that anterior lumbar interbody fusion (ALIF) is an effective primary procedure for spondylolisthesis.

Key Words. Spondylolisthesis, anterior interbody fusion, low back pain, sciatica

[1] Department of Orthopaedic Surgery, Kaohsiung Medical College, 100 Shith-Chuan 1st Road Kaohsiung, Taiwan

Introduction

Spondylolisthesis without separation of the pars interarticularis was first reported by Junghanns in 1930 [2]. Later, in 1932 Capener also reported anterior spinal fusion for cases of spondylolisthesis. Since then, this surgery has been accepted as one possible treatment for adult spondylolisthesis. There has been some disagreement among advocates of anterior spinal fusion regarding the success rate of the operation. Batchelor reported a 26% success rate [3], while Stauffer and Coventry reported 56% [4], Goldner et al. reported 80% [5], Freebody et al. reported 92% [6], and Harmon 95% [7]. Takahashi [8], who reported long-term results in 1990, suggests that clinical results will vary depending on the age of the patient, with the success rate declining from 80% to 50% as the age of the patient increases. There is also disagreement regarding the correlation of the clinical success rate with the fusion rate. van Rens and van Horn [9] reported a 96% fusion rate with a 93% satisfaction rate. Kim and Kim [10] reported a 77% fusion rate with an 87% satisfaction rate. Finally, Flynn and Hoque [11], although reporting only a 56% fusion rate, still had an 87% satisfaction rate. In recent years, the cases of spondylolisthesis treated by instrumentation from a posterior approach with interbody fusion or posterolateral fusion have been increasing rapidly as this procedure has a high satisfaction rate and is relatively safe. From a biomechanical point of view, however, anterior fusion provides the largest increase in stiffness [12,13] which is the main goal of treatment for instability of the spine. Both methods have the same high satisfaction rate. There are also, some different opinions about how often sterility and impotence occur in men following this procedure. Flynn and Hoque [11] had a survey of world authorities on anterior spine fusion which revealed only 16 patients with the sequela of retrograde ejaculation. So this complication may be over-exaggerated and our research also supports this finding.

Patients and Methods

We followed up 88 spondylolisthetic patients who received anterior lumbar interbody fusion (ALIF) from 1973 to 1990. The mean period of follow-up was 7 years. Their age distribution was from 13 to 74 years old, with a mean of 46.8 years. Female patients comprised 62 of the cases. Most of the spondylolisthesis were degenerative (n = 55) while the rest were isthmic (n = 33). In this series, L4 on L5 cases were most common (n = 59), but we also treated 20 cases of L5 on S1 and 9 cases of L3 on L4. Symptoms of the spondylolisthetic patients mostly complained of back pain, leg pain, and claudication. Medication and rest were the first recommendations for symptomatic spondylolisthetic patients. If this failed, we proceeded to surgery. By using a tricortical bone strut harvested from the iliac crest, the initial reduction and stability were achieved. During the postoperative course, the patients were completely restricted to bedrest for 6 weeks, instead of being fitted with a spica or brace. However, further protection with a corset for 3 more months after bedrest was still necessary.

Results

The mean preoperative Japan Orthopedic Association (JOA) score was 15.0 and at the final follow-up the mean JOA score was 24.3. From the evaluation of the score shown in Fig. 1 it can be seen that great improvement was made in leg pain, claudication, and sensory disturbances. There was also an increase in the MMT (manual muscle test) and a decrease of restriction from the ADL (activities of daily living). The extent of reduction by ALIF was significant postoperatively, but the continuation of the result was not so encouraging. From the X-ray studies of our series, 20 patients were reduced from Gr II to Gr I immediately postoperatively, but it was also the case that loss of reduction was significant during the final follow-up. Seventeen patients aggravated to Gr II from Gr I slippage and the correction of slippage was from 44% to 24%. From the data of mean disc height measured by the Dabbs method, we made a 38% increase of the original deranged disc height, but it collapsed to only a 27.7% increase by the final follow-up. Figure 2 shows a solid good fusion 8 years postoperatively. The mean disc height was 9.4 mm preoperatively, 13.0 mm postoperatively, and decreased to 12.0 mm during the follow-up. Preoperatively, the mean slip angle of our patients was 3.5 degrees. Immediately postoperatively, the mean slip angle was corrected to 11.7 degrees. During the follow-up, however, the mean slip angle narrowed to 10.5 degrees. Whether the slip angle might affect the clinical results remains unknown. We divided our cases into 2 groups, one with lordosis greater than 35 degrees and the other with lordosis less than 35 degrees. The postoperative lordosis analysis revealed that ALIF changed the original abnormal lordosis to a more physiological lordosis, approaching 35 degrees as shown in Fig. 3. The insertion of the iliac bone strut could correct some degree of scoliosis due to spondylolisthesis as shown in Fig. 4. Our satisfaction rate was 86%, 6% no change, and 8% complained that no operation would have been better. During follow-up, nearly 90% of our patients were capable of returning to work, but 35% of them changed jobs for lighter ones. We encountered some complications, such as 3 cases of vascular injuries, 2 cases of abdominal hernia, 2 cases of donor site infection, and many cases of lateral femoral cutaneous nerve injuries. Nevertheless, we did not encounter severe complications such as pulmonary embolism or retrograde ejaculation.

A questionnaire study showed that we did not have any complaints of severe aggravation of sexual function. Six patients had mild micturition difficulty postoperatively, but most were unaffected. Concerning long-term follow-up of adjacent motion segment problems, our study of disc height by Dabbs' measurement revealed this to be insignificant. Preoperatively, the superior and

Subjective Symptoms

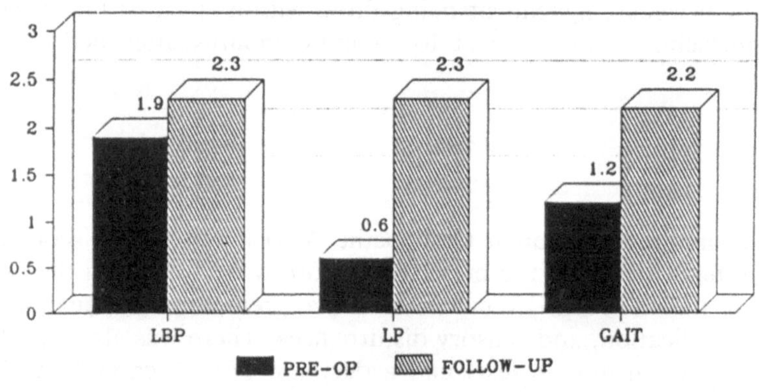

CLINICAL SIGNS

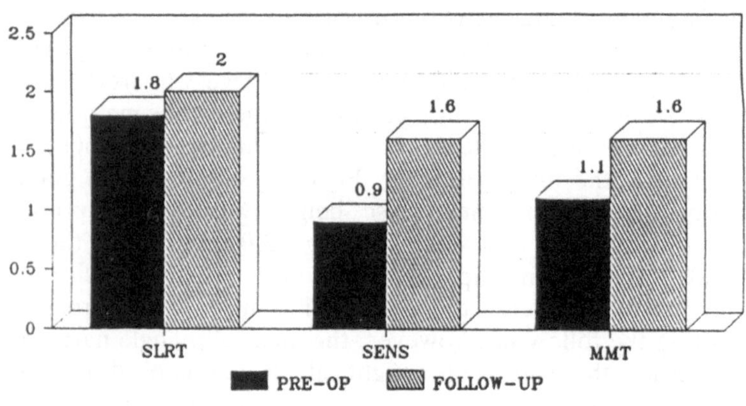

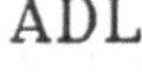

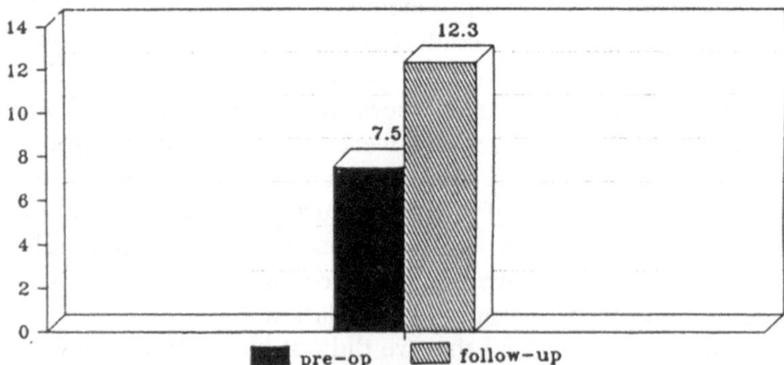

Fig. 1. The Japanese Orthopedic Association (JOA) score was evaluated preoperatively and during follow-up. *SLRT*, Straight leg raising test; *SENS*, sensory; *MMT*, manual muscle test; *ADL*, activities of daily living; *LBP*, low back pain; *LP*, leg pain

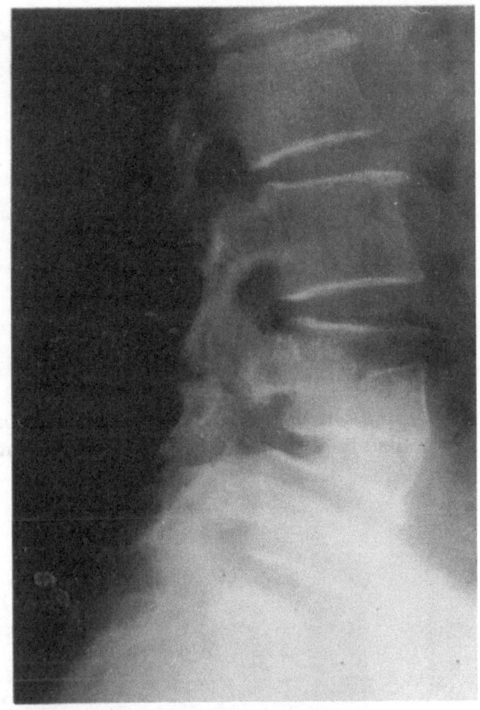

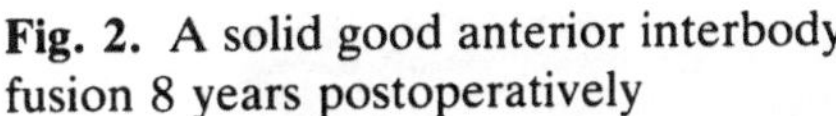

Fig. 2. A solid good anterior interbody fusion 8 years postoperatively

inferior mean disc height was 12.1 mm and 12.3 mm respectively. Immediately postoperatively, the superior and inferior mean disc height was 12.5 mm and 12.9 mm, respectively. During follow-up, the mean superior and inferior disc height was 12.4 mm and 12.9 mm, respectively. From a biomechanical point of view, Lee and Langrana [12] reported that fused segments will increase in stiffness and shift the center of rotation of the unfused segment. Loss of continuity in load transmission caused uneven stress distribution in motion segments. Bodsky and Hendricks [14] reported the clinical results from the same biomechanical view point; however, only 2.7% of his patients required a secondary operation. The biomechanical theory of Lee was not justified in our clinical results. Furthermore, the clinical results in our series also differed from the observations of Brodsky.

Discussion

Back pain, leg pain, and claudication caused by spondylolisthesis that can not be eradicated with medication was our criteria for surgery. The concern of circulatory complications and severe stenosis caused by facet joint hypertrophy occurring in patients of more than 60 years of age deterred us from choosing anterior spinal surgery for spondylolisthesis. Using this rationale, we chose

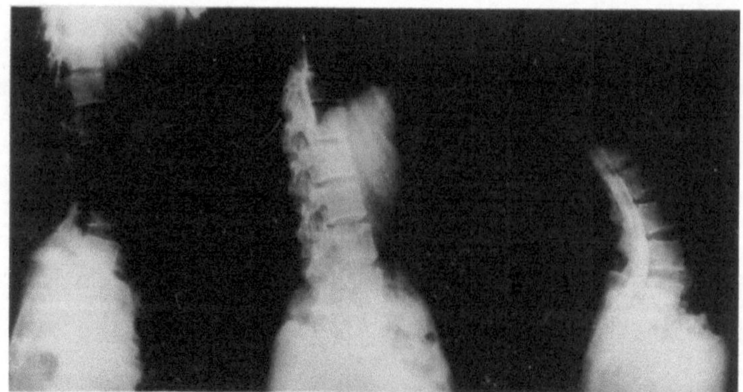

Fig. 3. *Right* X-ray showed hyperlordosis preoperatively, the *middle* one was immediately postoperative, the *left* one showed improvement of pathological lordosis

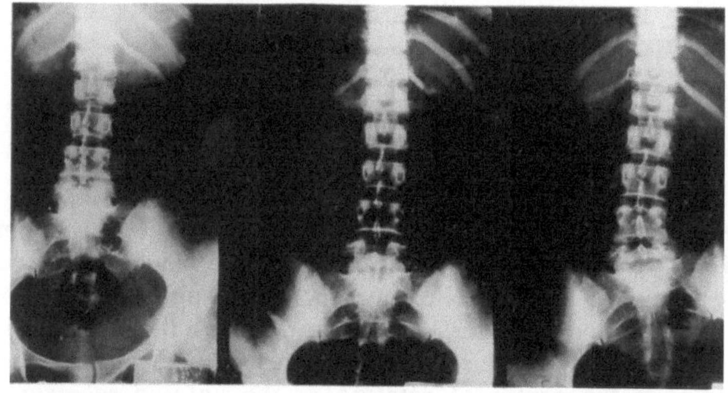

Fig. 4. *Right* X-ray showed a case of spondylolisthesis with scoliosis deformity. The *middle* one was immediately postoperative. *Left* X-ray showed fusion with correction of scoliosis

anterior lumbar interbody fusion as the primary procedure for younger spondylolisthetic patients, mostly below 60 years of age. The advantages of ALIF are the following: (1) excellent disc exposure; (2) complete disc excision and decompression of herniation; (3) some extent of immediate reduction by restoring disc height; (4) avoids violation of the spinal canal and its nerve roots; (5) ability to avoid prior area of neurogenic scarring; and (6) decreased occurrence of blood transfusions. Of course, the continuous challenge of avoiding damage to the great vessels and autonomic neural system during the retroperitoneal approach make this procedure stressful, but this undesirable situation is avoidable. It is possible that our relative lack of complications with pulmonary embolism is related to the ethnic make-up of our patients. The judgement on fusion by trabeculation is not controversial, but the union takes a long time to fuse. Flynn and Hoque reported that their iliac-graft fusion time was 2.54 years on average, although they did have one patient in whom union after iliac graft fusion was first evident 11 years postoperatively. So once pseudoarthrosis from grafting is observed, it does not necessarily mean "definite pseudoarthrosis" during only a limited years' observation after the operation. It might need a longer waiting period.

The value of ALIF in the surgical treatment for degenerative spondylolisthesis may be attributed to the resection of the diseased disc, the reduction of slippage, and some restoration of disc height, which will result in correction of malalignment, enlargement of the stenotic canal, and decompression of nerve tissue. Inoue reported his series in 1988. Under the 100% fusion rate, he had 59.6% mean correction rate of slippage [15]. In our series, we had a 44% slippage correction postoperatively, but only 24% correction during follow-up. Similar results were present in the disc height correction: We had a 38% increase of disc height postoperatively, but it declined to only 27.7% during follow-up. This phenomenon tells us that, during the course of fusion, stiffness of the graft will decrease with a resulting lose of some efficacy of its corrective power. Nevertheless, it might not reach the extent which would result in significant clinical aggravation.

It is commonly accepted to treat grade I and grade II spondylolisthesis by fusion in situ. We also agree that a minor degree of spondylolisthesis, once fused, may not induce clinical symptoms. Recently, many orthopedic surgeons have also taken notice of the correction of scoliosis and lordosis during their treatment of low back pain syndrome. With the insertion of an iliac graft, our patients progressed from hyperlordosis or hypolordosis to reach physiological lordosis, corresponding to normal adults' lumbar lordosis [16]. Whether in the future the tendency to treat spondylolisthesis with instrumentation persists. The high rigidity of this construct remains in dispute when compared with the semi-rigid anterior bone graft. By Dabbs measurement in our 88 cases, we did not induce significant narrowing of the adjacent disc height. An anterior interbody fusion for spondylolisthesis does not seem to provoke early deterioration of the adjacent discs, provided that the position of the adjacent vertebrae is normal.

References

1. Dabbs VM, Dabbs LG (1990) Correlation between disc height narrowing and low back pain. Spine 15(12):1366–1368
2. Junghanns H (1930) Spondylolisthesen ohne Spalt im Zwischengelenkstuck (Pseudospondylolisthesen) Arch Orthop Unfall Chiru 29:118–127
3. Batchelor JS (1963) Anterior interbody spinal fusion. Guy's Hosp Rep 112:61–65

4. Stauffer RN, Coventry MB (1972) Anterior interbody lumbar spine fusion. Analysis of Mayo Clinic series. J Bone Joint Surg 54-A:756–768
5. Goldner JL, McCollum DE, Urbaniak JR (1969) Anterior disc excision and interbody spine fusion for chronic low back pain. In: American Academy of Orthopaedic Surgeons, Symposium on the spine, St. Louis, C.V. Mosby, pp 111–131
6. Freebody D, Bendall R, Taylor RD (1971) Anterior transperitoneal lumbar fusion. J Bone Joint Surg 58-B:193–199
7. Harmon PH (1958) Anterior extraperitoneal lumbar disk excision and vertebral body fusion. Clin Orthop 18:169–198
8. Takahashi K (1990) Long-term results of anterior interbody fusion for treatment of degenerative spondylolisthesis. Spine 15(11):1211–1215
9. van Rens TH.JG, van Horn JR (1982) Long-term results in lumbosacral interbody fusion for spondylolisthesis. Acta Orthop Scandinavica 53:383–392
10. Kim NH, Kim DJ (1991) Anterior interbody fusion for spondylolisthesis. Orthopaedics 14(10):1069–1075
11. Flynn JC, Hoque MA (1979) Anterior fusion of the lumbar spine. J Bone Joint Surg 61-A(8):1143–1150
12. Lee CK, Langrana NA (1984) Lumbosacral spinal fusion, A biomechanical study. Spine 9(6):574–581
13. White AA, Panjabi M (1990) Clinical biomechanics of the spine, 2nd edn. Lippincott, Philadelphia, p 535
14. Brodsky AE, Hendricks RL (1989) Segmental ("floating") lumbar spine fusions. Spine 14(4):447–450
15. Inoue SI, Watanabe T, Goto S (1988) Degenerative spondylolisthesis. Clin Orthop 227:90–98
16. Lin RM, Jou IM (1992) Lumbar lordosis: Normal adults. J Formosan Assoc 91(3):329–333

Sagittal Splitting Laminoplasty for Spinal and Spinal Cord Surgery

TADASHI SHIMAMURA, MASATAKA ABE, KEN YAMAZAKI, YOSHIYUKI KAN, and MASAHIRO SUZUKI[1]

Key Words. Sagittal splitting laminoplasty, posterior spinal exposure, spinal reconstruction, spinal surgery, spinal cord surgery

Introduction

To attempt restoration of the posterior spinal elements, we have tried to use sagittal splitting laminoplasty (SSL) in spinal and spinal cord surgery, because laminectomy has some disadvantages reported by many authors [1–8]. For exposure of the spinal canal and reconstruction of the posterior spinal elements, SSL employs some procedures and improvements which have been added to Kurokawa's cervical spinal canal enlargement [9]. SSL is applicable to various disorders from the cervical to the lumbar spine. The purpose of this paper is to present the surgical technique and results of SSL.

Patients and Operation

Since 1983, 54 of 219 patients with disorders from the cervical to the lumbar spine have been operated on using SSL, excluding 165 cases with cervical myelopathy due to ossification of the posterior longitudinal ligament and multisegmental spondylosis. They were 27 males and 27 females, and the average age was 51 years, ranging from 20 to 70 years. The cases were spinal cord tumor (n = 29), syringomyelia (n = 1), dural granuloma (n = 1), epidural hematoma (n = 4), epidural abscess (n = 3), epidural scar (n = 1), cervical calcification (n = 3) and thoracic ossification (n = 5) of the yellow ligament,

[1] Department of Orthopaedic Surgery, Iwate Medical University School of Medicine, 19-1 Uchimaru, Morioka, 020 Japan

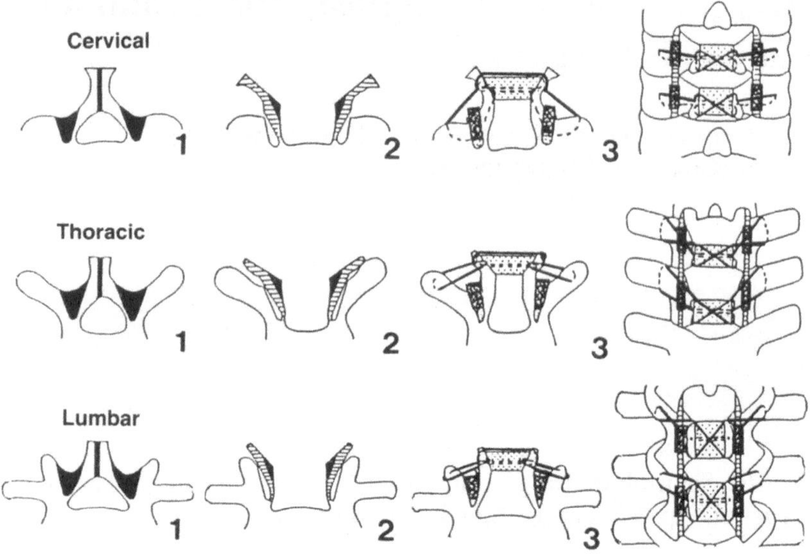

Fig. 1. Schematic drawing of the sagittal splitting laminoplasty for the cervical to the lumbar spine. For the exposure, bilateral wedge-shaped grooving (*1*) and cutting away the ventral corners of the split laminae (*2*) with suitable resection of the yellow ligament are necessary. In the reconstruction, bilateral wiring for stabilization of the split halves (cervical: the lower articular process, thoracic: the transverse process, and lumbar: the upper articular process) in addition to median double cross wiring for the bone block and fine corticocancellous bone block grafting in the bilateral grooves are performed (*3*) (with permission, from [11])

atypical lumbar disc herniation (n = 5), and lumbar spinal canal stenosis with instability due to degenerative spondylolisthesis (n = 2). In this series, the occurrence of the spinal levels was cervical (n = 10), cervicothoracic (n = 5), thoracic (n = 21), thoracolumbar (n = 2), and lumbar (n = 16 cases).

The SSL technical improvements added to the original method [9] are as follows: For the exposure, first there is bilateral wedge-shaped grooving and cutting away the ventral corners of the split laminae with suitable resection of the yellow ligament, and then there is firm stay suturing the split laminae to the paraspinal muscles. In the reconstruction, there is bilateral wiring to stabilize the split halves in addition to median double cross wiring for the median bone block and fine corticocancellous bone grafting in the bilateral grooves for stabilization (Fig. 1). When indicated, as a result of a focal location, unilateral SSL can be performed. At this time, no lateral wiring is necessary because the opposite site is intact and stable [10]. There was bilateral SSL in 43 cases and unilateral SSL in 11 cases. The average number of split laminae was 2.4 (range: 1–10) over all the levels. Details are provided in Table 1. The patients were kept in bed for an average of 1.5 weeks (range: 1–3 weeks) after surgery and then several kinds of spinal braces were applied for 3–4 months.

Table 1. The number of cases, the average number of split laminae, and the corresponding spinal levels.

Level	No. of cases Bilateral $n = 43$	Unilateral $n = 11$	Average No. of split laminae Bilateral $n = 43$	Unilateral $n = 11$
C	9	1	3.3	1.0
C-T	5		5.0	
T	16	5	2.0	2.0
T-L	2		4.0	
L	11	5	1.0	1.0
			(C to L: 2.6	1.5)

C, Cervical; *C-T*, cervicothoracic; *T*, thoracic; *T-L*, thoracolumbar; *L*, lumbar spine

Results

In 50 cases (93%), including two cases switched from unilateral to bilateral, SSL was performed successfully. However, laminectomy with facetectomy was required in four cases of dumbbell tumor and meningioma with remarkable ossification. In SSL, the depth of the operative field was slightly increased compared with laminectomy, so that there were some difficulties with the intracanal manipulation at the ventral site of the spinal canal where the spinal cord is present.

Reconstructive posterior spinal elements had good stability, because bilateral wiring was in the same segment, and fine bone blocks in the bilateral grooves worked as key stones. Therefore, the restoration of the posterior spinal elements was almost complete with retention of the enlarged spinal canal. The operative and adjacent facets were almost completely preserved, and postoperative instability and deformity of the spinal column were not found in any of the cases (Fig. 2) [11]. In 90% of the cases, postoperative spinal motion was kept in a good range with mroe than 50% of preoperative spinal motion. However, in five cases of bilateral SSL, postoperative severe restriction or disappearance of spinal motion was found. Although there was no problem in their activities of daily living, the restriction or disappearance of spinal motion indicated a disadvantage of SSL. No neurological deterioration due to SSL and no infection was found in any of the cases.

Discussion and Conclusion

SSL has several advantages and disadvantages. The advantages are restoration of the posterior spinal elements, retention of the enlarged spinal canal, prevention of postoperative instability and deformity, and protection of the

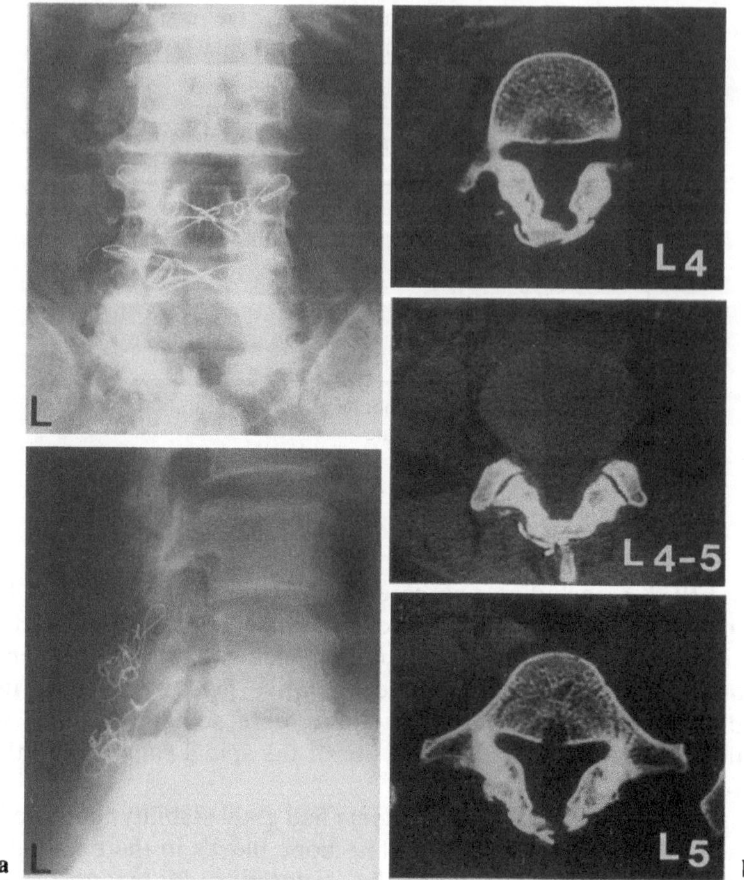

Fig. 2a,b. Postoperative roentgenograms **a** and computed tomograms **b** of the lumbar spine show almost complete restoration of the posterior spinal elements with retention of the enlarged spinal canal and no deformity of the spinal column. The facets are also almost completely preserved (with permission, from [11])

spinal cord and the cauda equina. On the other hand, the disadvantages are a longer operating time including the necessity for bone graft, necessity for external fixation, restriction of postoperative spinal motion, and some influence on the quality of postoperative magnetic resonance imaging films. To shorten the operating time and to prevent problems due to taking iliac bone, hydroxyapatite spacers for the median repair and the spinous process tips for the repair of bilateral grooves were employed 2 years ago. To decrease the metallic artifact on magnetic resonance imaging, titanium wire (0.4 mm) is recommended. Non-metallic materials, for example tekmiron suture [12] are ideal, but they can not be used at present because they can not be tightened repeatedly until the split laminae are stabilized. Postoperative restriction of spinal motion protects spinal stability in the operative portion. Therefore, a long-term follow-up study on the adjacent segments will be necessary.

In SSL, the depth from the split lamina to the ventral site of the spinal canal is slightly increased. Ultrasonic instruments should be used for the intracanal manipulation at the ventral site of the spinal canal where the spinal cord is present.

Even if there are lateral gutter fractures, bilateral wiring with fine bone block as key stones makes the split posterior spinal elements stable when combined with median repair. Although SSL has some disadvantages described above, this procedure, which produces a relatively good operative field and which can be changed into laminectomy when needed during surgery, is now taking the place of laminectomy in our institute and related hospitals.

First, it is important to treat the focus safely and correctly, but it is also necessary to consider operative destruction of the posterior spinal elements at the same time. Recently, some kinds of procedures for reconstruction and restoration of the posterior spinal elements have been reported in cases of spinal cord tumor [13–16].

We believe that in spinal and spinal cord surgery, laminectomy, which has some disadvantages, should be avoided as much as possible, because in most cases of various disorders from the cervical to the lumbar spine, laminectomy was not always necessary. The posterior spinal elements not only have a mechanical importance, but they also serve to protect the spinal cord and the cauda equina.

References

1. Cattel HS, Clark GL Jr (1967) Cervical kyphosis and instability following multiple laminectomies in children. J Bone Joint Surg 49-A:713–720
2. Arima T (1969) Postlaminectomy malalignments of the cervical spine (in Japanese). J Brain Nerve Trauma 1:71–78
3. Hirabayashi K, Sasaki T, Takeda T (1972) The posterior and anterior operation in treatment of cervical disc lesions including cervical spondylosis. A long-term follow-up study. Cent Jpn J Orthop Traum Surg 15:786–788
4. Jenkins DHR (1973) Extensive cervical laminectomy. Long-term results. Br J Surg 60:852–854
5. Sim FH, Svien HJ, Bickel WH, James JM (1974) Swan-neck deformity following extensive cervical laminectomy. A review of twenty-one cases. J Bone Joint Surg 56-A:564–580
6. Harada Y, Kaneda K, Echizenya T, Ohnishi H, Fujiya M (1974) Instability of the cervical spine after extensive laminectomy (in Japanese). Rinsho Seikeigeka 9:909–911
7. Yasuoka S, Peterson HA, MacCarty CS (1982) Incidence of spinal column deformity after multilevel laminectomy in children and adults. J Neurosurg 57:441–445

8. Yonenobu K, Juji T, Ono K, Okada K, Yamamoto T, Harada N (1985) Choice of surgical treatment for multisegmental cervical spondylotic myelopathy. Spine 10:710–716
9. Kurokawa T, Tsuyama N, Tanaka H, Kobayashi M, Machida H, Nakamura K, Iizuka T, Hoshino Y (1982) Cervical canal enlargement by sagittal splitting of the spinous process (in Japanese). Bessatsu Seikeigeka 2:234–240
10. Shimamura T, Hayashi T, Iizuka J, Namiki M, Abe M (1990) Hemilaminoplasty by sagittal splitting method (in Japanese). Operation 44:1917–1923
11. Shimamura T, Yamazaki K, Kan Y, Suzuki M, Okuda S, Abe M (1993) Sagittal splitting laminoplasty for the whole spine (in Japanese). East Jpn J Clin Orthop 5:110–114
12. Ueda Y, Nishiyama S, Tamai S, Iwasaki Y, Yokota H (1990) Tekmiron suture as a material for spinal fusion (in Japanese). Bessatsu Seikeigeka 18:201–206
13. Ohtake S, Tohno S, Harata S, Ohmi Y, Toh S, Nakano K, Okamura Y, Araki T, Nakamura R, Ichikawa S, Nishio M, Ueyama K, Shiono M (1985) Osteoplastic laminectomy for the spinal cord tumor (in Japanese). Orthop Surg Traumatol 28:829–832
14. Shimamura T, Yamazaki K, Yamataka H, Yasuda T (1988) Sagittal splitting laminoplastic exposure for spinal cord tumors (in Japanese). Operation 42:1825–1829
15. Shikata J, Shimizu K, Ono K, Saito T, Yamamuro T (1990) Prevention of spinal deformity after resection of the spinal cord tumor (in Japanese). Seikeigeka 41:163–172
16. Mitsuhashi T, Ikata T, Murase M, Fukushima T, Morita T, Nakamura T, Tamada H, Kashiwaguchi S (1992) Surgical approaches of spinal cord tumor (in Japanese). Rinsho Seikeigeka 27:111–116

Part V.

Pathogenesis and Treatment of Osteoporosis and Rheumatoid Arthritis

Paraplegia Caused by Nonunion After Fracture of Osteoporotic Spine

Tetsumori Cho[1], Yushin Ishii[2], Masataro Tani[2], Tetsuro Sato[3], Yasuhisa Tanaka[4], Shoichi Kokubun[1], and Minoru Sakurai[1]

Key Words. Paraplegia, spinal osteoporosis, fracture, posttraumatic vertebral collapse, nonunion

Introduction

Neurological compromise associated with vertebral fracture in senile osteoporotic patients is not uncommon. So far, several studies have been reported, especially in the last decade [1–7]. However, the pathological mechanism of progressive collapse of a vertebral body and developement of delayed paraplegia has not been clarified yet.

In this paper, we describe our experience of ten cases and propose a hypothesis on the mechanism of delayed-onset paraplegia.

Patients and Methods

Between 1986 and 1991, we treated ten patients who had developed paraplegia after the fractures of osteoporotic vertebrae. There were seven women and three men. The age at onset of paraplegia ranged from 55 to 80 years (average, 71 years). The fractured vertebrae were T10 in one patient, T12 in three, L1 in five, and L2 in one.

[1] Department of Orthopaedic Surgery, Tohoku University School of Medicine, 1-1 Seiryo-machi, Aoba-ku, Sendai, 980 Japan
[2] Department of Orthopaedic Surgery, National Nishitaga Hospital, 2-11-11 Kagitorihoncho, Taihaku-ku, Sendai, 982 Japan
[3] Department of Orthopaedic Surgery, Tohoku Rosai Hospital, 4-3-21 Dainohara, Aoba-ku, Sendai, 982 Japan
[4] Department of Orthopaedic Surgery, Shiogama Ekisaikai Hospital, 1-15-24 Niihama-cho, Shiogama, 983 Japan

Table 1. Patient data.

Case	Sex, Age (years)	Fractured vertebra	Degree of osteoporosis[a]	Cause of fracture	Gait disturbance	Urinary disturbance
1	F, 71	T12	2	Fall from bed	Weakness in left L/E	None
2	F, 70	L1	2	Fall on buttocks	Intermittent claudication	None
3	M, 72	L1	2	No trauma	Unable to walk	Urinary retention
4	F, 65	L1	1	No trauma	Unable to walk	Frequent urge
5	M, 69	L1	0.5	Fall from roof	Clumsy walk	Retarded miction
6	M, 79	T12	1	No trauma	Unable to walk	Retarded miction
7	F, 67	T12	2	No trauma	Need support	Incontinence
8	F, 80	T10	1	Fall on back	Unable to walk	None
9	F, 74	L1	2	Fall on buttocks	Unable to walk	Urinary retention
10	F, 65	L2	1	No trauma	Unable to walk	None

L/E, Lower extremity
[a] Classification of Jikei Medical College

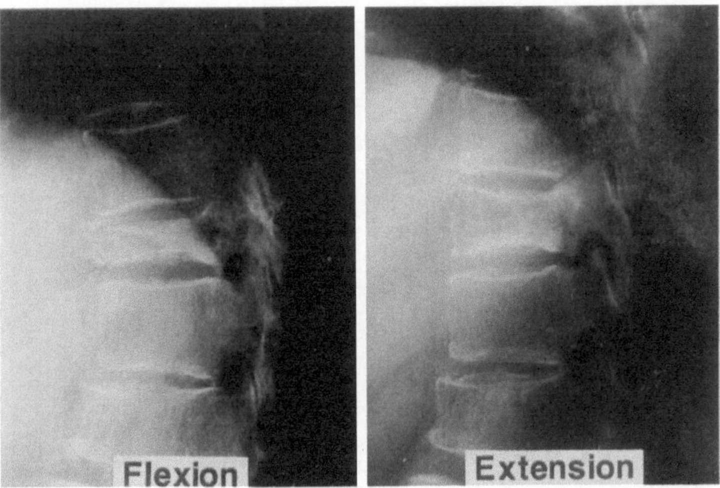

Fig. 1. Dynamic X-ray of a 80-year-old woman. Note the abnomal mobility at the fractured T10 vertebral body.

There was no history of causative trauma in five patients, in whom the initial symptom was acute backache. In eight patients, paraplegia appeared anywhere from 2 weeks to 58 months after the onset of backache or trauma. Initial treatment had been carried out on an outpatient basis in eight patients. They were advised to rest at home thoroughly, but they did not. In two cases, 3 and 6 weeks of hospitalization were prescribed, respectively.

Five patients were unable to walk due to weakness of their lower extremities. Six patients had urinary disturbance. All the patients complained of tingling or burning pain in their buttocks or legs. Laboratory examination revealed nothing remarkable (Table 1).

Plain X-rays showed a severe collapse of the vertebral body with retropulsion of its posterior wall in all the patients. Dynamic X-rays revealed an abnormal mobility at the fracture site in seven patients (Fig. 1). A vacuum phenomenon was observed in spinal extension in most of the patients. Myelograms showed compression of the dural sac by the retropulsed posterior wall of the vertebral body in all the patients. Progressive collapse of the vertebral body was confirmed in six patients (Fig. 2). The degree of osteoporosis, according to the classification of the Jikei Medical College [9], was grade 0.5 in one patient, grade 1 in four, and grade 2 in five. There was no cases of grade 3. Enhanced magnetic resonance imaging (MRI) with Gadolinium-DTPA, in four patients, showed positive enhancement in the posterior wall and periphery of the affected vertebral body, while enhancement was negative in the central portion (Fig. 3).

One patient was treated conservatively with 1 month of bed rest followed by an application of a hard corset. The other nine patients were treated operatively. In all the patients operated on, posterior decompression by means

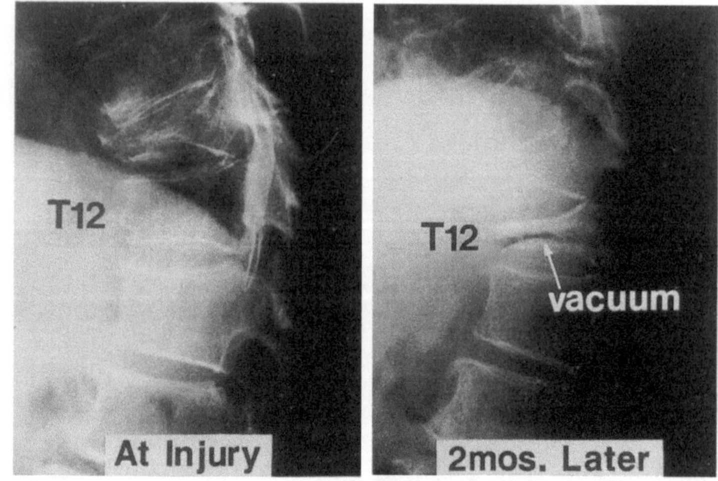

Fig. 2. Progressive collapse of the vertebral body in a 71-year-old woman.

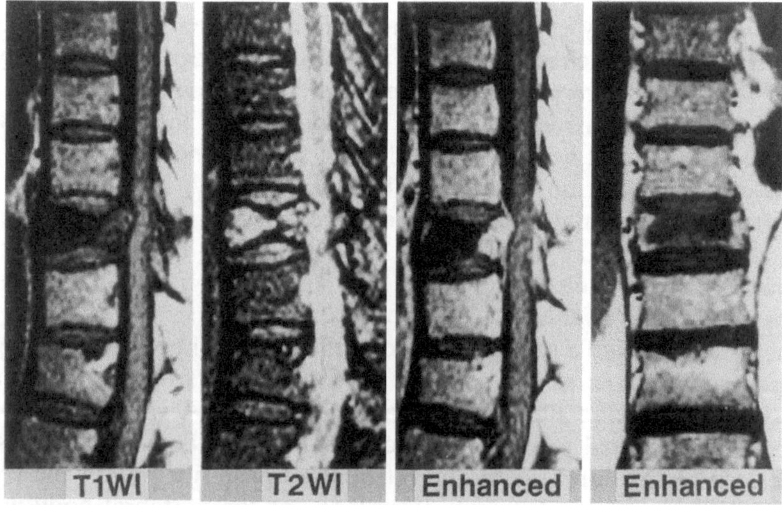

Fig. 3. Magnetic resonance imaging in a 80-year-old woman. Enhanced imaging shows positive enhancement in the posterior wall and periphery of the fractured vertebral body, while negative in the central portion.

Table 2. Operative treatment and result.

Case	Laminectomy	Instrumentation (pused leveis)	Treatment of retropulsion	Improvement of paraplegia	Complications
1	T12	Harrington (T7–L4)	None	+	None
2	T12, L1	Luque (T10–L3)	Reduction	–	Radicular pain, wire breakage
3	L1	Luque (T11–L3)	None	+	Wire breakage
4	T12, L1	Luque (T10–L3)	Removal	+	Wire breakage
5	T12, L1	Leque (T10–L3)	Removal	+	Exacerbation of dementia
6	T11, T12	Harrington (T8–L3)	Reduction	+	None
7	T11, T12, L1	Harrington (T8–L3)	Reduction	+	None
8	T9, T10	Luque (T5–L1)	None	+	Wire breakage
9	L1	Luque (T10–L4)	Removal	+	Wire breakage
10[a]				+	

[a] Conservatively treated case

of laminectomy and instrumentation was performed. The retropulsed posterior wall of the fractured vertebral body was removed in three cases, pushed back into the body in three cases, and left untouched in three cases. Harrington instrumentation was performed in the three earlier cases, and Luque instrumentation in the remaining six cases (Table 2). The postoperative follow-up ranged from 5 to 78 months (average, 20 months).

Results

The patient treated conservatively recovered completely from paraplegia. In the nine patients treated surgically, the paraplegia improved. Out of the five patients who had been unable to walk preoperatively, four had become ambulatory with a cane. The remaining patient, who had senile dementia, showed improvement of the weakness in his lower extremities. Out of the six patients who had had urinary disturbance before the operation, three recovered and three improved.

In five of the six cases with Luque instrumentation, a breakage of the sublaminar wire occurred 2–5 months postoperatively. There was no neurological complication caused by the breakage of the wires (Table 2).

Histopathological examination of the posterior part of the fractured vertebral body in two patients (cases 4 and 10), that was removed en bloc at operation, revealed no evidence of necrosis in the posterior wall. One case revealed the findings of nonunion.

Discussion

The following have been emphasised as possible mechanisms of delayed-onset paraplegia: Kyphotic deformity caused by progressive collapse of the vertebral body after the initial fracture [3], posterior extrusion of disc material [6], and instability and retropulsion of the vertebral body [5]. We observed retropulsion of the posterior wall of the fractured vetebral body in all of our cases. Progressive vertebral collapse was confirmed in six cases. Abnormal mobility at the fracture site was confirmed in seven patients who underwent dynamic X-ray examination, and nonunion was suspected. On enhanced MRI, the retropulsed posterior wall and periphery of the fractured vertebral body was enhanced positively, but the central part negatively. This fact indicates that vascularity was preserved in the posterior and peripheral parts, and in contrast, the central portion was ischemic. Based on these findings, we propose a possible mechanism of delayed-onset pareplegia as follows: Progressive collapse of the fractured vertebral body leads to kyhpotic deformity and retropulsion of the fractured vertebral body, which causes compression of the spinal cord or cauda equina. Vertebral fracture falls into nonunion, and abnormal mobility at the fracture site gives rise to chronic cyclic compression of the neural tissue. Consequently, the paraplegia develops.

References

1. Arciero R, Leung KYK, Pierce JM (1989) Spontaneous unstable burst fracture of the thoracolumbar spine in osteoporosis. Spine 14:114–117
2. Takemoto T, Kawabata M, Tukizawa H, Mikami Y, Tachibana S, Momoi Y, Totii S, Yoshino Y, Nakamichi K (1990) Three cases of vertebral burst fracture due to osteoporosis causing paraparesis. Orthopedic Surgery (Seikeigeka) 41:691–697
3. Kaneda K, Asano S, Hashimoto T, Abumi K, Yamamoto I, Shirado O, Fujiya M (1990) Delayed posttraumatic vertebral collapse in osteoporosis with spinal cord, cauda equina compression. J Jpn Orthop Assoc 64:S160
4. Shikata J, Yamamuro T, Iida H, Shimizu K, Yoshikawa K (1990) Surgical treatment for paraplegia resulting from vertebral fractures in senile osteoporosis. Spine 15:485–489
5. Nishimura T, Baba H, Takahashi K, Kawahara N, Tomita K, Umeda S (1990) Late paraplegia following vertebral body fracture in osteoporotic patients. Orthop Surg Traumatol 33:735–741
6. Ogata M, Fukuda S, Mochizuki K, Yamagishi N, Kokame M, Mizushima T, Yamada T (1983) Two cases of vertebral compression fracture causing paraparesis. Cent Jpn J Orthop Traumatol 26:625–627
7. Salomon C, Chopin D, Benoist M (1988) Spinal cord compression: An exceptional complication of spinal osteoporosis. Spine 13:222–224
8. Itami Y (1964) Epidemiology and clinical problem of osteoporosis. J Jpn Orthop Assoc 38:487–489

Occipito-Cervical Fusion in Rheumatoid Cervical Spine

TOKUICHI ARAKI, SEIKO HARATA, KAZUMASA UEYAMA, SHIRO ICHIKAWA, and JUNJI ITO[1]

Key Words. Rheumatoid spine, atlanto-axial instability, basilar impression, occipito-cervical fusion

Introduction

Upper cervical lesions are a relatively common problem in patients with rheumatoid arthritis. Surgical treatment is required in patients with severe instability of the atlanto-axial joint and basilar impression. We have reviewed 14 cases of rheumatoid disease of the cervical spine in patients who underwent occipito-cervical fusion. We studied fusion rate, maintenance of the reduced position, and subaxial changes in these cases.

Patients and Methods

We performed occipito-cervical fusion in 14 cases. There were 12 females and 2 males with a mean age of 60.8 years and a mean duration of disease of 16.3 years. The average length of follow-up period was 2.8 years. All cases were stage 4 according to Steinbrocker's classification (ARA), which includes both stages and classes. There were 9 cases with class 3 and 5 cases with class 4. The types were mutilans type in 8 cases and polyarticular type in 6. Eleven cases had recieved steroid therapy. Radiographically, 8 cases were atlanto-axial subluxation and 6 were basilar impression. Fusion levels were C0–C2 in 7 cases, C0–C4 in 1. C0–C5 in 2, C0–T1 in 1, and C0–T2 in 3. The operative procedures were Luque segmental spinal instrumentation (SSI) in 6 cases,

[1] Department of Orthopedic Surgery, Hirosaki University School of Medicine, Honcho 53, Hirosaki, Aomori, 036 Japan

Newman's method in 4, and wiring with bone grafts in 4. Halo-vests were used for 2–3 months in the cases without Luque instrumentation. Bone grafting of autogenous bone extended with hydroxyapatite granules was used in 4 cases.

Results

Union. Bony fusion was not achieved in one case. Radiograms showed no instability, but absorption of the grafted bone was found when a second operation was performed. In all other cases, including all four in which hydroxyapatite granules were used, bony union was achieved.

Change of Atlanto-Dental Interval. The atlanto-dental interval (ADI) changed from an average of 8.8 mm preoperatively to 4.5 mm postoperatively (Fig. 1). These reduced positions were maintained throughout the follow-up periods.

Changes Below the Fusion Level. Ten cases, with fusion levels of from C0–C2 to C0–C5, were followed up for more than 2 years (Table 1). Eight of these showed aggravated change of the subaxial area. Four of these had subaxial subluxation, two had narrowing of the disc space, and two had collapse of the vertebral body. Additional surgery (fusion to T1) was necessary in two of these cases due to myelopathy.

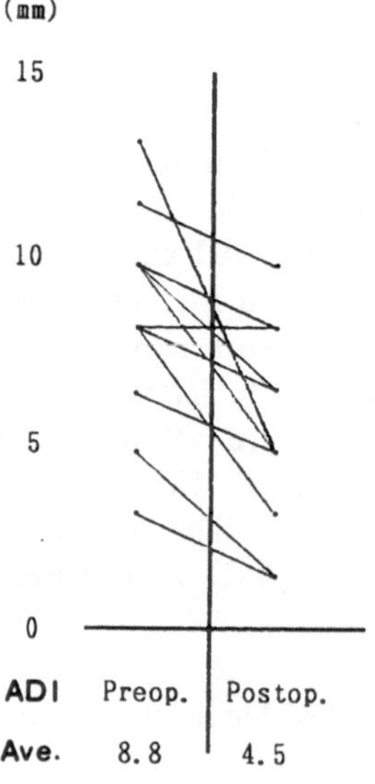

Fig. 1. Change in average (ave.) atlanto-dental interval (ADI)

Table 1. Changes below the fusion level.

Subaxial subluxation	4
Narrowing of the disc space	2
Collapse of the vertebral body	2
No change	2

Discussion

Newman's method [1] or wiring with bone grafts [2,3], can achieve solid fusion when external support such as a Halo-vest is used. Recently we have been using Luque rectangular rods with sublaminar wiring [4,5], in place of those methods, as this technique does not require any postoperative immobilization and facilitates early rehabilitation. There were no complications with either the drill burr holes in the basi-occiput or the sublaminar wiring.

Bone in rheumatoid patients is generally too weak for use in bone grafts because of osteoporosis due to steroid therapy. Hydroxyapatite granules are useful for increasing the volume of the grafted bone [6] (Fig. 3). There were no problems with fusion of the hydroxyapatite granules in this study.

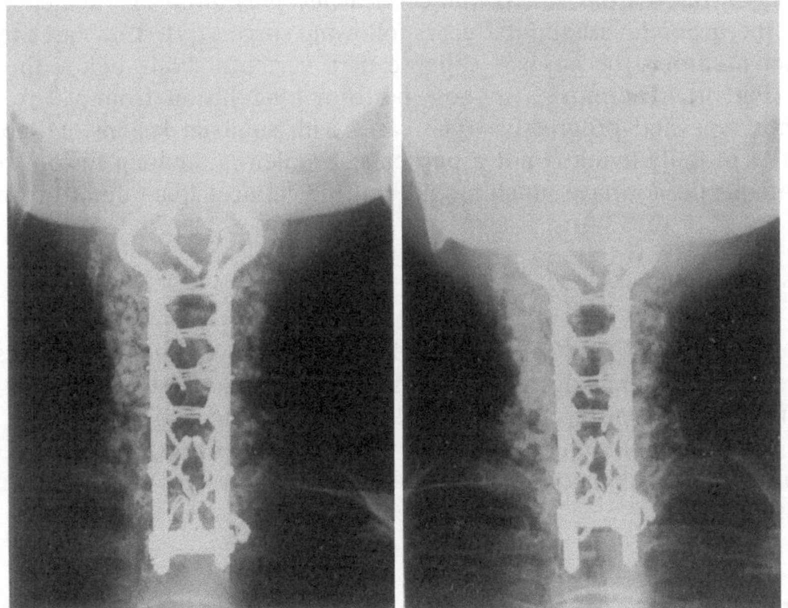

Fig. 2a,b. Radiograms of a 63-year-old woman. Posterior fusion using autogenous bone mixed with hydroxyapatite granules. **a** Plain radiogram soon after surgery. **b** Mixed bone has became homogeneous 1 year after surgery.

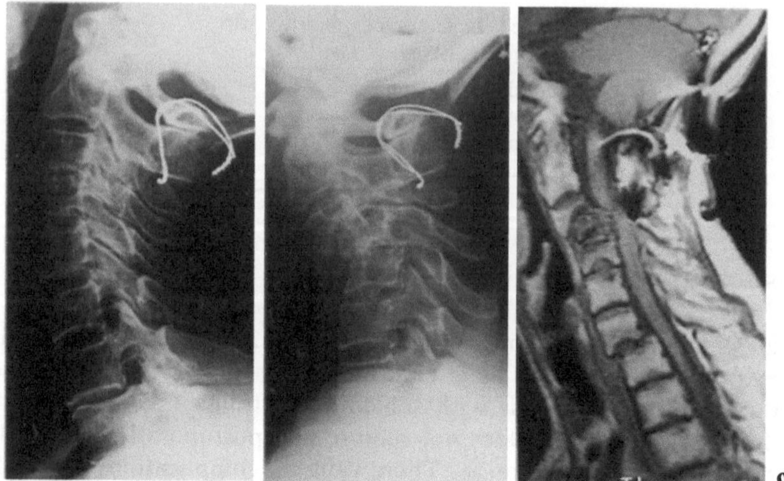

Fig. 3a–c. Radiograms of a 71-year-old woman. **a** Plain radiogram soon after C0–C3 fusion. **b** The C3 and C4 vertebral bodies collapsed 2 years 6 months after surgery. **c** MRI shows compression of the spinal cord at the C4 level

Short fusion is an ideal treatment for simple atlanto-axial subluxation, but most cases fused from C0 to mid-cervical levels showed aggravated changes below the fusion levels about 2 years following surgery [7]. Two cases required additional surgery because of collapse of a vertebral body below the fusion level (Fig. 4). Therefore, we now perform long fusion from C0 to T1 on mutilans type and progressive type cases with subaxial lesions. Disability in activities of daily living is not a particular problem after long fusion, because the patients do not have much mobility of the cervical spine due to pain.

Conclusion

Cases fused from C0 to mid-cervical levels showed aggravated changes (subaxial subluxation, narrowing of disc space, or collapse of a vertebral body) blow the fusion levels approximately 2 years following surgery.

We concluded that long fusion from C0 to the upper thoracic spine should be performed on mutilans type and probable progressive type cases with subaxial lesions.

References

1. Newman P, Sweetnam R (1969) Occipito-cervical fusion, an operative technique and its indication. J Bone Joint Surg 51B:423–431

2. Brooks AL, Jenkins EB (1978) Atlanto-axial arthrodesis by the wedge compression method. J Bone Joint Surg 60A:279–284
3. McGraw RW, Rusch RM (1973) Atlanto-axial arthrodesis. J Bone Joint Surg 55B: 482–489
4. Sakou T, Yoshikuni N, Morizono Y, Kawaida H, Tanaka S, Akamine T, Hamahata K, Oohira H, Hashiguchi M (1987) Application of the rods for atlanto-axial posterior fusion. J Jpn Orthop Assoc 61:S658
5. Toyama Y, Suzuki N, Hirabayashi K, Hujimura S, Satomi K, Ishige S, Kobayashi K (1989) Occipito-cervical fusion with a newly designed Luque rod for the upper cervical lesion (in Japanese). Rinsho Seikei Geka 24:1264–1272
6. Higashi S, Yamamuro T, Mikawa Y, Nakamura T, Shioide H (1982) Autogeneous bone grafting mixed with hydroxyapatite granules as an extender. An experimental study and a case report (in Japanese). Rinsho Seikei Geka 17:634–642
7. Horikawa T, Takahara M, Abe M, Nakayama H, Watanabe E, Kobayashi T, Yoshida S, Goto H, Sato H, Inomata Y, Chiba K (1985) Upper cervical spine fusion in rheumatoid arthritis, a radiological follow-up study. Cent Jpn J Orthop Traumatol 28:1604–1606

Posterior Fusion of the Cervical Spine in Rheumatoid Arthritis

Tadamasa Hanyu[1], Kiyoshi Nakazono[2], Akira Murasawa[2], Hajime Ishikawa[2], Takao Homma[1], and Hideaki E. Takahashi[1]

Key Words. Rheumatoid arthritis, posterior spinal fusion, Luque SSI, enlargement of spinal canal, cervical myelopathy

Introduction

The cervical spine is commonly involved in rheumatoid arthritis (RA). The deformities present are atlanto-axial subluxation (AAS), vertical subluxation (VS), and subaxial subluxation (SAS). Patients with these deformities generally also have severe osteoporosis, and the porotic bone is often a difficult problem to treat surgically.

This time, we review the cases of 21 patients with RA who had a posterior fusion for SAS between 1983 and 1992. This paper presents the results of posterior fusion with or without instrumentation in RA.

Patients and Methods

Of 21 patients, 4 were male and 17 were female. The average age at the time of surgery was 61 years old (range, 35–74 years), and the average duration of RA was 20 years. All patients had undergone treatment with corticosteroids. Mutilans type included 11 patients (about 52%).

The neurological status of each patient was rated according to the classification system of Ranawat et al. [1]. Only one case was rated class II

[1]Department of Orthopedic Surgery, Niigata University School of Medicine, Asahimachi-dori 1-757, Niigata, 951 Japan

[2]Niigata Prefectural Senami Hospital, Senami-onsen 2-4-15, Murakami, Niigata, 958 Japan

(subjective weakness with hyperreflexia and dysesthesia), 10 were rated class III-A (able to walk), and 10 were rated class III-B (quadriparetic).

SAS was defined as translation of one vertebrae in relation to an adjacent vertebrae of greater than 3.5 mm. Radiographically, a C3–4 subluxation was most prevalent.

Operation Technique

Achieving both decompression of the cord and fixation of vertebrae, enlargement of spinal canal (so-called laminoplasty) was performed in 14 of 21 patients, laminectomy with lateral bone graft in 1 patient, and posterior bone graft with wiring in 2 patients. Recently, Luque segmental spinal instrumentation (SSI) was done in 4 patients. Enlargement was carried out by sagittal splitting of the spinous processes, as described by Kurokawa et al. [2]. Bone graft was placed in the bilateral gutter and also between split spinous process. A halo-vest was used postoperatively for an average of about 3 months.

Fixation Areas

Figure 1 shows the relationship between AAS and VS. Four patients with mild AAS and mild or absent VS were underwent only enlargement. Five patients in which AAS was severe were operated on using the McGraw procedure between C1 and C2 and enlargement simultaneously. In the remaining 12 patients, VS was moderate or severe, and occipito-cervical fusion was indicated. In two patients, fixation of occiput-C2 was done previously. After that, new subluxation occurred at the subaxial level, and a second stage operation was applied. In four patients, Luque SSI was performed. In six patients, bone graft between the occiput and C2 and enlargement of the subaxial level was done simultaneously.

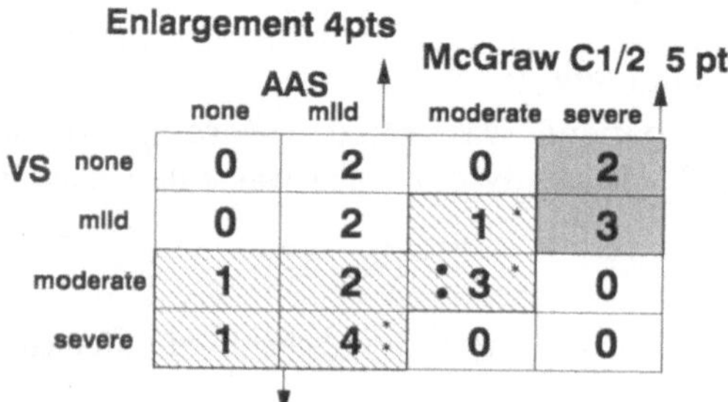

Fig. 1. Relationship between atlanto-axial subluxation (*AAS*) and vertical subluxation (*VS*). *Closed circle*, fixation of occiput-C2 was done previously; *, Luque SSI

Results

All patients had head or neck pain more than moderate preoperatively, and with the exception one patient, had mild or no pain on follow-up. At follow-up, neural deficits in 4 patients were class II, in 12 were class III-A, and in 5 were class III-B. Eight patients improved and 13 remained unchanged. One of the 6 patients who underwent enlargement of a subaxial level and occiput-C2 fusion died during the early postoperative period, and this case was excluded from radiographical examination. Additionally, there were 5 additional unrelated deaths.

In 4 of the 14 patients who underwent enlargement at the subaxial level, bone graft was placed only in the bilateral gutter. However, pseudoarthrosis was found in two patients. In the remaining ten patients, bone graft was done not only in the lateral gutter but also between split spinous processes. Pseudoarthrosis was only found in one case. Finally, the failure rate of the enlargement at the level of subaxial lesions was 21%. Next, pseudoarthrosis rates for the 10 patients who underwent an additional operation for a subsequent upper cervical lesion were as follow: 60% with fusion of C1–C2 and 40% with fusion of occiput-C2, but none occurred with Luque SSI.

Case Reports

Case 1

A 67-year-old female had pain in the neck and could not walk for 3 months due to meylopathy. Roentgenogram revealed severe VS and anterior subluxation of C3 and C4. Myelogram showed a complete block at the interspace between C4 and C5. Enlargement of C4–C7, laminectomy of C3, and a McGraw procedure were done. A halo-vest was applied for 3 months. Roentgenograms taken 3 years after operation showed good alignment and good fixation (Fig. 2). Currently, she can ambulate with the aid of crutches.

Case 2

A 62-year-old female with a history of RA for 44 years had severe neck pain and weakness of the upper and lower extremities. Laminectomy of C3 and enlargement of C4–C7 was scheduled, but unfortunately a lamina of C4 was broken and it was no longer possible to perform a bone graft for posterior fusion. Roentgenogram revealed instability of C4-5 (Fig. 3). She started having pain in the neck and quadriparesis.

Case 3

A 38-year-old female had AAS and a stepladder formation from C4 to C6. A McGraw procedure and enlargement of C3–C7 was carried out. However,

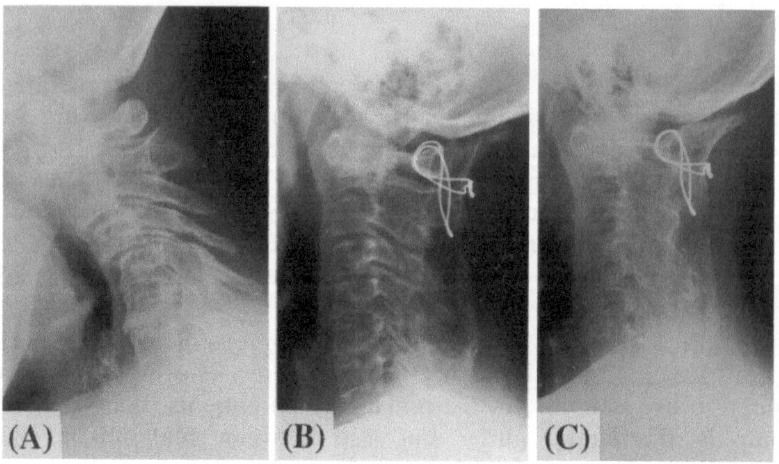

Fig. 2A–C. Case 1: A 67-year-old female. **A** Roentgenogram reveals severe vertical subluxation (VS) and anterior subluxation of C3 and C4. **B** Enlargement of C4–C7, laminectomy of C3 and McGraw procedure were done. **C** Three years after operation, good alignment and good fixation was achieved

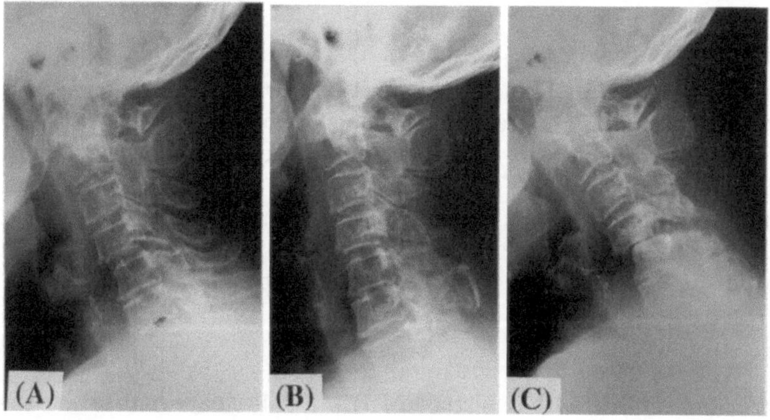

Fig. 3A–C. Case 2: A 62-year-old female. **A** Anterior subluxation of C4. **B** Lamina of C4 was broken and enough bone graft was available for posterior fusion. **C** Roentgenogram reveals instability of C4–5

bone graft between split spinous processes was omitted in this case. Roentgenogram revealed a fracture at the grafted bone of C1–C2, recurrence of AAS, and kyphosis of the subaxial level (X-ray not shown). Again, she had moderate pain in the neck.

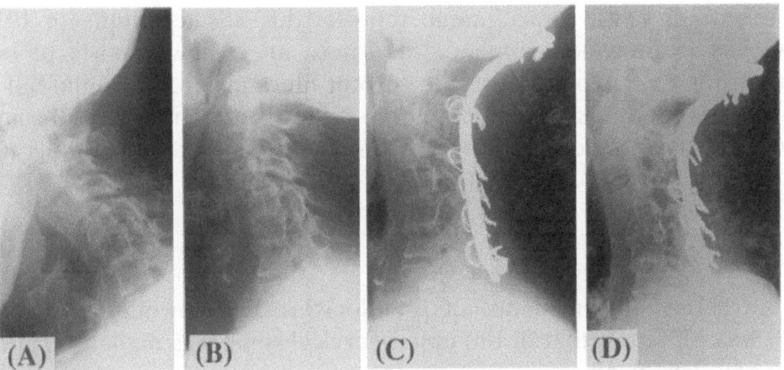

Fig. 4A–D. Case 4: A 57-year-old female. **A,B** Roentgenogram reveals VS and anterior subluxation of C4. **C** Laminectomy was carried out at C1 and C3, and Luque SSI was used for internal fixation. **D** Two years after operation, she maintained good alignment and bony fusion, although a little shortening occurred

Case 4

A 57-year-old female had VS and anterior subluxation of C4. Laminectomy was carried out at C1 and C3, and Luque SSI was used for internal fixation. A roentgenogram taken 2 years postoperatively shows she maintained good alignment and bony fusion, although a little shortening occurred (Fig. 4).

Discussion

Ranawat et al. [1] described, in rheumatoid patients, anterior decompression of the spinal cord often fails because of vertebral osteoporosis. We also had many similar experiences. Santavirta et al. [3] reported 16 cases of SAS. They have performed laminectomies and fusions as short as possible. During 4 years' follow-up, 20% or more of their patients had new subluxations at other levels. Kraus et al. [4] noted that, of the occiput-C2 fusion patients, 36% developed SAS requiring surgery an average of 2.6 years later. Only 5.5% of those patients with atlanto-axial fusions developed SAS. When occipito-cervical fusion is required, careful evaluation of the subaxial joints should be performed. If early SAS is already present, longer occipito-cervical fusion or occipito-thoratic fusions should be seriously considered.

In our patients, the failure rate of posterior fusion for SAS was 21%. As methods of bone graft are improved, this failure will decrease but the pseudoarthrosis rate of occiput-C2 or C1–C2 that was operated simultaneously was high in spite of the long halo-vest used. When upper cervical fusion is indicated, we should select a more stable fixation than wiring.

On the other hand, since Luque reported his SSI technique in 1977, this method has been widely applied [5]. There are a few reports of occipito-cervical fusion in RA patients in the current literature [6,7]. Luque SSI in four patients had good results although the follow-up period is still short. No pseudoarthrosis occurred. The loop technique provided a more stable fixation.

Conclusion

1. In our series, the incidence of pseudoarthrosis following enlargement for SAS was 21%, but that of the upper cervical spine was higher in spite of the long halo-vest used.
2. Results of posterior fusion using Luque SSI were satisfactory.
3. When occipito-cervical fusion is required, we should seriously consider both decompression of the cord by laminectomy and a more stable fixation by the loop technique.

References

1. Ranawat CS, O'Leary P, Pellicci P, Tsairis P, Marchisello P, Dorr L (1979) Cervical spine fusion in rheumatoid arthritis. J Bone Joint Surg 61-A:1003–1010
2. Kurokawa T, Tsuyama T, Tanaka H, Kobayashi M, Machida H, Nakamura K, Iizuka T, Hoshino Y (1983) Enlargement of spinal canal using sagittal splitting of spinous process (in Japanese). Bessatsu Seikei Geka 2:234–240
3. Santavirta S, Konttinen YT, Sandelin J, Slatis P (1990) Operations for the unstable cervical spine in rheumatoid arthritis. Acta Orthop Scand 61:106–110
4. Kraus D, Peppelman WC, Agarwal AK, Deleeuw HW, Donaldson WF (1991) Incidence of subaxial subluxation in patients with generalized rheumatoid arthritis who have had previous occipital cervical fusions. Spine 16:S486–S489
5. Luque ER (1982) Segmental spinal instrumentation for correction of scoliosis. Clin Orthop 163:192–198
6. Crockard HA, Essigman WK, Stevens JM, Pozo JL, Ransford AO, Kendall BE (1985) Surgical treatment of cervical cord compression in rheumatoid arthritis. Ann Rheum Dis 44:809–816
7. Itoh T, Tsuji H, Katoh Y, Yonezawa T, Kitagawa H (1988) Occipito-cervical fusion reinforced by Luque's segmental spinal instrumentation for rheumatoid diseases. Spine 13:1234–1238

Part VI.

Appendicular Manifestations of Spinal Disorders

Problems in Functional Reconstruction of a Myelopathy Hand

Hidehiko Saito, Minoru Shibata, and Yasuhiro Iwabuchi[1]

Key Words. Myelopathy hand, tendon transfer, spastic hand

Introduction

Clumsiness in finger motion and loss of power in pinch and grasp are common complaints of patients with compression cervical myelopathy. Very little attention, however, has been paid to the functional reconstruction of a hand paralyzed by this spinal disorder, that is, a myelopathy hand.

We have been reconstructing myelopathy hands since a few years ago and found some important points which are completely different from reconstruction of hands paralyzed by peripheral nerve lesions.

What Is a Myelopathy Hand?

One was the first to coin the term "myelopathy hand" [1]. In his paper published in 1987, he emphasized two clinical signs, the finger escape sign and the inability to repeat grasping and opening the hand rapidly.

Typical symptoms of a myelopathy hand were seen in the case of a 53-year-old man. On extending or flexing the fingers of his right hand, the patient bends the wrist down or up excessively (Fig. 1). This trick motion can be missed easily but the abduction of the little finger (a finger escape sign or Wartenberg's sign) cannot be missed (Fig. 2). When the patient is asked to extend his fingers up with the wrist immobilized in a neutral position, his inability to extend the metacarpophalangeal (MP) joints becomes apparent as

[1] Department of Orhthopedic Surgery, Niigata University School of Medicine, Asahimachi-dori 1-757, Niigata, 951 Japan

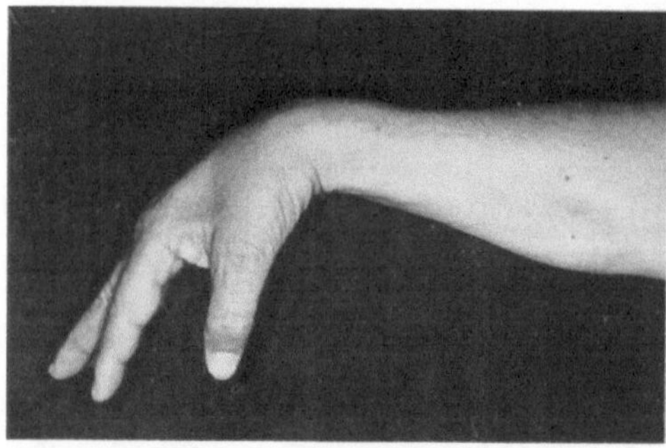
a

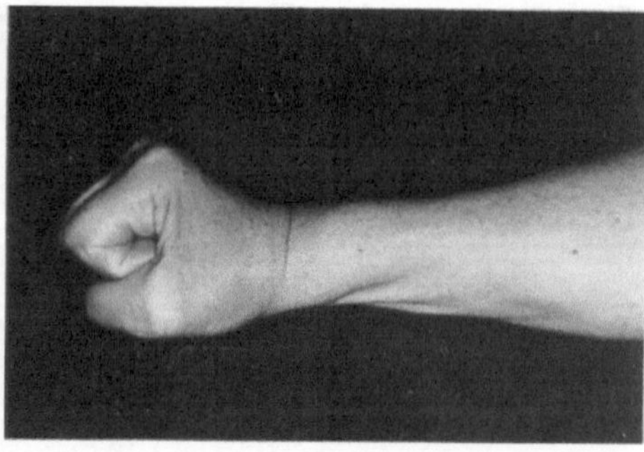
b

Fig. 1a,b. Trick motions to compensate loss of the function of finger extensors or flexors. **a** The patient extends the fingers using a tenodesis effect of the finger extensors exerted by palmar flexion of the wrist joint. **b** He bends the fingers fully by augmenting the finger flexion with a tenodesis effect exerted by excessive dorsiflexion of the wrist joint

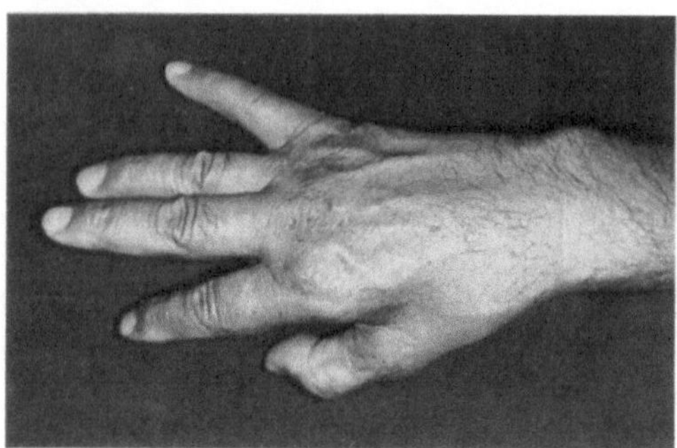

Fig. 2. Persistent abduction of the little finger (Wartenberg's sign). Adduction of the little finger is not feasible because of paralysis of the third palmar interosseous muscle

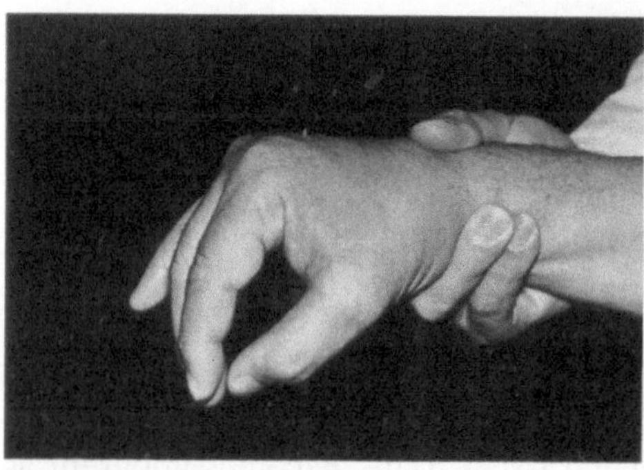
a

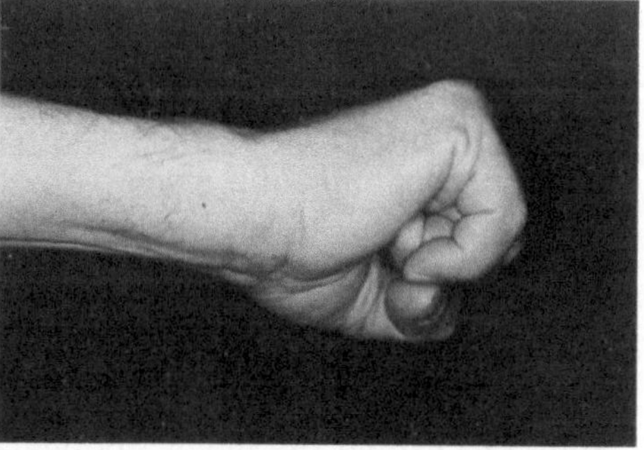
b

Fig. 3a,b. Paralysis of the finger extensors or flexors. **a** Inability to extend the metacarpophalangeal (MP) joints becomes evident by immobilizing the wrist in a neutral position or in dorsiflexion. **b** Inability to flex the fingers fully is demonstrated by immobilizing the wrist in a neutral position or in slight palmar flexion

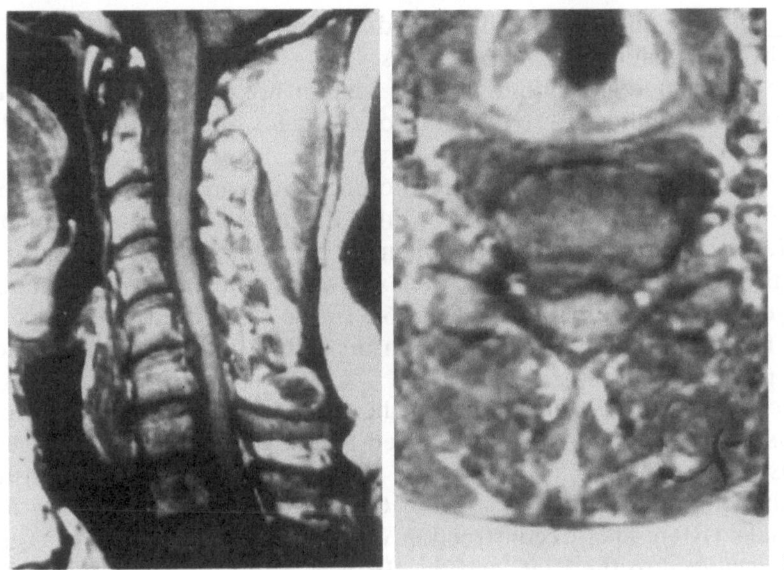

Fig. 4a,b. Magnetic resonance imaging (MRI) of the cervical spine and the spinal cord. **a** A sagittal section reveals anterior compression on the spial cord between C5 and C6. **b** An axial section reveals compression located mainly on the right side

shown in Fig. 3a. Another inconspicuous symptom is limitation in flexion of the little finger (Fig. 3b).

An X-ray film revealed narrowing of the intervertebral space and posterior osteophytes at the levels of C5/6 and C6/7. In magnetic resonance imaging (MRI), anterior compression on the spinal cord was seen at between C5 and C6 (Fig. 4a,b). So, paralysis of this hand is ascribed to this spinal cord compression.

Operated Cases

We treated five hands of four patients, including three men and one woman over the last 3 years. The age at the time of reconstruction ranged from 24 to 60 years. The etiology was cervical spondylotic myelopathy in one patient and anterior cord compression on flexion of the neck, so-called flexion myelopathy, in three patients who are in their 20's or early 30's.

Case S.O. is a 60-year-old man who had undergone anterior spinal fusion from C5 to C7 for extensor paralysis of the index and long fingers due to cervical spondylotic myelopathy. He had been followed at the spine clinic without any noticeable recovery of finger extensors until 1 year after the operation when he was referred to us because of the inability to extend the index and long fingers of his right hand. Examination revealed marked intrinsic atrophy and weakness of finger flexors.

The extensor digiti minimi (EDM) tendon was transferred to the extensor digitorum communis (EDC) tendons of the index and long finger, and this the function of extension returned in those fingers.

Case M.S. is a 25-year-old man who underwent anterior spinal fusion at the level of C5 through C7 2 years ago with a diagnosis of flexion myelopathy (Fig. 5). He was referred to us for treatment of paralysis of both hands.

In the left hand, the intrinsics, the extensors of the index and thumb, and the thenar muscles were paralyzed (Fig. 6). In the right hand, the thenar muscles were functioning but weak. The extensors of the index, ring, and little fingers were paralyzed (Fig. 6).

Reconstruction was first done on the left hand. The extensor carpiradialis longus (ECRL) tendon was transferred to the extensor pollicis longus (EPL) and EDC of the index using the "Y" principle. The EDM was transferred to the abductor pollicis longus (APL). Opponoplasty was performed using the brachialis (BR). Then reconstruction was done on the right hand. The ECRL was transferred to the EDC and the BR was used for the opponoplasty.

The patient resumed the function of finger extension in both hands and of palmar abduction in the left hand (Fig. 7), and eventually powerful pinch and opposition of the thumb in both hands (Fig. 8).

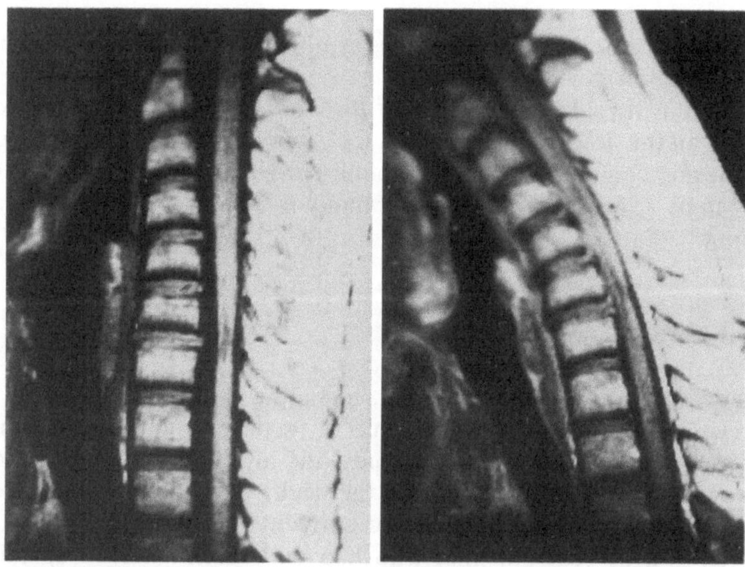

Fig. 5a,b. MRI of Case M.S. **a** A mild compression on the cervical cord is seen at the level of C5 through C7 in an upright position. There is an area of low intensity in the cord between C6 and C7. **b** The compression increases at the level of C5 through C7 by flexion

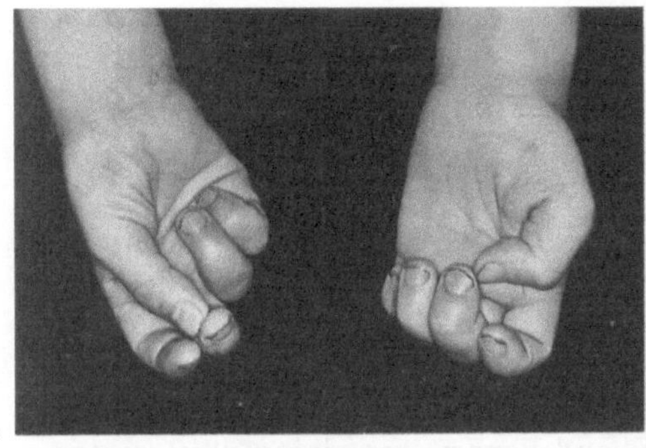
a

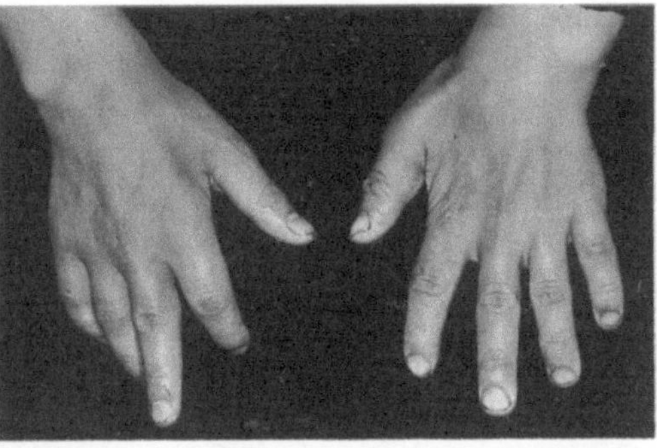
b

Fig. 6a,b. Preoperative views of hands of Case M.S. **a** The thenar muscles of the left hand were paralyzed while those of the right were functioning but weak. **b** The extensors of the left thumb and index finger were functioning but weak while the extensors of the right index, ring, and little fingers were paralyzed

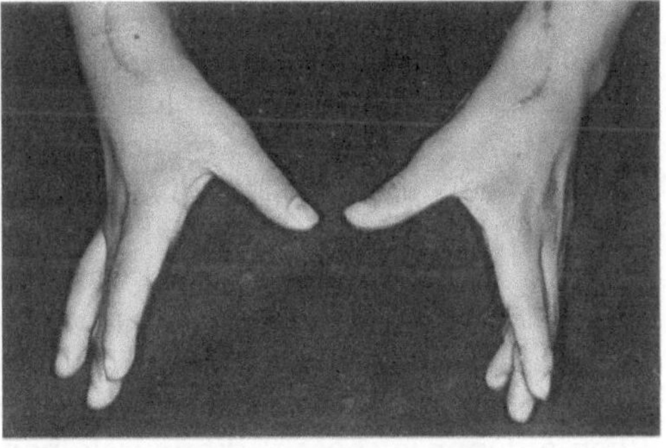

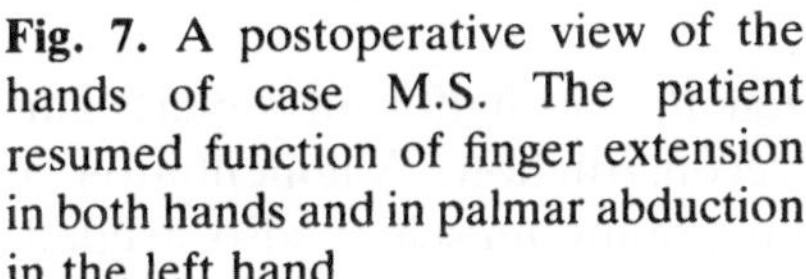
Fig. 7. A postoperative view of the hands of case M.S. The patient resumed function of finger extension in both hands and in palmar abduction in the left hand

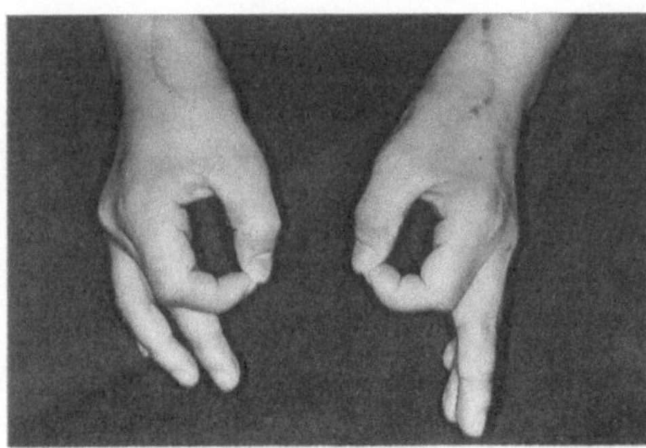
a

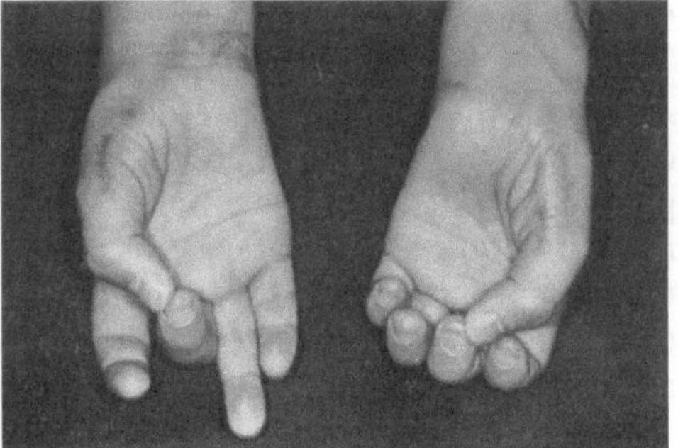
b

Fig. 8a,b. Postoperative views of the hands of Case M.S. He resumed function of **a** powerful pinch and **b** opposition in both hands

Discussion

Ono emphasized two clinical signs, the finger escape sign and inability to repeat grasping and opening of the hand rapidly. According to his description, the little finger stays abducted because of paralysis of the palmar interosseous and the extensors of ulnar fingers become paralyzed as the severity increases while the extensors of the radial fingers and thumb are preserved. Slow and difficult repetition of grasping is ascribed to loss of coordination and to spasticity of the muscles.

A myelopathy hand is characterized by paralysis of intrinsic muscles, simultaneous involvement of finger extensors and flexors, remaining wrist motors and spasticity of muscles. However, our observations of the progression of extensor paralysis is different from Ono's. In almost all cases, the extensors of the radial fingers or thumb are paralyzed while those of the ulnar digits are preserved (Figs. 2, 6b). The segmental level of compression seems to be directly related to which finger is involved. This pattern of paralysis of the finger extensors can also be observed in tetraplegics. Zancoll's group 3 with functioning finger extensors is subdivided into 3-A and 3-B depending on the extent of finger extension [2]. In 3-A, extension of the ulnar fingers is complete but that of the index and the thumb is incomplete. In 3-B, extension of all fingers and the thumb is complete.

Donor muscles available for tendon transfer are limited in number because the finger flexors, especially the flexor superficialis, are involved as well as the extensors. The ECRL and BR are almost always available for transfer, whereas the ECU and EDM can be used occasionally.

Tenodesis and "lasso" transfer of paralyzed flexor digitorum superficialis (FDS) are sometimes needed for functional reconstruction. Augmentation of incompletely paralyzed muscles with a well-functioning muscle is also needed. When a donor is chosen, the muscle power of the antagonist of the muscle to be reconstructed should be taken into consideration to avoid a reverse deformity.

Conclusion

A myelopathy hand is characterized by involvement of the intrinsics, finger extensors, and flexors while the wrist motors are preserved. Because a myelopathy hand is caused by compression on the spinal cord, principles used in the reconstruction of a tetraplegic hand can be applied to its reconstruction. Since the number of donors is limited, tenodesis or "lasso" transfer should be combined. Spasticity in involved muscles deteriorates the coordination of muscles. Therefore, dexterity of the hand is not well restored.

References

1. Ono K, Ebara S, Fuji T, Yonenobu K, Fujiwara K, Yamashita K (1987) Myelopathy hand; New clinical signs of cervical cord damage. J Bone Joint Surg 69-B:215–219
2. Zancolli E (1979) Structural and dynamic bases of hand surgery, 2nd edn. Lippincott, Philadelphia, pp 229–262

Ulnar Nerve Palsy in Elderly Patients

Minoru Shibata, Hidehiko Saito, Eiji Shiraishi, Yoshiro Hatano, and Yasuhiro Iwabuchi[1]

Introduction

Cubital tunnel syndrome with intrinsic muscle atrophy in elderly patients occasionally fails to respond to surgical decompression of the entrapped nerve. It is believed that severe irreversible changes due to prolonged nerve entrapment or insufficient decompression of the nerve are frequently responsible for the persistent symptoms and occasional cervical radiculopathy. However, magnetic resonance imaging (MRI) often reveals spinal cord segment compression at the C5/6 intervertebral space, where the C8 spinal cord segment is located, instead of C8 root compression at the C7/T1 intervertebral level in patients with persistent ulnar entrapment neuropathy. We studied ulnar nerve palsy with cervical spinal cord compression utilizing various kinds of evaluation methods to assess whether the cubital or cervical lesion was more responsible for the symptom.

Materials and Methods

We evaluated nine patients (eight men and one woman) with sensory changes in the ulnar digits and intrinsic muscle atrophy from both cervical and cubital lesions.

The patients' ages ranged from 42 to 77 years with an average of 59.1 years.

For imaging assessment of the cervical spondylosis, we used MRI and computed tomography (CT) as well as plain X-ray films. MRI was considered the most reliable imaging method for diagnosing cervical compression, and was used in all patients.

[1]Department of Orthopedic Surgery, Niigata University School of Medicine, Asahimachi-dori 1-757, Niigata, 951 Japan

Both physicians and occupational therapists assessed sensory change by evaluating hypesthesia, paresthesia, and static and moving two-point discrimination pre- and postoperatively.

Electrophysiological examination included measurement of nerve conduction velocities (NCV) including motor nerve conduction velocity (MCV) and sensory nerve conduction velocity (SCV), the inching method, somatosensory evoked potential (SEP), and distribution of motor nerve conduction velocity (DCV). Evaluations using NCV measurements and the inching method were regarded as the most reliable means of detecting the cubital tunnel syndrome.

Physical examination consisted of evaluations of ulnar nerve Tinel's sign, hyperreflexia, and the head compression test. Both hand and spine surgeons evaluated these findings, and surgical indications were determined based on preoperative discussion. Eight patients were operated and one was scheduled for surgery.

Results

We operated on eight patients, three of whom had a history of ulnar tunnel release (Table 1). One patient remained under close observation and was also scheduled for cervical spinal surgery.

Ulnar nerve surgery was carried out by senior hand surgeons and cervical spinal surgery by senior spinal surgeons. Modified King's procedure or Learmonth procedure was selected for ulnar nerve decompression and anterior spinal fusion or spinal canal enlargement for decompression of the spinal cord.

We carried out decompression of the ulnar nerve in five cases, one of which had a history of cubital tunnel release. MCV was delayed with a wide range of severity in these patients. Compared to MCV, there was a significant delay in SCV; however, NCV was unmeasurable in three of these patients. One of the five patients had undergone King's procedure at another hospital without improvement. The Learmonth procedure was chosen for this particular case as the reoperation procedure.

The ulnar nerve decompression procedure produced notable improvement soon after surgery but there were some residual or recurrent symptoms in these five cases. In contrast, no distinct change was obtained for the two patients who also had a history of ulnar tunnel release. They underwent spinal fusion secondarily. These two patients, whose decompression of the ulnar nerve did not relieve their symptom, showed discernible improvement after the secondary procedure, suggesting double lesions with a dominant cervical lesion. Preoperative head compression test elicited clear shooting pain and/or additional numbness precisely at the ulnar one-and-a-half digits in the five patients who underwent ulnar nerve decompression. This test strongly suggested crushing of cervical and cubital lesions in these patients. One of the five patients had bilateral symptoms with right dominant bilateral intrinsic muscle atrophy as well as neck pain and discomfort, which also suggested double crush syndrome.

Table 1. Results of evaluations, operative procedures and their results.

Case	MRI	Sensory change	I-M atrophy	MCV m/s	SCV m/s	SEP	Inch. meth.	Hyp.-ref.	H-C test	Operation performed	Postop. improve	Diagnosis
T.T.	C5/6	uln. 1.5	+	23.2	NM	CL	+	–	+	uln. nerve	+	Pro. doub
U.K.	C4/5/6	uln. 1.5	+	15.0	NM	WNL	+	–	+	uln. nerve	+	Pro. doub
I.S.	C5/6/7	uln. 1.5	+	NM	NM	NM	+	–	+	uln. nerve	+	Pro. doub
I.Y.	C5/6	uln. 1.5	+	44.0	NA	NA	+	–	+	uln. nerve	+	Pro. doub
S.H.	C5/6/7	uln. 1.5	+	42.0	38.4	WNL	+	–	+	uln. nerve	+	Pro. doub
H.I.	C5/6	uln. 1.5	+	46.2	NM	CL	+	+	–	SF	+	Double
Y.M.	C4/5/6	uln. 1.5	+	17.8	NM	CL	+	+	–	SF	+	Double
S.K.	C5/6/7	uln. 3	+	62.0	67.8	CL	–	–	–	SCE	+	CSM
N.T.	C4/5/6	uln. 2	±	62.7	77.1	CL	–	–	+	NO		CSM

MRI, Level of spinal compression by MRI; *I-M atrophy*, intrinsic muscle atrophy; *NM*, not measurable; *NA*, not available; *CL*, cervical lesion; *WNL*, within normal limits; *uln*, ulnar; *Inch. meth.*, delay more than 0.5 m/s at elbow by inching method; *Hyp.-ref.*, hyperreflexia in upper limb; *H-C test*, head compression test; *SF*, spinal fusion; *SCE*, spinal canal enlargement; *Pro. doub.*, probable double crush; *CSM*, cervical spondylotic myelopathy (compression myelopath)

A preoperative diagnosis of the ulnar nerve palsy simulated by compression myelopathy was made in two patients with normal nerve conduction. One of them underwent 3–7 spinal canal enlargement with marked postoperative improvement in his symptoms; the other patient has been closely observed and spinal surgery is being considered.

These results suggest that the nine patients can be classified into three groups: group I, five with provable double crush syndrome; group II, two with double crush syndrome; and group III, two with compression myelopathy.

Discussion

In 1966 Crandall and Batzdorf [1] classified "central cord syndrome" as a type of cervical spondylotic myelopathy in which motor and sensory deficit affect the upper limb more severely than the lower. Hattori et al. [2] divided cervical spondylosis into three types in 1975 and defined type I as cases with a segmental sign in an upper limb. Neurological localization and the level of cervical spondylosis have been studied clinically [3,4] and anatomically [5]. In this cervical spondylotic meylopathy, a limited segmental sign of the upper limb may not demonstrate a long tract sign.

Recently, it has been widely accepted that there is a discrepancy between the level of spinal cord segment and that of the spine. The C8 sensory spinal cord segment is located at the C5/6 intervertebral space, and the C8 motor segment at a slightly higher level in the majority of the cases. C5/6 cervical spondylosis often accompanies similar lesions at adjacent levels. Image analysis using MRI and CT scan has provided more detailed information on spinal cord compression. Considering the level discrepancy between the spinal cord segment and the spine, we believe that cervical spondylotic myelopathy involving C5/6 can simulate ulnar nerve palsy. With this type of injury, cervical compression lesion is proximal to the sensory ganglion and theoretically SCV has to be normal.

Cubital tunnel syndrome, on the other hand, is one of the most common of the entrapment neuropathies. Osteophytes, or ganglia associated with osteoarthritis of the elbow joint which narrows the tunnel, are known to directly induce cubital tunnel syndrome, often in elderly patients. Cubital tunnel entrapment is characterized by delays in NCVs, among which SCV is usually more susceptible than MCV.

Overlapping of cervical spondylotic myelopathy and cubital tunnel entrapment may be encountered occasionally because both lesions are relatively common in elderly people and could affect each other, resulting in the manifestation of ulnar nerve palsy. If C8 segment compression is involved in the spondylotic lesions, vulnerability of the ulnar nerve may increase in the case of double lesions of cervical spondylosis and cubital tunnel syndrome.

Upton and McComas [6] hypothesized the occurrence of double crush nerve entrapment syndromes in which cervical radiculopathy rather than myelopathy is considered the upper lesion. (Because of the one-level discrepancy between spinal bone segment and root, C8 spinal root lies at the C7T1 intervertebral level.) On the basis of their hypothesis, C8 root is involved in the double crush syndrome of cervical spondylosis and cubital tunnel syndrome, but root compression lesions at the C7T1 level are rarely identified. Instead of this rare root lesion, spinal cord segment compression at the C5/6 intervertebral space occasionally simulates ulnar nerve palsy. Based on these findings, we postulated a new type of double crush syndrome which manifests itself as ulnar nerve palsy.

In this study, we divided nine cases into three groups utilizing many evaluations which included the effectivity of surgical procedures. As shown in these cases, C8 compression myelopathy may well simulate ulnar entrapment syndrome and may overlap with cubital tunnel syndrome. Regarding the severity of both lesions, each can be labeled as either subclinical or manifestive. A lesion is classified as "subclinical" if it is not severe enough to be clinically symptomatic and only the electrophysiological data are abnormal. If there are clinical symptoms, the lesion is termed "manifestive"; this category also includes double subclinical lesions, which are sometimes clinically symptomatic. These lesions can also be accompanied by various combinations of symptoms. Care is required for the evaluation of ulnar nerve palsy in elderly patients.

References

1. Crandall PH, Batzdorf U (1966) Cervical spondylotic myelopathy. J Neurosurg 25:57–66
2. Hattori S, Koyama M, Hayakawa H, Kawai S, Saiki K, Sigematu A (1975) Cervical spondylotic myelopathy: Pathology and types. Rinsyoseikeigeka (Clin Orthop Surg) 10:48–56
3. Hirabayashi K, Satomi K, Wakano K (1983) Level diagnostic neurology of cervical spondylotic myelopathy—Retrospective observation in cases treated by anterior spinal fusion at a single level. Rinshoseikeigeka (Clin Orthop Surg) 19:409–415
4. Kokubunn S (1984) Neurological localization of the symptomatic level of lesion in cervical spondylotic myelopathy. Rinsyoseikeigeka 19:417–424
5. Tsuzuki N, Honda H, Tanaka Y (1983) Morhological variations of human cervical spinal cord segment and roots and their clinical significance. Rinshoseikeigeka (Clin Orthop Surg) 34:229–235
6. Upton AR, McComas AJ (1973) The double crush in nerve entrapment syndromes. Lancet 2:359–361

Operative Treatment for Vertebral Fracture in Osteoporotic Patients

HIDEAKI E. TAKAHASHI, TERUO HABA, AKIYOSHI YAMAZAKI, SEIJI UCHIYAMA, and TAKAO HOMMA[1]

Key Words. Osteoporosis, paraplegia, nonunion

Introduction

In involutional osteoporosis, vertebral fracture often occurs in the thoracolumber region, precipitated by the minor stress of such actions as bending and lifting. Sudden pain may be incapacitating, but it will eventually subside spontaneously as the fracture heals. It was believed that vertebral fracture due to osteoporosis had no risk of spinal cord involvement and was purely compressive. It has been reported, however, that vertebral fracture due to involutional osteoporosis may be not only compressive but also a burst fracture, resulting in kyphosis, occasionally associated with incomplete paraplegia and prolonged back pain due to delayed or nonunion of a fracture of a vertebral body. The purpose of this study is to describe operative treatment for fracture of the vertebra in osteoporotic patients with neurological complication or prolonged back pain due to disturbed healing of vertebral fracture.

Patients and Methods

Between 1982 and 1992, 27 patients (7 men and 20 women) were operated on at the Niigata University Hospital and affiliated hospitals. The age range of the patients at the time of surgery was 53 to 80 years, and 20 were above 65 years of age. The preoperative symptoms were incomplete paraplegia in 22 cases (classified Frankel scale C in 14 cases and D in 8 cases) and prolonged pain in 5

[1] Department of Orthopedic Surgery, Niigata University School of Medicine, Asahimachi-dori 1-757, Niigata, 951 Japan

cases due to delayed union of intravertebral fracture. Paraplegia with onset delayed more than 4 weeks after the appearance of initial symptoms occurred in 20 patients and acute onset in 2. The postoperative follow-up period was 2 years 6 months on average, ranging from 4 months to 6 years 9 months.

Decompression and correction of kyphosis through an anterior approach was performed without instrumentation in 3 cases and with a Kaneda device in 1 [1]. Posterior decompression or posterior and anterior decompression were performed through the posterior approach in 23 cases. In 18 patients with paraplegia, 9 had more than 4 vertebrae fixed, a Harrington instrument was used on 5, and 4 were fixed with Harrington and Luque rods together with segmental sublaminar wiring. In the other 9 patients, three vertebrae, including two intervertebral disc spaces, were fixed with a Steffee variable screw placement (VSP). In the 5 patients with prolonged back pain without paraplegia, 3 were operated on without instrumentation, 1 with a Harrington instrument, and 1 with a Steffee VSP. Hydroxyapatite (Bonfil, Mitsubishi Materials, Tokyo, Japan) together with autogenous iliac bone was implanted into the fractured vertebral body in 3 cases of prolonged back pain and in 1 case of paraplegia. Implantation was performed through a posterior approach via the inferiolateral quarter of the pedicle bilaterally.

Results

Of the 22 cases of incomplete paraplegia, 13 rated as Frankel scale C improved to D; 1 case rated C became an E; and 4 cases rated D improved to E. Four cases rated preoperatively as D remained D postoperatively, though all improved within the D scale.

In the four patients operated on through the anterior approach, bone union was obtained without any complication. Of the 23 patients operated on using the posterior approach, 3 were operated on without instrumentation using intravertebral implantation of hydroxyapatite with autogenous iliac bone. Leakage of hydroxyapatite from the anterior wall of the vertebral body was observed in 2 cases. In 9 cases, long instrumentation was applied; in 6 of these, the wire pulled out of the laminae, needing reoperation in 4 cases. Loosening of the instrument occurred in 4 of 11 cases using short instrumentation.

Protrusion of the posterior wall of the burst vertebra into the spinal canal and angular kyphosis formation at the level of the wedged vertebra were causes of paraplegia (Fig. 1). Other causes were vertebral fracture associated with a bone spur or ossification of the yellow ligament in one case and a herniated disc in another case.

Although neurological findings improved, additional compression fractures occurred in the lowest segment of the fused vertebra in three cases and in either the four upper or five lower adjacent vertebra in five cases. The additional compression fractures were painless or produced temporary mild pain, but did not give rise to new neurological symptoms.

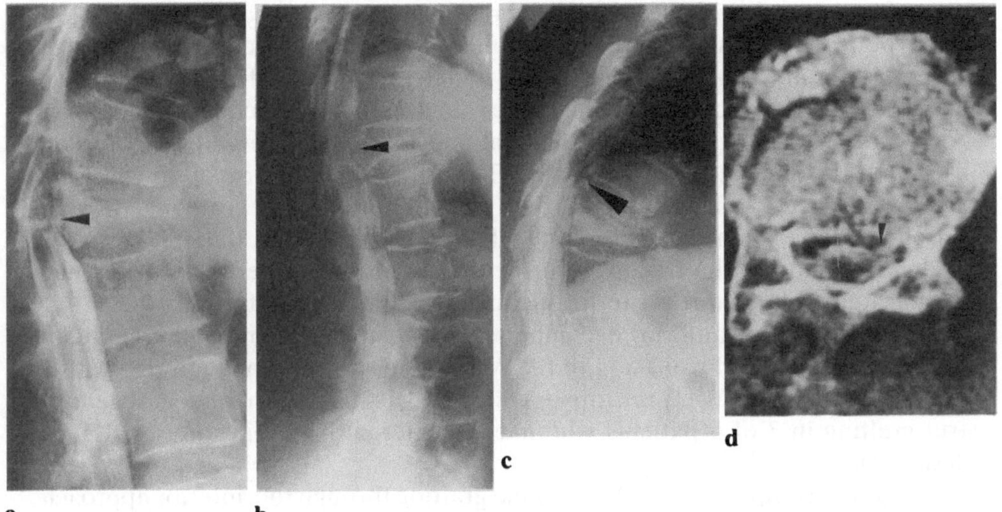

Fig. 1a–d. Causes of narrowing of the spinal canal (*arrows*): **a** sharp angulation at the posterior wall; **b** mild angulation at the posterior wall; **c** sharp angulation at the disc level; **d** bursting fragment of the posterior wall

Discussion

It had been believed that neurological complications such as paraplegia would not occur in a compression fracture of the vertebra due to involutional osteoporosis. Since Kempinsky [2] reported a case with neurological complication and Suda et al. [3] reported the first case complicated with paraplegia in Japan, more than 100 cases have been reported.

A vertebral fracture may be precipitated by minor stress and is a cause of pain that may be severe and of sudden onset. However, vertebral fractures are completely painless in many cases. Parfitt and Duncan [4] described the mechanisms of back pain after vertebral fracture. The first type of pain from vertebral fracture may be severe, but it will eventually subside spontaneously as the fracture heals, usually in 2 to 3 months. The second type of pain may develop in the lower back from increased lumbar lordosis as compensetion for the increased kyphosis of the thoracic or thoracolumber region. This type of pain usually subsides in 3 to 6 months. In patients with multiple fractures, the third type of pain may occur in the lower and mid back and may be related to continued stress on ligaments, muscles, and intervertebral joints due to a change of curvature of the spinal column. The fourth type of pain, i.e., true bone pain, is often associated with sensitivity to percussion and may occur in osteoporotic patients. The pain might be related to a microscopic crack or trabecular microfracture.

The fifth type of pain occurs in vertebral fracture in osteoporotic patients [5]. This type of pain may last more than 6 months due to delayed or nonunion of vertebral fracture. This is demonstrated by lateral views of the fracture site on both maximal flexion and extension of the spinal column. A vacuum phenomeon, a dark area within the fractured vertebral body, may be observed on extension or even in the neutral position (Fig. 2). The dark area was a cavity in which no bleeding occurred on currettage. If it is considered to be osteonecrosis of cancellous bone of the fracture body, then decortication of the cavity wall is needed for union of the fracture. Furthermore, posterior interbody fusion may be indicated with a short posterior instrument such as a Steffee VSP.

Kaneda advocated anterior decompression and implantation of glass ceramics containing apatite and wollastonite (A-W) and autogenous bone grafting with a Kaneda device [6]. We performed anterior decompression and autogenous strut grafting in 3 of 4 patients who needed external immobilization such as a plaster cast.

Anterior decompression and strut bone grafting through the anterior approach with or without instrumentation and ceremics may be indicated in cases of kyphosis and relatively mild osteoporosis. Anterior decompression and bone grafting through the posterior approach with posterior instrumentation and posterior or posterolateral bone grafting may be indicated in even older patients

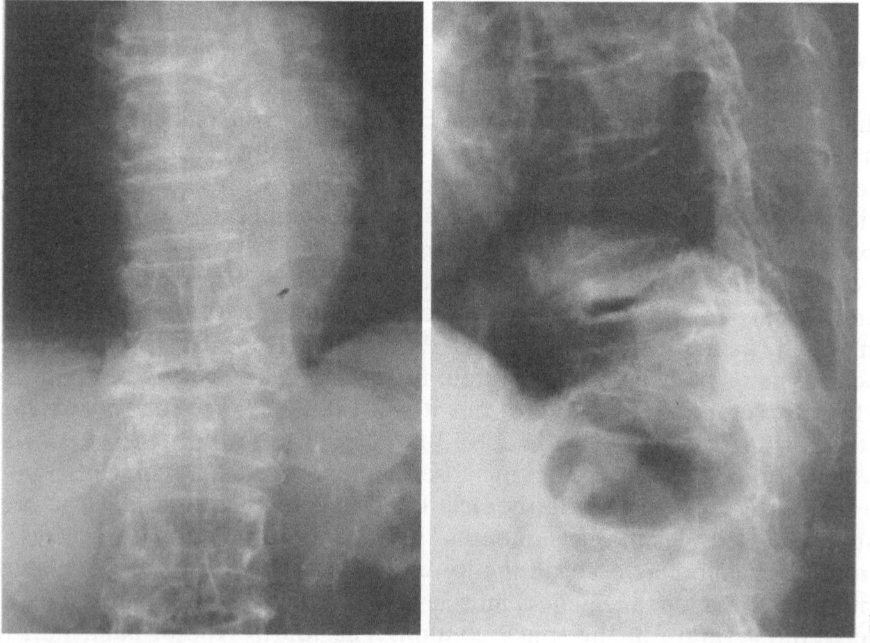

Fig. 2a,b. A 75-year-old woman with fracture of T11 treated with a short posterior instrument. A vacuum sign is shown in the middle of fractured vertebral body. **a** anterior-posterior view, **b** lateral view of X-ray of thoracolumbar region

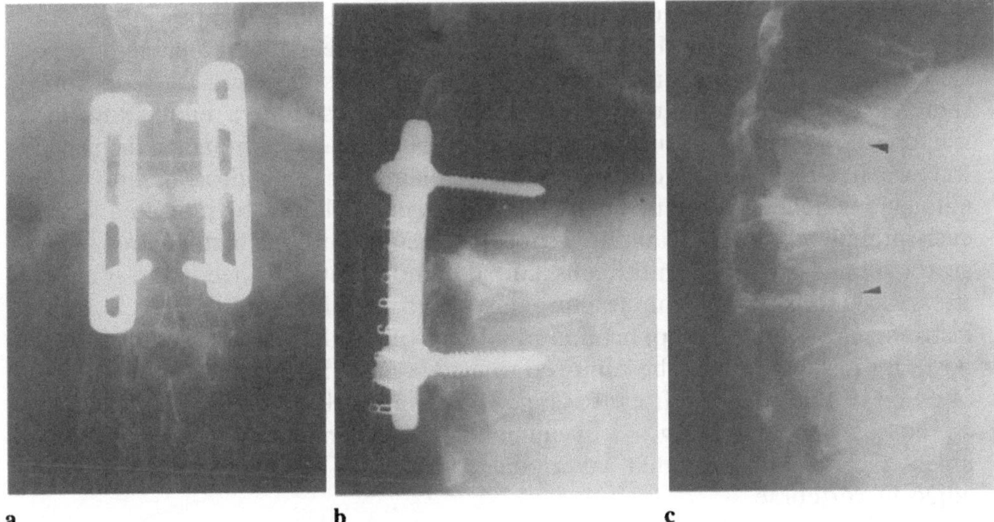

Fig. 3a–c. A 63-year-old female with paraplegia due to severe angulation at the upper disc level of T12. Correction of angular kyphosis and fixation with Steffee variable screw placement (VSP) were performed, together with packing using synthesized hydroxyapatite granules (HAP) sintered at 1000°C and autogenous iliac bone chips. **a** Anterior-posterior view, **b** lateral view of X-ray taken immediately after surgery, **c** lateral view twelve months after surgery. The insturments were removed and HAP was packed into the four pedicular screw holes (*arrows*)

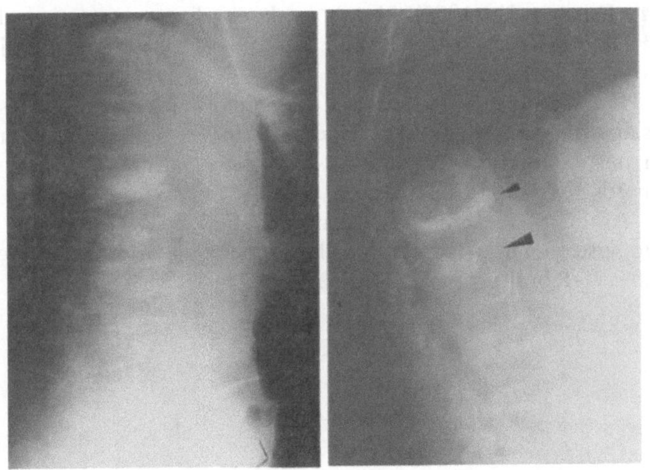

Fig. 4a,b. A 70-year-old woman with prolonged back pain treated with a packing of synthesized hydroxyapatite granules without instrumentation. **a** HAP granules sintered at 900°C were packed into L1 and L2 to prevent further compression. **b** Twelve months later, a small amount of HAP protruded from the L1 vertebra, and a compression fracture occurred at L2. HAP ensured compression was of mild degree than those indicated through the anterior approach.. Since fixation of two or three laminae above and below the fractured vertebra with Harrington or Luque rods using hooks or sublaminar wiring becomes loose in an osteoporotic spine, a short instrument with pedicular screws just above and below the fracture may be more useful. In cases of prolonged back pain due to disturbed fracture healing of the vertebral body, implantation of hydroxyapatite with autogenous bone grafting through a posterior approach may be indicated, since each granule of hydroxyapatite is incompressible and the autogenous bone graft contains osteoprogenitor cells. Initial immobilization is needed to prevent stress accumulation at the fracture level and can be achieved by a short instrument and external application of a brace or a light plaster cast. The short posterior instrument may be removed to avoid stress shielding after completion of union of the vertebral fracture (Fig. 3). It is advisable to maintain flexibility of the spinal column (Fig. 4) by minimizing the number of fused segments, unless there is concern that additional compression fractures may occur in adjacent vertebrae.

References

1. Kaneda K, Abumi K, Fujiya M (1984) Burst fractures with neurologic deficits of the thoracolumbar spine. Spine 9:788–795
2. Kempinsky WH (1958) Osteoporotic kyphosis with paraplegia. Neurology 8:181–186
3. Suda K, Ikeda A, Tokida Y (1974) A case of paraplegia due to pathological fracture of spinal osteoporosis (in Japanese). Clin Orthop Surg 9:346–350
4. Parfitt AM, Duncan H (1975) Metabolic bone disease affecting the spine. In: Rothman RH, Simeone FA (eds) The spine, vol II. Saunders, Philadelphia, pp 599–720
5. Takahashi HE, Homma TT, Haba T, Matsumoto M (1987) Transplantation of autogenous iliac bone and hydroxy-apatite into compression and comminuted fracture of spine in postmenopausal or senile osteoporotic patients (in Japanese). Orthop Surg Traumatol 30:1445–1452
6. Kaneda K, Asano S, Hashimoto T, Satoh S, Fujiya M (1992) The treatment of osteoporotic-posttraumatic vertebral collapse using the Kaneda device and a bioactive ceramic vertebral prosthesis. Spine 17:S295–S303

Key Word Index